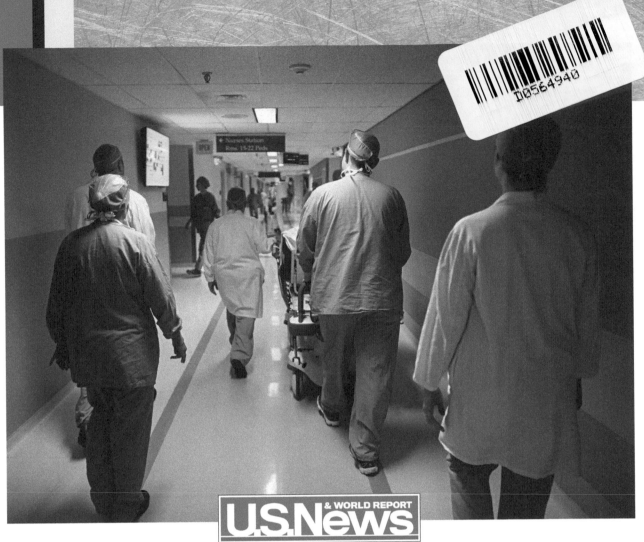

U.S.News & WORLD REPORT

2020 EDITION

Best Hospitals

ON THE WAY TO SURGERY AT MAYO CLINIC
BRETT ZIEGLER FOR USN&WR

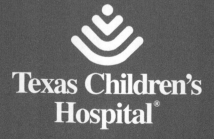

BEST CHILDREN'S HOSPITALS

U.S.News & WORLD REPORT

HONOR ROLL
2019-20

#1 Cardiology &
Heart Surgery

#1 Pulmonology &
Lung Surgery

#2 Gastroenterology &
GI Surgery

#2 Nephrology

#3 Cancer

#3 Neurology &
Neurosurgery

Texas Children's
Hospital®

CONTENTS

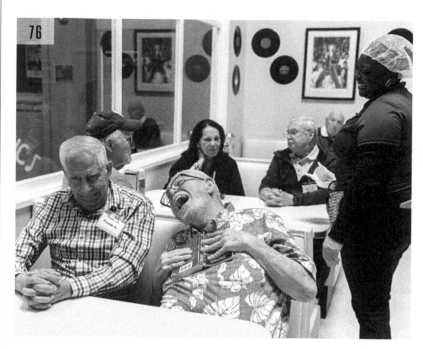

76

CHAPTER ONE
On Medicine's Front Lines

CHAPTER TWO
Patient Power

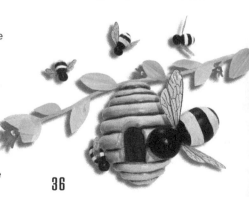

36

FROM TOP: JENNIFER EMERLING FOR USN&WR; ILLUSTRATION BY PUSHART FOR USN&WR
COVERS: GETTY IMAGES (2)

CONTENTS CONTINUED ON PAGE 4

ONE OF THE
NATION'S
BEST

TEXAS'
OWN

At Texas Children's Hospital, we're proud to be in the top 10 in all 10 specialties ranked by *U.S. News & World Report*, and to be the only children's hospital in Texas listed on the prestigious Best Children's Hospitals Honor Roll for the 11th year in a row. It's an honor to be recognized for helping improve the lives of kids across Texas and beyond.

Learn what makes us the best at **texaschildrens.org/best**.

Texas Children's
Hospital®

CONTENTS

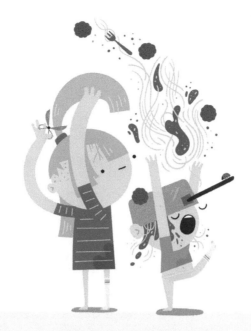

The U.S. News Rankings

BEST HOSPITALS
U.S.News & WORLD REPORT
2019-20

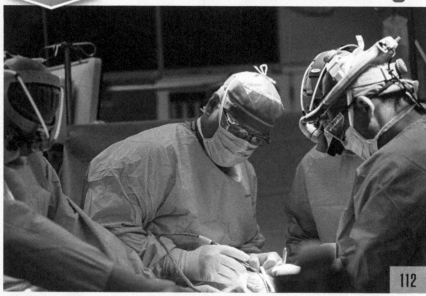

112

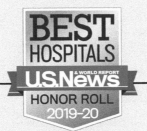

AMAZING THINGS ARE HAPPENING HERE

Amazing is **being top 5** in a nation with 5,000+ hospitals

This honor would not be possible without all our team members, nurses, Weill Cornell Medicine and Columbia physicians, Board of Trustees, donors, volunteers and friends. And to our patients — thank you for your continuing trust in our care.

⌐⌐NewYork-Presbyterian

New York's #1 hospital for a reason

Ranked by *U.S. News & World Report* 2019–20

Weill Cornell Medicine | ⌐⌐NewYork-Presbyterian | COLUMBIA

@ USNEWS.COM

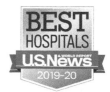

NUTRITION & LIFESTYLE

Best Diets

A look at some of the most popular and most researched diets, with reviews by a panel of health experts. Discover the top diets for weight loss, diabetes management and heart health, as well as the best plant-based and commercial diets.
usnews.com/bestdiets

Eat + Run

Doing what it takes to stay in shape can be tough to manage. We serve up expert advice daily.
usnews.com/eat-run

INSURANCE

Best Medicare Advantage Plans

State-by-state ratings of insurers offering Medicare Advantage and Medicare Part D plans, plus tips on choosing one of these plans vs. original Medicare.
usnews.com/medicare

Health Insurance Guide

Your marketplace: a state-by-state guide. Plus answers to frequently asked questions.
usnews.com/healthinsurance

MEDICAL CARE

Health Care of Tomorrow

Health reform, technological innovation and big data are transforming hospitals and care delivery. U.S. News explores how the industry is adapting.
usnews.com/healthcareoftomorrow

BEST HOSPITALS HONOR ROLL

A Visual Tour of the Top 21

See the best of the Best Hospitals – 21 medical centers that lead the pack in a host of specialties, procedures and conditions, excelling in both breadth and depth of care.
usnews.com/hospitalphototour

BEST HOSPITALS

In Specialties, Procedures & Conditions

We've evaluated more than 4,500 hospitals in up to nine common procedures and conditions, including hip replacement, knee replacement, heart bypass surgery, and COPD, as well as 16 medical specialties, including cancer care.
usnews.com/best-hospitals

SENIOR CARE

Best Nursing Homes

We've analyzed government data and published ratings of more than 15,000 facilities nationwide.
usnews.com/nursinghomes

PHARMACIST PICKS

Top Recommended Health Products

Which over-the-counter products do pharmacists prefer? Check out Top Recommended Health Products to make your next trip to the drugstore easier.
usnews.com/tophealthproducts

PHYSICIAN SEARCH TOOL

Doctor Finder

A searchable directory of more than 900,000 doctors. Patients can find and research doctors who have the training, certification, practical experience and hospital affiliation they want – and can see ratings based on other patients' experiences. With free registration, physicians can expand or update the profile patients see.
usnews.com/doctors

Saint Barnabas Medical Center: One of America's Best Hospitals

Continuing a tradition of delivering healthcare excellence, Saint Barnabas Medical Center (SBMC) was recently named a Best Hospital nationally for Diabetes & Endocrinology and Gynecology by *U.S.News and World Report*.

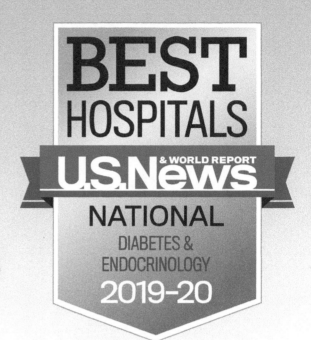

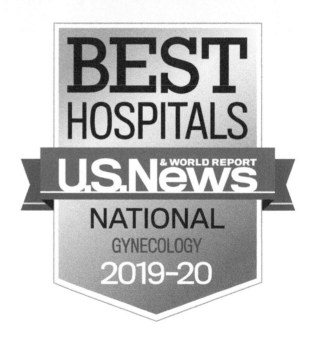

Saint Barnabas Medical Center | **RWJBarnabas HEALTH**

Let's be healthy together.

Livingston, New Jersey

rwjbh.org/saintbarnabas

Once Again, Top 10 in the Nation

UCSF Medical Center is ranked among the nation's best hospitals.

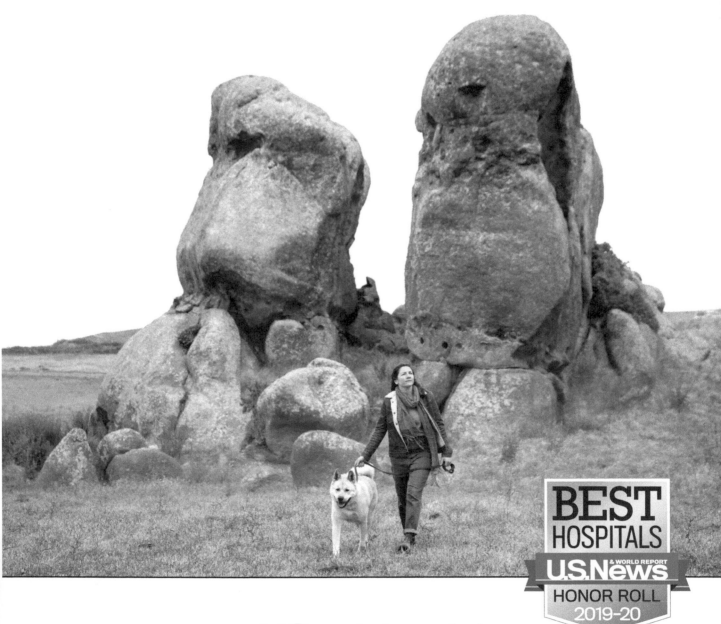

UCSF Health

Redefining possible.™

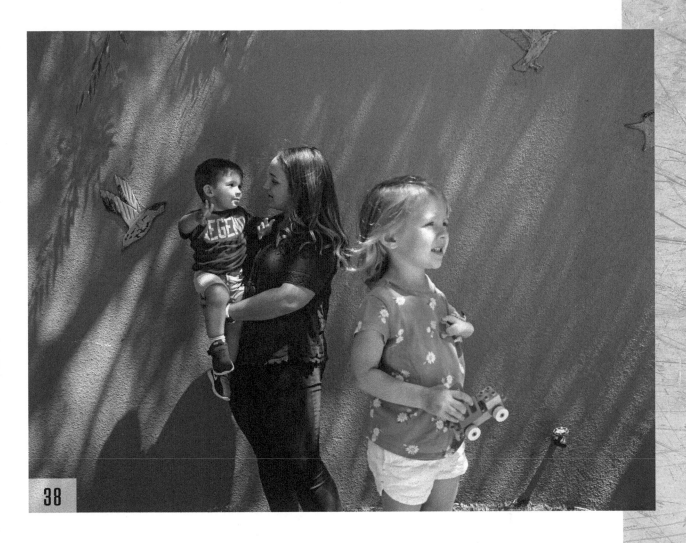

38

On Medicine's Front Lines

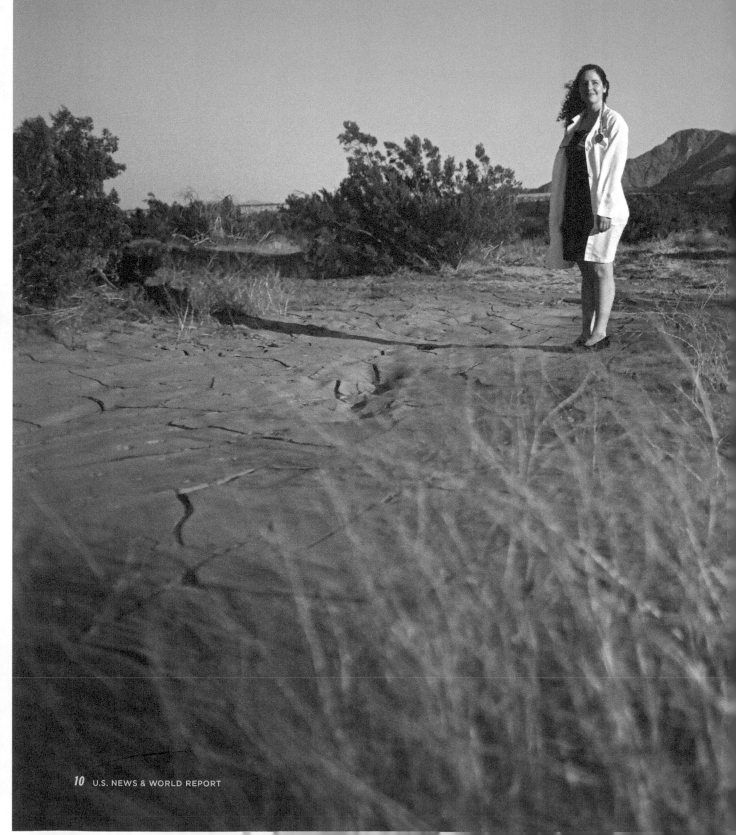

Doctors Wanted

A looming physician shortfall – of up to
120,000 doctors by 2030 – has hospitals
compensating in creative ways

by **Linda Marsa**

SARAH GÓMEZ went into the family business. Inspired by her father, a doctor who devoted his life to caring for the underserved, the third-year family medicine resident works at the Desert Regional Medical Center hospital and the UCR Health Family Medicine Center in a part of Palm Springs, California, that seems light years from the plush playgrounds of Hollywood golden-era icons like Bob Hope and Frank Sinatra. Many of her hospital patients are homeless, living in their cars or crammed into tiny apartments with relatives, with little protection from the blazing 120-degree heat in summer. They suffer from uncontrolled diabetes, heart disease, high blood pressure, and some from the ravages of addiction. "This is my community and I wanted to take care of the people in it," says Gómez, 30, who emigrated with her family from Mexico at age 6 and grew up in nearby Corona.

That's why she chose to pursue her medical education at the University of California–Riverside, about 60 miles east of Los Angeles. UCR School of Medicine, which opened its doors six years ago with a mission of serving the underserved, was deliberately located in "the other California" – the hardscrabble towns far removed from the affluent coastal enclaves – and recruits aggressively in economically disadvantaged areas; a large proportion of current students come from populations woefully underrepresented in medicine.

The strategy seems to be working: Roughly one-third of

'Half of the country's counties lack an ob-gyn.'

recent graduates now practice locally. "That's a remarkable outcome," says Paul Lyons, former chair of its department of family medicine. "I can hear in their voices and see in the eyes of these students a sense of commitment to these communities that you can't manufacture."

This is a bit of good news in an otherwise worrisome landscape. A growing physician shortage nationwide, which is hitting impoverished urban and rural regions hardest, is projected to create a deficit of up to 120,000 doctors by 2030 and seriously undermine patient care, according to a 2018 report by the Association of American Medical Colleges. Not surprisingly, mortality rates are lower in counties with more family doctors, and life expectancy is longer: almost two months for each 10 additional primary care physicians per 100,000 people, according to a 2019 study in JAMA Internal Medicine.

At the same time, the shuttering of struggling hospitals in rural America has exacerbated shortages in many communities. Since 2010, nearly 90 rural hospitals have closed and as many as 430 other hospitals across 43 states are at high risk of shutting their doors. When hospitals close, family doctors may be forced to leave, too. "Do doctors have the ability to do an X-ray or a mammogram in their offices when the closest hospital or ER is 100 miles away? These are all questions that can play into whether you can keep a physician in the community," says Suzanne Allen, vice dean for academic, rural and regional affairs at the University of Washington School of Medicine.

Specialist shortfall. The dearth of specialists is even more pronounced. To cite just one example, half of the country's 3,143 counties lack a single obstetrician-gynecologist, according to a 2017 report by the American College of Obstetricians and Gynecologists. More than 10 million women live in these predominantly rural communities, and at least half of them must drive 30 minutes or longer to receive perinatal services.

When obstetric specialists are widely available, maternal deaths can be significantly reduced, according to Medical University of South Carolina research. Without adequate prenatal care, on the other hand, more babies are premature, and women in labor may end up in emergency rooms or find themselves driving 100 miles or more in the middle of the night through rough terrain to get to a hospital.

The strains on the system are spurring hospitals to change traditional ways of doing business. In addition to launching training and residency programs in rural towns and impoverished inner cities, they're developing innovative approaches to serving patients and finding ways to take better care of doctors already in practice so physicians stay on the job rather than retire early. Here are some snapshots of the more pioneering programs around the country:

Expanding the team. In October of 2018, when victims of the Tree of Life Congregation shooting were rushed to UPMC hospitals in Pittsburgh, it was "all hands on deck" to deal with the crisis.

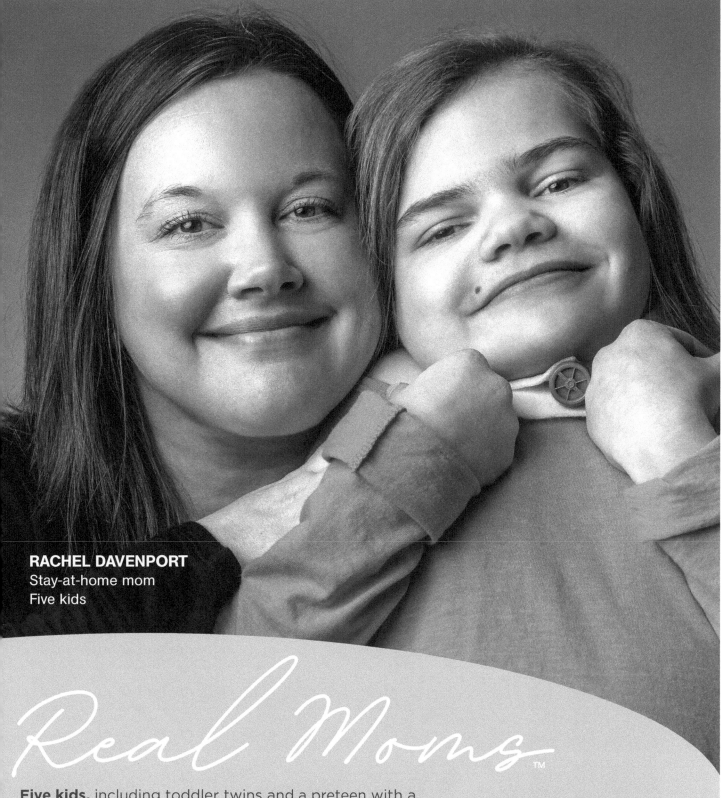

RACHEL DAVENPORT
Stay-at-home mom
Five kids

Real Moms ™

Five kids, including toddler twins and a preteen with a long list of health challenges, a husband's pending military deployment and scary health issues of her own. How does she do it? Find out on **Real Moms**, a new reality series featuring moms connected by the common bond of raising kids with medical challenges.
Watch at **RealMoms.org.**

@byrealmoms

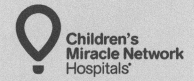

Children's
Miracle Network
Hospitals®

CHANGE KIDS' HEALTH
CHANGE THE FUTURE

Working side by side with the ER docs and the trauma surgeons were teams of nurse practitioners and physician assistants. "When someone comes in with a gunshot wound or even a car accident or a fall with an elderly patient, they are the first responders in the trauma bay," says Ben Reynolds, a physician assistant and chief advanced practice officer who oversees the UPMC Office of Advanced Practice Providers and was part of the trauma team that day.

UPMC operates over 40 hospitals and 600 medical offices across western Pennsylvania. The system's workforce of more than 2,600 physician assistants, nurse practitioners, nurse anesthetists and nurse midwives – numbers making these APP groups among the largest in the country – is a core part of the team in every facet of medicine, from anesthesiology, surgery and the ICU to cancer care.

Since the implementation of the Affordable Care Act, the ranks of advanced practice providers, who earn at least a master's and often a doctoral degree and can diagnose and treat patients and write prescriptions in all 50 states, have swelled, fueled by the influx of patients into an already overcrowded system. Their numbers are expected to grow by more than 30 percent between 2016 and 2026,

according to the Bureau of Labor Statistics. Health systems across the country, from Atrium Health in North and South Carolina to Utah's Intermountain Healthcare and Northwell Health in New York, employ large forces of advanced practice professionals. Nurse anesthetists, who beginning in 2022 will be required to earn a doctoral degree when they choose to enter the field, are the primary providers of anesthesia for surgical, therapeutic and diagnostic procedures in rural hospitals. "This is definitely a trend, and it's growing rapidly," says Stanley Marks, chairman of the UPMC Hillman Cancer Center. "We have difficulty filling our positions because we're competing with institutions all over the country."

Multiple studies indicate that the use of PAs reduces hospital readmission rates, lengths of stay and infection rates, and lowers overall costs and increases access to care. In the future, expanding the use of advanced practice professionals could greatly ease the country's shortages of primary care doctors: A 2018 analysis by UnitedHealth Group found that the number of people living in a county with a primary care shortage would decline from 44 million to fewer than 13 million by using nurse practitioners.

"It's a comfort knowing if I have a problem, I'll get an immediate answer," says Erin McCarty, 38, a UPMC patient who has ovarian cancer. McCarty had her surgery in

ERIN MCCARTY GETS CARE FOR CANCER NEAR HOME FROM UPMC NURSE PRACTITIONER SHARON BURGERT, RIGHT.

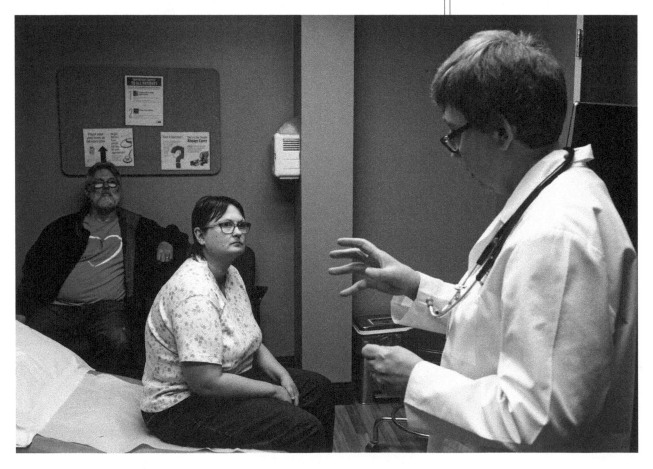

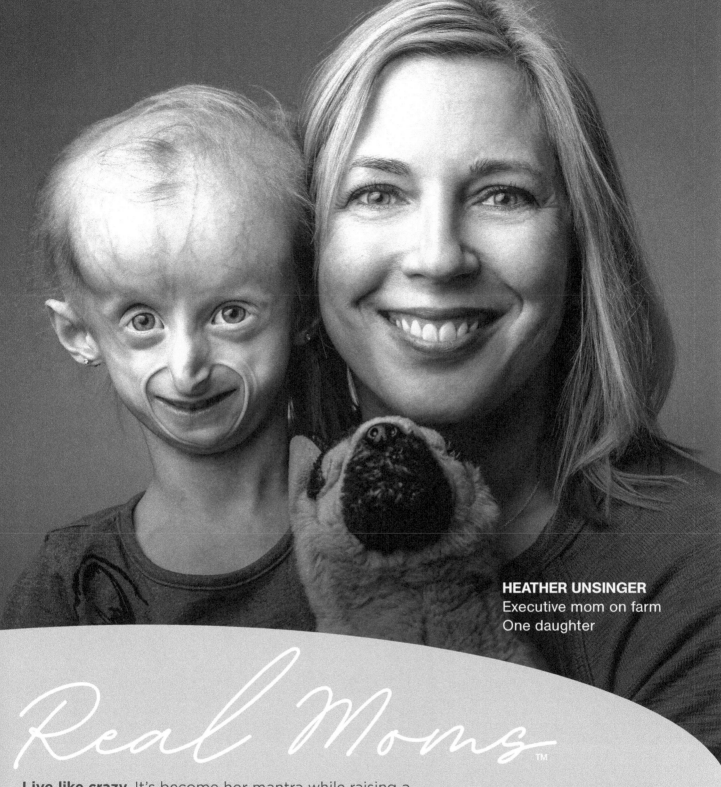

HEATHER UNSINGER
Executive mom on farm
One daughter

Real Moms™

Live like crazy. It's become her mantra while raising a daughter with progeria, a rare disease with no cure. Can it keep her going as she balances a demanding job, a farm and a newly blended family? Find out on **Real Moms**, a new reality series featuring moms connected by the common bond of raising kids with medical challenges.
Watch at **RealMoms.org.**

@byrealmoms

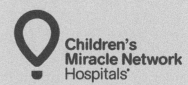

Children's
Miracle Network
Hospitals®

CHANGE KIDS' HEALTH
CHANGE THE FUTURE

Pittsburgh but gets her regular cancer care from a nurse practitioner 120 miles closer to her home, at one of the cancer center's 60 community clinics, many of which are in rural areas where it's tough to recruit oncologists. Even in smaller cities like Erie, where McCarty lives, oncologists often have 1,000 patients or more in their caseload.

When McCarty recently noticed blood in her urine, she gave her nurse practitioner, Sharon Burgert, a quick call. Within 24 hours, she had blood and urine tests, and was ushered in the next day for a transfusion. "She's really good at keeping in contact, which gives me an extra sense of personal connection," McCarty says.

Remote control. In the case of a stroke, where the mantra is "time is brain," administering the proper treatment swiftly can prevent long-term disability or even death (story, Page 22). Yet in South Carolina, known as the "buckle" of the stroke belt, a third of counties don't have a neurologist.

To minimize the time lost between symptom onset and treatment, Prisma Health, with 18 hospitals and 300 medical offices serving 1.2 million patients throughout the state, ensures that patients are "seen" by specialists immediately. In their local ER, stroke victims are examined in real time and monitored remotely by neurologists at telestroke hubs in Columbia and Greenville. Patients who need it can then be given the clot-busting drug tPA, which can reduce the severity of the stroke but must be administered within a few hours of the onset of symptoms to be effective. For surgery to deal with more severe blockages, which can be performed within a wider 24-hour time frame, patients may be transported to a stroke center.

"This allows me to log in to the bedside, see this patient live and interview them myself to make a diagnosis," says Anil Yallapragada, a vascular neurologist and medical director of Prisma Health–Midlands Stroke Center in Columbia. Prisma Health treated more than 3,500 stroke patients and did some 700 of these types of remote consults in 2018.

In addition, the system offers a school-based telehealth program for children;

> 'Doctors put twice as much time into paperwork as they spend on patient care.'

a program called Delivery Buddy that connects community hospitals with neonatologists; and SmartExam, an online service providing patients medical guidance for over 150 common conditions. When Hurricane Florence hit in 2018, causing massive flooding, more than 240 patients were able to receive essential care through SmartExam.

Prisma Health's comprehensive telehealth program is one of many across the country bringing care to underserved areas. One pioneering hub-and-spoke model developed at the University of New Mexico Health Sciences Center, Project ECHO (short for Extension for Community Healthcare Outcomes), provides frontline doctors – the spokes – with advice and mentoring from specialists in academic hubs, including regular virtual grand rounds, so they can manage complex cases locally. This model is now used in 46 states to manage a wide array of conditions from cancer to cardiology.

Arkansas, where 73 of 75 counties are medically underserved, is home to a widely lauded statewide maternal telemedicine program of the University of Arkansas for Medical Sciences, known as UAMS ANGELS (for Antenatal and Neonatal Guidelines, Education and Learning). It offers real-time long-distance consultation by maternal-fetal medicine specialists to family doctors, obstetricians, neonatologists and pediatricians at more than 55 hospitals, community clinics and local health units in outlying areas.

"It's hard to get physicians to go to the rural areas, and even in cities, there are health care deserts," says Curtis Lowery, director of the UAMS Institute for Digital Health & Innovation, who helped found UAMS ANGELS. "Telemedicine is one way of bridging this gap."

Combating burnout. A 2017 National Academy of Medicine report found that more than half of the nation's doctors were emotionally exhausted and felt unsatisfied professionally. This is more than a personal problem: Doctors suffering from burnout retire early or leave the profession, and studies suggest their stress can compromise patient safety. "Burnout has a huge im-

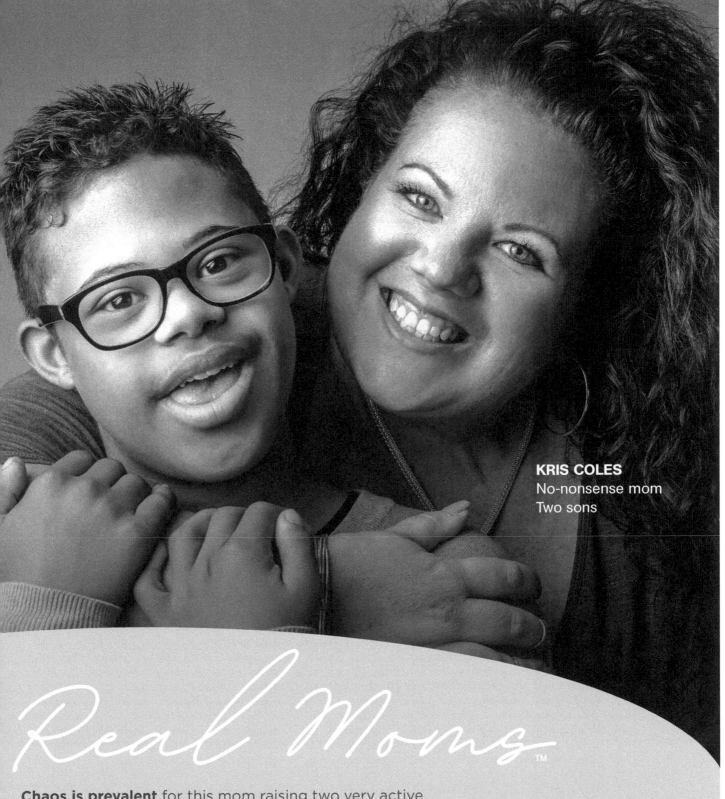

KRIS COLES
No-nonsense mom
Two sons

Real Moms™

Chaos is prevalent for this mom raising two very active boys, one with Down syndrome. Can she manage it while working full time? Find out on **Real Moms**, a new reality series featuring moms connected by the common bond of raising kids with medical challenges. Watch at **RealMoms.org.**

Children's Miracle Network Hospitals®

CHANGE KIDS' HEALTH
CHANGE THE FUTURE

@byrealmoms

Lifesaving Measures

ONE MINUTE completely altered Hannah Holbrooks' life. Early one evening in April of 2018, she was chatting with her 2-year-old daughter when she was suddenly gripped with searing pain. "I felt like my appendix had burst," says the 30-year-old resident of Walhalla, South Carolina, a town in the foothills of the Blue Ridge Mountains.

Because she was 27 weeks pregnant, Holbrooks' first thought was for her unborn child. She made a decision that may have saved both their lives: Instead of calling 911 and waiting for an ambulance, she made the 15-minute drive herself to Prisma Health's Oconee Memorial Hospital – which fortuitously has access via telemedicine to neonatal specialists considerably farther away. Doctors later told Holbrooks that her internal hemorrhaging was so severe – a ruptured vessel filled her abdomen with blood – that five more minutes could have been fatal for her and her baby.

The ob-gyn at the hospital made another lifesaving call: Holbrooks was immediately wheeled into the operating room for a cesarean section while Dad, Thomas "Casey" Mcguffin, who had frantically raced to the hospital, anxiously waited. Shortly thereafter, Hannah delivered tiny 2-pound, 6-ounce Isaiah.

Guided from afar. Because physicians at the small community hospital didn't have the expertise to care for a newborn who was three months premature, the on-call neonatal telemedicine team at Prisma Health Children's Hospital–Upstate, 40 miles away in Greenville, swung into action. They were "there" in the operating room at Oconee Memorial, guiding doctors and nurses via a telerobot, whose advanced high-resolution camera allowed the team to zoom in on the infant and provide instructions as the on-site team worked. Under the supervision of neonatologist Michael Stewart and neonatal nurse practitioner

pact on recruitment and retention," says Jonathan Ripp, an internist and chief wellness officer at the Mount Sinai Health System in New York and senior associate dean for well-being and resilience. Mount Sinai, like many systems, has made addressing burnout an urgent priority.

Doctors there have been surveyed to identify the key factors that lead to burnout; results are still being analyzed. The major suspected culprits include a heavy clerical burden – having to seek prior authorization for prescriptions and spending hours entering data into patients' electronic health records (or EHRs) and filling out all the forms required by insurance companies – that prevents doctors from doing what they were trained to do: namely, take care of patients. Physicians now put twice as much time into paperwork as they spend on patient care.

The health system has instituted initiatives to relieve the burden – by rethinking workflows, optimizing the EHR system and providing advanced speech-to-text software, to name three examples. Doctors can now dictate their notes directly into electronic records or use "scribes," people who accompany them on their rounds and write up patient notes. The hope, Ripp says, is that the various initiatives will eventually save doctors at least an hour a day.

"The issue of burnout has been around for a long time, but we've reached an inflection point where we realize we need to take a more structured approach," he says. "It's not about simply making doctors tougher to withstand the stressors." Mount Sinai has also introduced programs promoting personal physical and mental well-being, such as workshops that teach stress-reduction techniques like yoga and mindfulness meditation.

Hospitals and systems across the country, including Johns Hopkins Medicine, University of Alabama–Birmingham Medicine, Stanford Health Care, Massachusetts General Hospital, Boston Medical Center and Mayo Clinic, have launched programs to unburden and otherwise aid demoralized doctors. In addition, the Collaborative for Healing and Renewal in Medicine (known as CHARM), a national network of educators, researchers and leaders at academic medical centers with expertise in burnout and practices designed to promote wellness, has developed guidelines to help physicians find a renewed sense of meaning, social support and community at work, and to more easily access mental health resources.

Training doctors where they're needed. While most medical students and residents train at teaching hospitals affiliated with (and

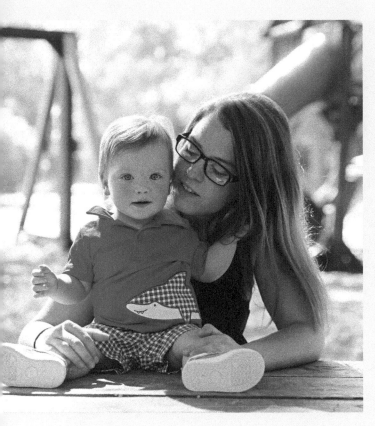

Melissa Dunham, doctors were coached on how to position a critical breathing tube and insert a catheter into the baby's umbilical vein – he was so tiny they couldn't thread an IV into his arm – to be certain he would be getting enough nutrients. "We make sure all these pieces are in place and that the baby is wrapped in plastic wrap – they actually got plastic wrap from the cafeteria – to keep him warm," Dunham says.

At the same time, a transport team, which included a neonatal nurse and respiratory therapist traveling in an ambulance equipped with a transport isolette and ventilator, was dispatched from Greenville to pick up Isaiah and bring him to the neonatal intensive care unit. Within 24 hours, Holbrooks was transferred to Greenville, too. Once she was released two weeks later, the family bunked at the nearby Ronald McDonald House during Isaiah's 76-day hospital stay. Today, despite some motor delays and lung weakness, Isaiah is a relatively healthy 18-month-old. "He's the happiest baby, and he's accomplished so much," Holbrooks says. "In 10 years, you won't be able to tell anything is wrong with him." *-L.M.*

HANNAH HOLBROOKS' SON, ISAIAH, WAS THREE MONTHS PREMATURE.

near) their medical schools, the University of California–Riverside program is an attempt at a different model. In a similar vein, the University of Wisconsin–Madison department of obstetrics and gynecology has developed a rural residency track to encourage doctors to practice in underserved areas. Over their four-year training, residents will spend about 20% of their time practicing at three rural sites in Wisconsin. The University of Alabama–Birmingham School of Medicine just launched a new family medicine residency that will place seven residents in an underserved urban community and five at its rural clinic in Centerville.

In Hettinger, North Dakota, a tiny hamlet in the southwestern part of the state with a population of about 1,200, the University of North Dakota School of Medicine & Health Sciences runs a well-regarded rural training program in family medicine. Medical residents spend two years getting hands-on experience working at West River Health Services' regional medical center. There are three dozen of these types of programs across the country, and they do genuinely increase the supply of doctors for the underserved: One study demonstrated that more than 35% of program participants were practicing in rural areas.

"Training in the sticks sticks," says David Schmitz, chair of the department of family and community medicine at the University of North Dakota School of Medicine & Health Sciences and a past president of the National Rural Health Association.

The University of Washington School of Medicine's WWAMI program, which has been around since 1971, is a multi-state medical education program; WWAMI stands for Washington, Wyoming, Alaska, Montana and Idaho. The program educates medical students in a variety of settings ranging from busy trauma centers in Seattle to small clinics in Libby, Montana, and Nome, Alaska, where they work with native populations in remote villages up to 150 miles away from the nearest town.

Randy Richter, a 74-year-old retired machine shop owner, feels that he enjoys excellent medical care because of WWAMI. He lives in Newport, a town of about 2,000 some 40 miles from Spokane, which has a small community hospital staffed by WWAMI graduates, including his family doctor, Geoff Jones, who is now also an assistant dean at the medical school. Aside from a mild case of glaucoma, Richter is "disgustingly healthy," he says. Still, he finds comfort in knowing that garden-variety ills can be treated so close to home. "If we need something deeper," he says, it can be handled in Spokane. ●

America's Healthiest Communities

What makes Douglas County, Colorado, shine?

IN AN ERA WHERE THE FOCUS is increasingly on population health, it's become clear that many of the factors affecting people's well-being and longevity have more to do with where they live and their economic status than with their medical care. Recognizing the importance of understanding and tackling these social determinants of health, U.S. News presents the second annual Healthiest Communities rankings, undertaken in collaboration with the Aetna Foundation. Winning top honors this year in the overall ranking of nearly 3,000 counties is Douglas County, Colorado, located within easy reach of Denver and Colorado Springs and blessed with opportunities for outdoor recreation. On these pages, you'll find other leading performers in four peer groups, distinguished by their economic strength and how rural or urban they are: urban high performing (where Douglas County also sits at No. 1), urban up-and-coming, rural high performing and rural up-and-coming.

Besides the metrics typically associated with health – obesity rate and access to doctors, parks and fresh produce, for example – U.S. News gathered data on dozens of measures that matter, from income and employment to affordability of housing, educational attainment and exposure to crime. Guided by a framework developed by a committee appointed to advise the U.S. Department of Health and Human Services, the rankings team assigned scores to counties on 81 indicators in the following categories: community vitality, equity, economy, education, environment, food and nutrition, population health, housing, public safety and infrastructure. Population health experts from the University of Missouri Center for Applied Research and Engagement Systems helped develop the methodology and did the analysis. Full details on the project can be found at usnews.com/healthiestcommunities.

The goal? To inform health leaders, policymakers and the public. Knowing how such factors interact to create a healthier community is an important first step toward targeting resources where they'll do the most good and improving health outcomes for all. ●

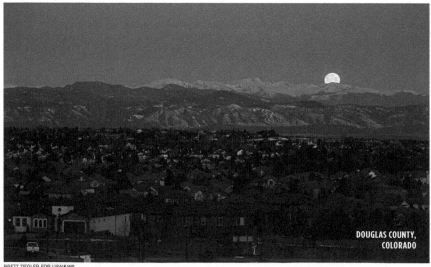

DOUGLAS COUNTY, COLORADO

BRETT ZIEGLER FOR USN&WR

40 Star Performers

Peer group rank	Community	Overall score (out of 100)
URBAN, HIGH PERFORMING		
1	Douglas County, Colorado	100.0
2	Los Alamos County, New Mexico	99.6
3	Falls Church city, Virginia	98.5
4	Loudoun County, Virginia	93.0
5	Broomfield County, Colorado	91.0
6	Hamilton County, Indiana	86.6
7	Carver County, Minnesota	85.7
8	Delaware County, Ohio*	84.9
9	Howard County, Maryland*	84.9
10	Fairfax County, Virginia	84.3
URBAN, UP-AND-COMING		
1	Houston County, Minnesota	72.8
2	Hood River County, Oregon	68.1
3	Bennington County, Vermont	66.2
4	Island County, Washington	65.3
5	Marquette County, Michigan	62.9
6	Giles County, Virginia*	62.6
7	Benzie County, Michigan*	62.6
8	Fillmore County, Minnesota	62.3
9	Freeborn County, Minnesota	60.9
10	Dickinson County, Michigan	60.6
RURAL, HIGH PERFORMING		
1	Teton County, Wyoming	87.3
2	Chaffee County, Colorado	84.6
3	Morgan County, Utah	84.4
4	Routt County, Colorado	84.2
5	Jefferson County, Montana	84.1
6	San Miguel County, Colorado	83.4
7	Pitkin County, Colorado	83.3
8	Sioux County, Iowa	80.7
9	Hardin County, Iowa	79.4
10	Lincoln County, Wyoming	79.1
RURAL, UP-AND-COMING		
1	Wallowa County, Oregon	67.8
2	Lincoln County, Washington	65.6
3	Calhoun County, Iowa	63.4
4	Iron County, Wisconsin	61.9
5	Baylor County, Texas	59.8
6	Grant County, Oregon	58.6
7	Curry County, Oregon	58.5
8	Yancey County, North Carolina	58.4
9	Rio Grande County, Colorado	58.2
10	Walworth County, South Dakota	58.0

NA = Not available. *Apparent ties are due to rounding.
[1]Percentage of Medicare beneficiaries with heart disease (2016).

Besides creating an overall ranking of Healthiest Communities, U.S. News measured counties against their peers based on how rural or urban they are and their economic strength. See how the top 10 in each of four peer groups stack up on a sampling of key metrics. To find out how your community fared, visit **usnews.com/healthiestcommunities.**

Years of life expectancy	Heart disease prevalence[1]	Obesity prevalence (adults)	Walkability index (20=best)	Adults who don't get exercise[2]	Population within 0.5 mile of a park	Preventable hospital admissions[3]	Population with no health insurance	High school graduation rate	Adults with advanced degree[4]	Unemployment rate	Poverty rate	Median household income	Home-ownership rate	Voter participation rate[5]	Violent crime rate[6]
83.72	21.0%	18.3%	9.0	9.6%	57.4%	2,771	3.7%	90.0%	65.6%	2.4%	3.8%	$105,759	79.6%	87.4%	82.3
83.49	16.0%	21.2%	5.4	12.0%	91.1%	2,297	3.2%	83.0%	72.4%	3.8%	5.1%	$105,902	72.6%	80.5%	281.0
81.81	20.0%	27.8%	16.2	20.0%	88.7%	3,203	3.7%	97.5%	83.2%	2.7%	2.7%	$115,244	59.7%	84.5%	134.3
83.19	22.0%	22.4%	8.0	16.1%	34.2%	4,533	6.9%	92.0%	64.9%	3.0%	4.0%	$125,672	77.4%	84.4%	85.0
80.02	22.0%	18.6%	10.4	11.3%	87.8%	2,606	5.1%	85.4%	60.4%	2.6%	5.9%	$83,334	67.7%	86.8%	52.7
81.78	26.0%	25.6%	7.8	13.9%	12.1%	3,451	5.3%	96.0%	62.9%	2.7%	5.1%	$87,782	77.7%	76.5%	56.0
82.80	19.0%	23.0%	7.3	14.2%	46.1%	6,516	2.9%	92.9%	56.8%	2.9%	4.1%	$88,638	79.8%	83.1%	62.1
81.43	26.0%	26.1%	7.1	16.9%	27.5%	3,849	3.9%	96.1%	59.2%	3.5%	4.9%	$94,234	81.2%	77.2%	80.9
82.98	24.0%	23.9%	10.1	15.4%	36.6%	3,752	4.4%	93.0%	66.6%	3.1%	4.9%	$113,800	73.4%	71.3%	200.5
83.73	20.0%	22.9%	12.0	16.2%	87.4%	3,287	9.3%	87.0%	65.6%	3.0%	6.0%	$114,329	67.5%	76.2%	89.4
81.74	20.0%	28.4%	7.9	21.9%	100.0%	2,867	4.7%	63.0%	37.1%	3.4%	10.3%	$55,550	80.8%	71.7%	86.5
80.34	17.0%	26.7%	8.7	14.8%	34.1%	2,776	10.6%	81.0%	36.6%	3.6%	13.3%	$56,581	64.6%	71.6%	193.7
79.49	23.0%	27.8%	6.5	19.1%	37.1%	4,050	5.0%	90.0%	42.0%	3.6%	13.4%	$51,489	72.9%	56.1%	133.5
81.93	18.0%	30.3%	8.7	15.7%	27.4%	2,633	6.3%	87.8%	43.7%	5.2%	9.5%	$60,261	67.1%	68.2%	111.6
79.31	25.0%	34.1%	6.4	19.2%	12.0%	3,084	5.4%	86.1%	39.1%	5.7%	16.6%	$46,822	70.1%	60.0%	141.7
75.91	28.0%	32.0%	5.3	25.0%	21.3%	3,817	11.1%	82.0%	24.3%	4.7%	11.8%	$47,675	75.0%	61.5%	125.5
79.66	24.0%	29.1%	5.1	24.3%	5.7%	3,296	7.5%	75.0%	35.8%	6.6%	11.2%	$48,694	86.5%	73.5%	107.0
81.16	20.0%	26.7%	5.6	24.4%	80.5%	4,095	7.6%	94.3%	32.0%	3.5%	12.1%	$54,358	78.9%	69.8%	57.3
80.76	22.0%	34.1%	6.5	20.5%	59.4%	5,629	5.6%	80.1%	28.9%	3.7%	11.2%	$48,827	75.6%	68.1%	123.1
79.73	25.0%	27.9%	7.4	18.0%	15.3%	2,842	5.7%	82.9%	32.8%	4.9%	14.6%	$43,373	79.5%	63.7%	564.2
83.46	18.0%	13.5%	6.8	12.0%	33.0%	2,693	15.0%	97.5%	60.0%	3.0%	7.3%	$75,594	59.8%	74.4%	502.7
81.22	17.0%	16.7%	7.7	14.3%	73.4%	2,339	8.9%	82.1%	43.6%	2.3%	9.6%	$50,993	75.9%	72.4%	81.3
81.47	21.0%	20.5%	6.0	12.9%	45.6%	2,231	6.5%	92.0%	48.3%	2.9%	4.1%	$80,865	84.8%	78.7%	49.7
82.73	18.0%	13.9%	6.6	9.8%	30.7%	2,786	8.4%	91.5%	56.8%	2.4%	10.2%	$63,505	67.4%	76.4%	171.3
78.88	18.0%	25.9%	6.1	15.0%	17.2%	3,071	8.6%	NA	41.6%	4.3%	8.6%	$62,939	84.5%	73.0%	191.4
83.73	15.0%	17.3%	6.7	11.9%	69.6%	3,064	11.5%	91.6%	60.7%	2.9%	11.9%	$58,170	59.3%	73.0%	90.9
86.52	23.0%	15.0%	7.0	10.3%	56.5%	2,266	12.1%	90.0%	65.9%	3.1%	8.6%	$69,789	62.8%	78.5%	99.5
82.86	20.0%	27.9%	7.1	18.2%	49.9%	2,678	5.7%	95.5%	39.7%	2.0%	7.6%	$63,466	79.4%	75.5%	109.6
79.74	24.0%	35.9%	6.4	19.1%	51.2%	2,817	5.2%	93.5%	34.4%	3.2%	8.1%	$51,821	76.1%	63.2%	139.4
80.03	18.0%	26.6%	5.8	20.2%	28.0%	2,868	13.3%	92.3%	30.7%	3.7%	8.8%	$64,579	79.1%	64.3%	72.0
80.42	19.0%	27.6%	6.3	16.2%	11.1%	3,431	6.9%	82.2%	34.8%	5.6%	14.6%	$42,349	67.9%	75.1%	31.9
80.03	20.0%	30.3%	6.5	22.4%	46.0%	3,079	6.8%	87.7%	33.1%	4.9%	14.8%	$47,676	78.2%	71.2%	83.1
79.85	23.0%	34.7%	6.7	26.9%	30.0%	3,311	5.2%	95.4%	30.8%	3.1%	14.8%	$44,635	76.1%	64.9%	44.2
79.27	24.0%	28.9%	6.1	19.4%	14.8%	3,730	7.2%	92.9%	32.6%	6.2%	12.8%	$41,270	77.6%	70.1%	253.1
76.33	32.0%	28.7%	7.2	24.8%	0.0%	5,698	16.8%	95.0%	35.5%	3.4%	12.7%	$34,382	77.0%	52.6%	299.5
79.74	19.0%	32.1%	6.3	20.8%	20.9%	2,867	8.6%	87.7%	32.1%	6.8%	14.9%	$40,193	72.8%	70.9%	22.7
76.80	20.0%	32.0%	8.5	16.7%	23.6%	2,751	8.8%	74.0%	32.6%	6.1%	15.2%	$38,661	66.0%	65.6%	107.5
78.08	21.0%	29.5%	4.9	23.4%	100.0%	2,366	14.4%	92.0%	29.9%	4.6%	21.3%	$36,993	75.2%	71.1%	71.6
77.71	17.0%	23.1%	6.3	14.2%	43.2%	4,058	12.2%	80.3%	28.4%	4.3%	19.2%	$40,177	66.7%	64.7%	153.1
78.14	24.0%	31.8%	8.3	22.7%	49.9%	5,859	12.5%	91.9%	30.9%	5.1%	10.8%	$46,526	68.6%	60.0%	149.8

[2]Percentage of adults who did not get leisure-time physical activity in past month (2015).

[3]Among Medicare beneficiaries per 100,000 population (2016).
[4]Age 25 and up with at least an associate degree (2012-2016).

[5]Share voting in 2016 presidential election.
[6]Per 100,000 population (2012-2014).

When Time Is a Matter of Life or Death

Some medical centers are now bringing the ER to stroke patients

by **Stacey Colino**

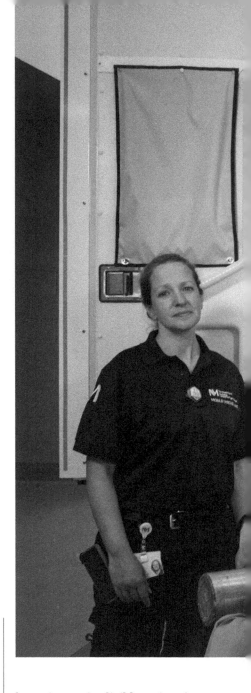

WHEN SOMEONE HAS A STROKE, a race against the clock begins. The average patient loses 1.9 million brain cells each minute that an ischemic stroke, in which a clot blocks blood flow in the brain, goes untreated. The first challenge is to get people to recognize the signs of stroke and act quickly. The next is to transport them to the right medical center fast enough. Not all hospitals are equipped to handle stroke, so many patients don't get the treatment that can save their lives and prevent disability.

Some medical centers are taking a new route to better results: They're bringing the emergency room to the patient. Specially equipped ambulances known as mobile stroke units, or MSUs, typically are staffed with a nurse, a CT technician, a paramedic and an emergency medical technician, and contain a CT scanner, the capacity to perform lab tests, access to a vascular neurologist via telemedicine and essential medications. These services make it possible for patients to be fully evaluated and for treatment to start well before they're wheeled into the hospital. "We have all the capabilities for treating the stroke on the scene," says Andrew Russman, medical director of the Comprehensive Stroke Center at the Cleveland Clinic.

The arsenal. Besides the equipment and telemedical expertise needed for accurate diagnosis, this arsenal includes the powerful clot-dissolving drug tPA, which, when administered intravenously within three hours of the onset of an ischemic stroke (and possibly up to 4.5

hours in certain eligible patients), can make all the difference in the outcome. For a hemorrhagic stroke, which occurs when a weakened blood vessel ruptures, the MSU team would immediately administer a different medication to control bleeding and blood pressure before transporting the patient to the hospital. Should an evaluation lead to tPA being administered on the spot and if the patient has a large vessel occlusion, a blockage in one of the major arteries of the brain, then the patient will bypass the ER and go straight to the interventional lab to have the clot extracted, explains Harish Shownkeen, medical director of neurointerventional surgery and of the comprehensive stroke center at Northwestern Medicine Central

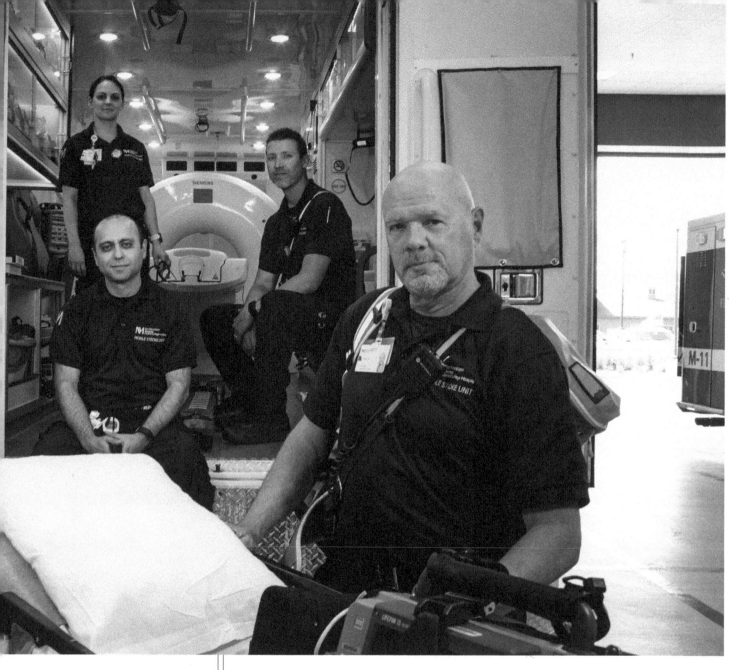

DuPage Hospital and co-medical director of the hospital's mobile stroke unit.

"I realized I wasn't making any sense, and when I tried to write a note, my right arm wasn't working properly," recalls Kevin Loughney of La Grange, Illinois, who was at work making sales calls in 2018 when he noticed he was slurring his words while leaving a voicemail message. When he stood up, his balance was way off. The owner of the company saw him looking wobbly and asked if he was OK. Loughney said he thought he might be having a stroke, so another employee called 911. Within minutes, a regular ambulance was dispatched by emergency medical services; suspecting a stroke, first responders also arranged for an MSU from Northwestern Medicine.

Right in the parking lot, the stroke unit team gave Loughney a CT scan, determined that he had a blood clot in the left side of his brain and gave him tPA. "It was 29 minutes from the 911 call to the tPA administration. I started feeling better immediately," recalls Loughney, 45, a father of three boys. After spending four days at Northwestern Medicine Central DuPage Hospital, Loughney went back to work and his usual activities – riding his mountain bike, playing golf and walking the dog – without any lingering effects. "It's like it never even happened," says Loughney, though he now takes a baby aspirin and a statin daily to prevent another stroke.

Seconds count. "Every minute earlier makes a tremendous difference," Shownkeen says – not just in outcome but also in the need for rehabilitation and time out of work. Research from the University of California–Los Angeles underscores the point, suggesting that patients who receive the clot-busting drug tPA before they get to the hospital may have less disability compared to those who receive it after arriving. Research from Germany found that MSUs reduced the symptom-to-treatment

MEMBERS OF THE MOBILE STROKE UNIT TEAM AND THEIR EQUIPMENT, AT NORTHWESTERN MEDICINE CENTRAL DUPAGE HOSPITAL

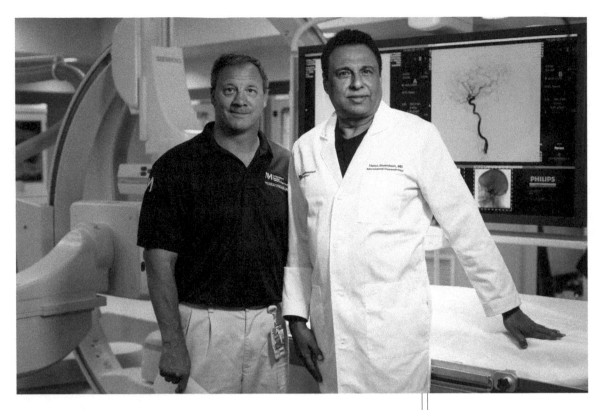

window by more than 50 percent. And a 2015 German study found that the proportion of patients with ischemic stroke who received treatment within the "golden hour" – the first 60 minutes after symptoms begin – was sixfold higher with an MSU than with regular care.

In fact, Germany pioneered the MSU concept in 2003. Then in 2014, the first MSU was introduced in the U.S. at the McGovern Medical School at the University of Texas Health Science Center–Houston, in partnership with Memorial Hermann-Texas Medical Center. More than a dozen are now in use, including in Denver, Phoenix, Memphis, Los Angeles, New York City and Trenton.

If someone having a stroke is outside a particular MSU

STEPHEN GRAHAM (LEFT) AND HARISH SHOWNKEEN, WHO DIRECT THE CENTRAL DUPAGE HOSPITAL MSU

radius area (usually 20 miles), there's potential for an ambulance to meet the stroke unit at an intermediate point where the patient can still get care more rapidly than otherwise. Recently, the University of Texas team met a man in trouble halfway between his location and theirs, gave him tPA, and alerted the nearest stroke center that he was en route. "The cath lab was ready for us, and we bypassed the ER," explains Stephanie Parker, nurse manager and program director of the MSU. "He was significantly better the next day."

Cynthia Reid, 49, had a massive ischemic stroke at home in Glen Ellyn, Illinois, in early 2017, and within 20 minutes was getting tPA in her driveway. Treatment by the MSU team "saved my life," says Reid, who recovered almost completely except for limited use of her left hand. "Given how massive my stroke was, it could have been so much worse."

Right now, the main downside is financial. Because there's limited reimbursement for treatment by an MSU, the hospitals that run these units bear the cost or they are financed through philanthropic donations. "The reimbursement model hasn't caught up yet – that's an impediment to the growth process for MSUs," Russman says. As more research supports the benefits, experts expect – or at least hope – that this will change. "With anything that's new, it takes time," Shownkeen says. "I think this is going to catch on because it makes a phenomenal difference." ●

Stroke Signals

Because seconds matter when treating a stroke, it's critical to seek help as soon as possible after you notice the symptoms:

- Confusion or trouble speaking

- Difficulty walking

- Sudden weakness or paralysis in the limbs or face, often just on one side

- Blurry or double vision involving one or both eyes

- Sudden severe headache, perhaps in concert with nausea or dizziness

The #1 hospital in the nation.

Once again, U.S. News & World Report has recognized Mayo Clinic as the #1 hospital in the nation. With the world's top doctors all working together across specialties to give patients the unparalleled care they deserve, Mayo Clinic is a destination for all who may need certainty, options and hope. When you need answers, **You Know Where to Go.**

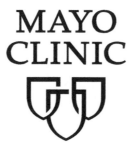

MAYO CLINIC

You Know Where to Go.

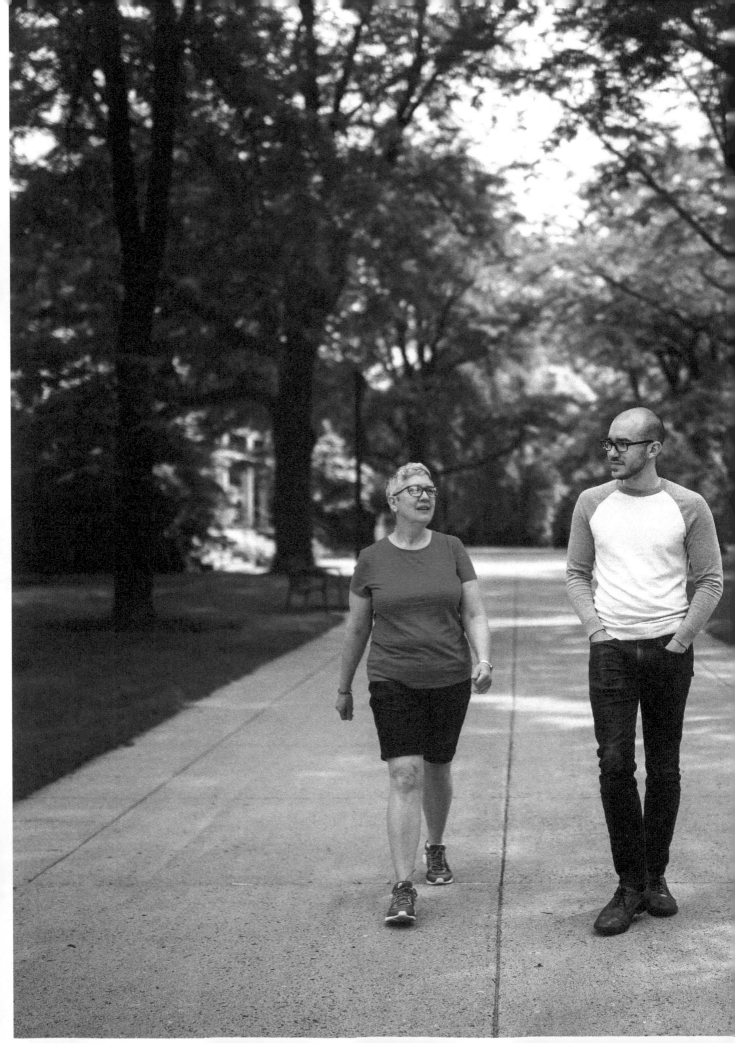

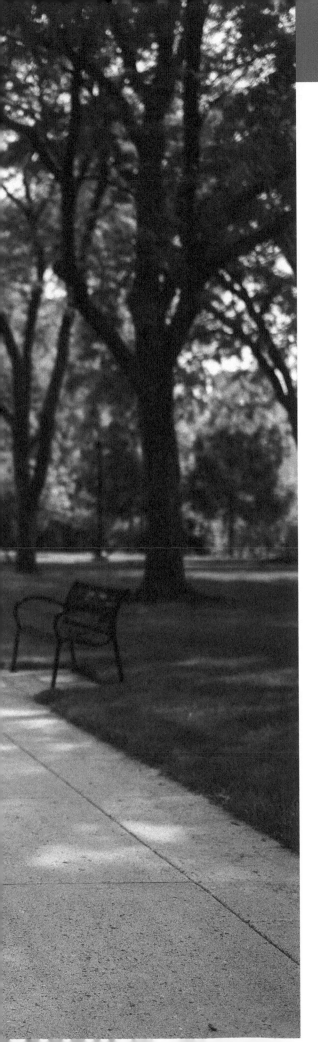

DNA Testing For All?

Healthy people are beginning to get notice of their risk of disease

by **Arlene Weintraub**

DURING A ROUTINE PHYSICAL in 2018, Matthew Farley of State College, Pennsylvania, was offered the opportunity to have his genome sequenced. As part of a research effort by his health system, Geisinger, he would learn of any disease-related gene mutations that were "actionable," meaning he'd be able to take steps to protect himself. Farley was 28 and healthy, so he figured he had nothing to lose.

Then, almost a year later, "someone from Geisinger called and said, 'We found something,'" Farley recalls. That something was a mutation in the BRCA2 gene, long tied to an increased risk of breast and ovarian cancer and more recently to a raised risk of prostate and pancreatic cancer. "My great-grandmother on my mom's side, as well as her mother, both had pancreatic cancer," says Farley, who works for Pennsylvania State University's online education arm, Penn State World Campus. After consulting with a genetic counselor and his physician, Farley is likely to start routine screening for prostate cancer around age 40 – a full 10 years earlier than a man of average risk would be advised to consider screening.

Genetic testing has been widely used for several years to guide treatment strategies, particularly in oncology, where several drugs targeting cancer-causing mutations have been approved by the Food and Drug Administration. But as the cost of whole-genome sequencing falls, the next phase of this push into precision medicine aims to hit a goal of precision health: By incorporating genetic testing into primary care, it might be possible not only to detect diseases and treat them early, but also to fend them off altogether.

Geisinger has enrolled more than 230,000 patients in its MyCode study, and the health

MATTHEW FARLEY AND HIS MOM, DIANE, BOTH HAVE A BRCA2 MUTATION.

system has completed sequencing of over 92,000 of them so far. The response has been so positive that the system has announced a goal of offering the testing to all of its patients as part of their routine care. Other institutions exploring the benefits of widespread genomic testing include Weill Cornell Medicine in New York and the Yale School of Medicine. "Someday we will all have our genomes sequenced, and it will drive our care. It's definitely on the horizon," says Michael Murray, director for clinical operations in the Center for Genomic Health at Yale. At the same time, consumers are finding more and more opportunities to seek out testing on their own from players like 23andMe and Helix, a startup that began offering its service directly to consumers in April.

Most of the genetic testing options offered to healthy people today are designed to detect 59 abnormalities that have been deemed actionable by the American College of Medical Genetics and Genomics. Those gene variants are correlated with about 30 diseases, half of which are cancers. Another third have been tied to cardiovascular disorders like abnormal heart rhythms or early heart attacks and strokes, while the rest are associated with conditions like cystic fibrosis and Fabry disease, an enzyme disorder. Patients with genes that are associated with actionable variants can pursue strategies to mitigate their risk of serious illness. Early or more frequent cancer screenings, for example, can pick up tumors when they're easy to treat.

Only about 2% of healthy people who are screened for actionable mutations end up having any of them – a hit rate that's so low some experts have questioned whether populationwide genetic testing is cost effective. David Ledbetter, executive vice president and chief scientific officer at Geisinger, says that after a decade or more of experience, his system will have enough data to prove cost-effectiveness, but that the opportunity to improve patient wellness now is so promising that it wouldn't make sense to wait for those answers before offering it to everyone.

"We think there's enough medical evidence to show that genetic testing is clearly clinically useful," Ledbetter says.

> # Gene variants that are "actionable" correlate with about 30 diseases.'

For those patients who have genetic risk factors, he adds, "it's a program that has profound implications." Geisinger predicts that the proportion of the population of patients with actionable genetic findings will expand to between 5% and 10% as more disease-related genes are discovered and the number of patients volunteering to learn about their risk grows.

From cancer to heart disease

In addition to BRCA mutations, flaws in several other genes have been implicated in cancer. Lynch syndrome, which is caused by alterations in five genes, increases the risk of colorectal cancer and nearly a dozen other types, including stomach, liver and bile duct cancers. Li-Fraumeni syndrome is caused by a mutation in TP53, a gene that normally is known to suppress cancer. People with this mutation face an elevated risk of multiple cancers, including leukemia, brain cancer and soft tissue sarcoma.

Early detection of many of these diseases can be a lifesaver: Colon cancer that's discovered before it spreads has a 90% five-year survival rate, but that falls to 71% once it starts to metastasize, according to the American Cancer Society. A 2014 study found that women with a BRCA1 or BRCA2 mutation who elect to have their ovaries removed reduce the risk of ovarian, peritoneal and fallopian tube cancer by 80%.

When it comes to heart disease, screening can uncover disorders that have no obvious symptoms. Several inherited mutations raise the risk of arrhythmias, irregular heartbeats that can cause sudden heart attacks. Long QT syndrome, which has been tied to mutations in several genes, raises one's risk of fainting, seizures and sudden death. And the chances of heart disease jump fivefold for people with familial hypercholesterolemia, an inherited form of high cholesterol that's caused by mutations in the gene responsible for making LDL, the "bad" cholesterol.

In 2017, concerned about her healthy 52-year-old aunt's sudden cardiac death years earlier, Hannah Bayer consulted

Cancer is smart... and relentless. At Dana-Farber, we are too. Each year, we conduct over 1,100 clinical trials

THINK LIKE

giving patients access to the latest advances. And, in partnership with Brigham and Women's Hospital

CANCER

and Boston Children's Hospital, we're mapping out the genetic weaknesses of 25,000+ tumors to create

TO BEAT

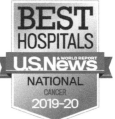

precision treatments that destroy cancer. These are just a few reasons why U.S. News & World Report

CANCER

has recognized us as a national leader in cancer for 19 years straight. It's also why, here, cancer is quickly losing ground.

DANA-FARBER
CANCER INSTITUTE

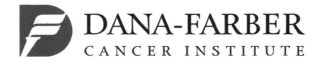

a cardiologist specializing in genetics at Stanford Health Care. "There were no electrical issues in my heart, no signs of structural issues, so as a Hail Mary, I was sent for genetic testing," says Bayer, 33, who works at a health care technology firm in San Francisco.

TESTING FOUND A MUTATION THAT COULD CAUSE HANNAH BAYER'S HEART TO STALL OR STOP. SHE HAD A DEFIBRILLATOR INSERTED.

That's when she learned she has a mutation in a gene called FLNC, which causes structural changes to the heart muscle that can cause it to stall or suddenly stop altogether. Bayer elected to have an automatic defibrillator inserted that can detect if her heart is about to stop and "jump-start" it, she says. The device also collects data on her heart rhythms and periodically transmits the information to her physician. "It's my insurance policy," Bayer says. "I have peace of mind knowing I don't face as high a risk that I might suddenly die." Her mother, who discovered she also has the mutation, had a similar device inserted.

As more disease-causing genes are uncovered, some geneticists are working toward developing "polygenic risk scores," algorithms that will calculate the danger of developing particular diseases based on all of the gene variants that are tied to them. "If you inherit one gene variant that's linked to cardiovascular disease, it's unlikely you'll get the disease," says Olivier Elemento, director of the Caryl and Israel Englander Institute for Precision Medicine at Weill Cornell Medicine. "But some people inherit 40 or 50 gene variants. Polygenic risk scores will identify those patients facing an extreme risk." People with high scores for cardiovascular disease could be put on cholesterol-lowering statins, for example.

One of the newest branches of genetic medicine is "pharmacogenomics," based on an increasing understanding of how certain genes affect the way people respond to drugs. The gene CYP2D6, for example, makes a liver enzyme involved in the metabolism of a quarter of the drugs on the market. Some people have extra copies of the gene, which causes them to process drugs very quickly – so fast that the typical dose might not be safe for them. Other people have a variant of the gene that makes an ineffective enzyme, so they are unable to metabolize some drugs properly. "It might mean that you need a higher or a lower dose of a certain medication," says Amy Sturm, co-director of the MyCode Genomic Screening and Counseling Program at Geisinger's Genomic Medicine Institute. "You might need a different medication altogether."

Geisinger's Ledbetter estimates that with the discovery of more genes that are related to drug metabolism, pharmacogenomic data could ultimately be useful for up to 90% of patients.

The "Achilles' heel" of gene testing

Is the medical community moving too quickly to incorporate genomics into the routine care of healthy people? That's a question that worries Joseph Wu, director of the Stanford Cardiovascular Institute and a professor of cardiovascular medicine at the medical school there. Often when patients undergo unnecessary genetic testing, they are found to have "variants of uncertain or unknown significance," meaning a gene may be abnormal, but its function isn't understood and it's not clearly linked to risk of disease. "That's the big Achilles' heel of genetic testing in healthy patients," Wu says. "Physicians can't interpret variants of uncertain significance. If they just look at those at face value, it could scare the heck out of patients."

The National Institutes of Health wants to contribute to the expanding knowledge base. To that end, it launched the All of Us Research Program nationally in 2018, with the goal of sequencing the genomes of 1 million

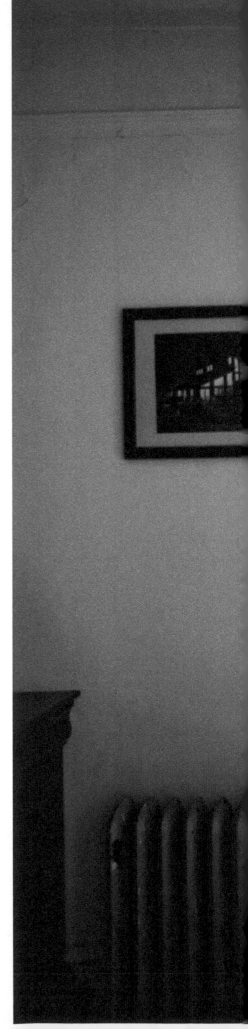

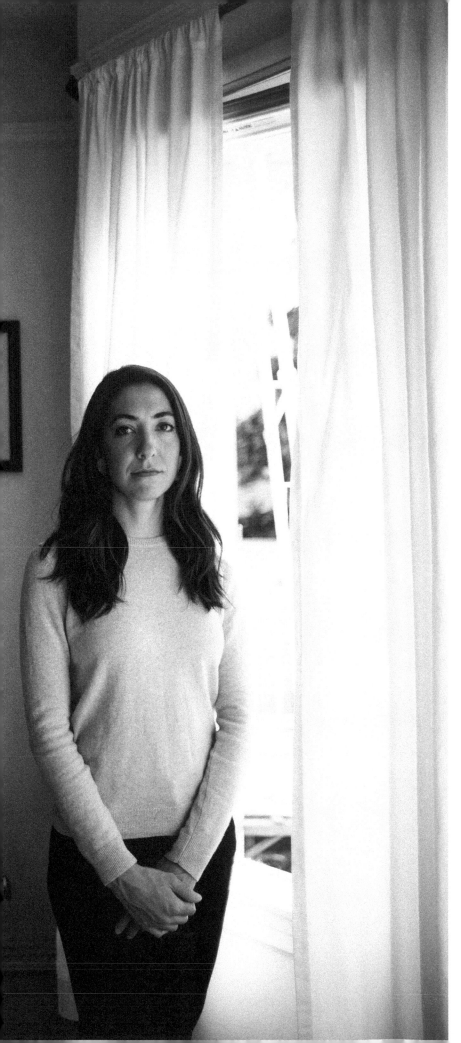

volunteers. Participation is free, and more than 190,000 people have enrolled so far, says Stephanie Devaney, deputy director of All of Us. Anyone can sign up at joinallofus.org.

The program hopes to start informing participants if they have likely disease-causing mutations in any of the 59 genes in 2020, Devaney says. The NIH will also report pharmacogenomic results to those who participate. And the program has started collecting data on exercise and sleep habits from participants who wear Fitbit activity trackers and who volunteer to share their data with the NIH. "We are interested in understanding how physical activity or sleep might affect health outcomes, and how all this data might fit together," she says.

For those who are willing to pay to have their genomes sequenced, Helix and diagnostics technology company PerkinElmer have partnered to offer a $300 test called GenePrism. Unlike 23andMe's direct-to-consumer kits, which are one-off tests for certain mutations, GenePrism includes all 59 actionable genes in one test. After customers get their results, they can consult with a genetic counselor free of charge. "We hold their hand through the entire process. We're not leaving them in the lurch," says Madhuri Hegde, vice president and chief scientific officer of PerkinElmer Genomics.

For Geisinger patient Matthew Farley, a benefit of talking to a genetic counselor was that it helped him communicate with his family about his BRCA2 mutation. His mother and grandfather decided to get tested, and they, too, carry the mutation. "For my mom, this was meaningful," Farley says. She had surgery to remove her ovaries and has increased the frequency of her breast exams. Her mammography appointments now sometimes include breast MRIs. "It really benefited her health care," he says. "She had a much higher risk of ovarian cancer than the average woman, and she was able to remove that risk."

Farley admits that having his genome sequenced made him anxious at first, because that's just how he is when it comes to his health. "But being able to help my family members made it really worth it," he says. "We have a lot of cousins, and we're now encouraging them all to get tested." ●

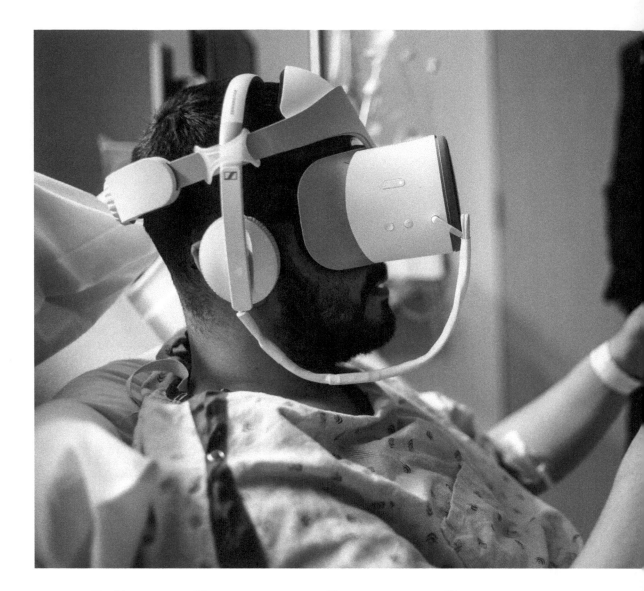

The Case for a Course
of Virtual Reality

It may help ease conditions from pain to phobias to PTSD

by **Katherine Hobson**

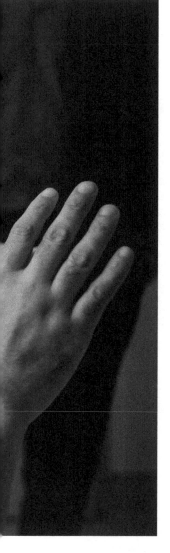

CROHN'S DISEASE and the pain it causes had landed Harmon Clarke in the hospital – again. This time, however, his treatment had a twist: a "flight" over waterfalls in Iceland in a helicopter. "I could almost feel the sun and hear the birds," he says.

When Clarke was first offered a spot in a clinical trial of virtual reality at Cedars-Sinai Medical Center in Los Angeles, he was skeptical but figured he had little to lose. "They told me it might be able to help me manage my symptoms, feel a bit better and sleep," he says. Indeed, as soon as Clarke put the VR headset on, he says, he felt elation that quickly turned to relaxation. In fact, Clarke, now 35, was so preoccupied by his altered reality that he missed a dose of his pain medication; usually, he was counting down the minutes. During that hospital stay, Clarke continued to use the headset to help him sleep, during IV insertions, and to cope with post-surgical pain. "It didn't take the pain away, but it allowed those moments to be more manageable," he says.

"People think of VR as a gaming technology," says Brennan Spiegel, director of health services research for Cedars-Sinai, who led the trial. But the computer-generated interactive, immersive worlds typically accessed by a headset and sometimes hand controls are also being used all over medicine. Besides pain management, researchers and clinicians are investigating how VR can be applied to everything from treating phobias to physical rehabilitation.

A review of randomized trials of inpatient VR applications published in 2017 found that the evidence suggests efficacy, but noted the need for larger, vigorous studies to nail down the degree of benefit as well as cost-effectiveness. "It's not like VR has magical properties," cautions Albert "Skip" Rizzo, a research professor and director for Medical Virtual Reality at the University of Southern California's Institute for Creative Technologies. But a growing body of evidence suggests it can improve on or expand access to certain treatments already known to work in the real world, he says.

Reliving trauma – safely. Take exposure therapy, for instance. This technique helps people confront situations they're scared of in the context of therapy, so their anxiety and distress can ease over time. It can be hard to fully replicate those scary situations, whether it's flying in a plane, speaking in front of a big crowd, or reliving a trauma that has contributed to post-traumatic stress disorder, says Barbara Rothbaum, a professor of psychiatry

and behavioral sciences at Emory University School of Medicine in Atlanta. VR can make the experience feel realistic, but also keeps it controllable. A therapist can add turbulence to a virtual flight only when the patient is ready for the exposure to intensify, for example.

Finding normal. Exposure therapy enhanced with VR is what finally helped Chris Merkle, a Marine veteran whose multiple tours of Afghanistan and Iraq left him struggling with PTSD. He tried traditional psychotherapy, but found it hard to open up about his experiences, which limited his progress. During a 10-week trial led by Rizzo, he discovered that recreating a traumatic day in Iraq, when his unit took heavy fire while stuck on a two-lane road, was so engaging in virtual reality that it prompted long-forgotten details to pop into his head. It wasn't pleasant to relive the day – but he survived it, over and over again. "It didn't kill me to talk about it. It normalized it," he says. Now he can smell a tire burning after a traffic accident on the highway and recognize it for what it is, rather than feel his stress and anxiety surge. Merkle is now in a clinical psychology doctoral program and works full time at a center for veterans that offers readjustment counseling.

Pain is likely alleviated through different mechanisms – at least three, Spiegel says. There's the distraction component: The VR "overwhelms the brain with visual stimuli and a sense of presence" elsewhere, he says, which can swing the spotlight of attention away from the physical experience of pain. (An offline example: blowing bubbles during kids' vaccinations to distract them from the shot.) An engaging experience can also make time seem to fly by, which reduces the perceived time spent in pain. And the pleasant, immersive experience is thought to block the "gates" in the spinal cord from receiving pain signals.

That can come in handy during labor. A pilot study published recently looked at the pain perceptions of 27 women giving birth for the first time, assigning them to either a period of unmedicated labor followed by a period of unmedicated labor plus VR, or the reverse. Women experienced a scuba diving simulation with manatees, set to relaxation-inducing

A CEDARS-SINAI PATIENT RECOVERING FROM GASTROINTESTINAL SURGERY TRIES OUT THE VIRTUAL REALITY TECHNIQUE.

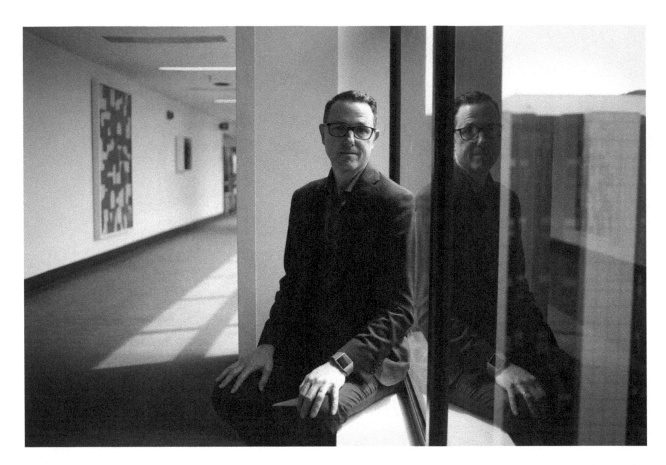

music, with an option to take virtual photos of the scene using a hand controller, says David Frey, an obstetric anesthesiologist now practicing in Orlando, Florida, and an author of the study, which was conducted at the University of Michigan. Their ratings for pain and anxiety were lower in the VR setting, no matter whether they entered the virtual world at the outset or later, and 82% said they very much or completely enjoyed using the technology during labor.

Anxiety can magnify pain and discomfort, so at Lucile Packard Children's Hospital Stanford, kids use VR to calm down before surgery, during nasal endoscopies and when they're getting casts or sutures removed, for example, says pediatric anesthesiologist Thomas Caruso. Child life specialists meet with the children beforehand to see what kind of content they're interested in – something active, like picking up pebbles, or passive, like watching fish float by. (That choice also gives them autonomy, which is often lost in the hospital.)

Side effects. Kids at Stanford are screened for risk factors that might make VR unsuitable, like a history of seizure disorders, nausea or motion sickness. The most common side effect of VR is "cybersickness," when a disconnect between what the eye is seeing and the inner ear is sensing can cause dizziness, nausea and vertigo, though that's less of a problem as VR technology has

THE PERCEPTION OF PAIN SEEMS TO BE EASED BY THE IMMERSIVE EXPERIENCE, SAYS CEDARS-SINAI RESEARCHER BRENNAN SPIEGEL.

improved, Spiegel says. Some people may also be susceptible to the equivalent of a VR bad trip, where the mind feels dissociated from the body, he says.

For those who can participate, VR can also be a motivating force. Many patients in rehab, for example, don't always perform exercises as frequently or with the intensity that's prescribed, says Danielle Levac, assistant professor in the department of physical therapy, movement and rehabilitation sciences at Northeastern University and director of the rehabilitation games and virtual reality lab. A VR scene that lets the patient virtually ski, say, shifting weight from foot to foot and losing points for missing a gate, can make it more entertaining to use, potentially leading to better results and a quicker recovery, she says. Rehab is also about learning new skills, and VR helps there, too; the idea is that the more engaged and motivated people are, the more enhanced their learning, possibly by better consolidating memories.

VR can be used to engage patients in other ways, too. At Lucile Packard, parents of kids with congenital heart defects can put on a headset and explore a virtual heart from the inside out. Chronic pain patients like Clarke can use VR to learn real-world coping or relaxation techniques such as yoga. That's what Clarke did after leaving the hospital, and he's now a certified instructor. ●

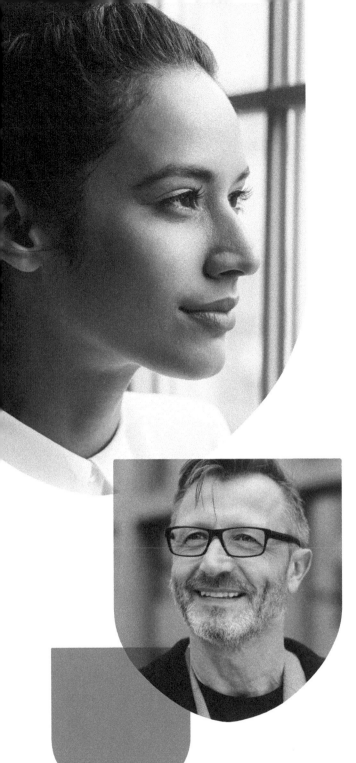

Giving our patients hope for a brighter tomorrow

Named in the top 10 for 30 consecutive years

Accurate assessment to personalized treatment. Intensive hospital care to outpatient therapy. Experts who care to better outcomes. We walk with each patient on their journey when they need it most. Recognized as one of America's Best Hospitals in psychiatry for 30 consecutive years, The Menninger Clinic strives to improve our patients' lives day after day, year after year.

To refer or to get more information, call 713-275-5400 or visit MenningerClinic.org

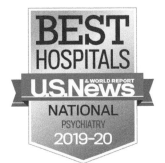

BEST HOSPITALS
U.S.News & WORLD REPORT
NATIONAL
PSYCHIATRY
2019-20

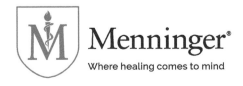

Menninger®
Where healing comes to mind

Affiliated with Baylor College of Medicine

Cleaner & Greener

Hospitals are pumping the brakes on their eco-unfriendly ways

by **Lindsay Cates** *and* **Ann Claire Carnahan**

NEWS FLASH: If the U.S. health care system were its own country, it would be 13th on the list of global polluters, ahead of the entire United Kingdom. In fact, the health care sector is to blame for nearly 10% of this country's total greenhouse gas emissions, known drivers of climate change. Hospital facilities traditionally require constant electricity for lighting and high-tech equipment. They generate a lot of waste (29 pounds per bed per day). Plus, certain gases used for anesthesia, coupled with emissions from hospital vehicles and patient travel, add to toxic air pollution.

But many hospitals are changing their ways. Big health systems are advertising ambitious goals like Cleveland Clinic's plan to be carbon-neutral by 2027 and Kaiser Permanente's aim to be carbon-positive by 2025, meaning its clean energy initiatives will result in removing more greenhouse gases from the atmosphere than the organization emits. Read up on how hospitals are working toward a healthier planet.

WATER WISDOM

Parkland Health & Hospital System in Dallas **washes all linens** in-house rather than outsourc-

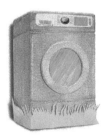

ing the task, and uses a water reclamation system that saves **almost 1 million gallons monthly,** or about **78%** of the water it needs. **Heating costs go down,** too: Thermal energy is trapped in the reused water, providing warmth.

PLASTIC MAGIC

The University of Vermont Medical Center has **recycled more than 50 tons** of the **blue plastic** wrap used to seal sterile equipment. The blue wrap is sent offsite, melted down and shaped into new patient care items like **bed pans** and **wash basins** for the hospital. The effort helps reduce the 30 million pounds of blue wrap tossed in U.S. landfills annually and is being adopted by other hospitals.

CLEAN COMMUTES

Seattle Children's Hospital is paying employees **$4.50 per day** to get to work by **train, bus, carpool, bike or on foot,** and is offering discounted transit passes and **free shuttle services** that connect to regional transit hubs. Solo commutes are down **50%** from two decades ago. For bikers, there's an onsite service center and **two free annual tune-ups.**

SOLAR POWER AND FRESH FISH

Boston Medical Center wants to become New England's first carbon-neutral hospital with new initiatives like a solar power purchasing agreement that will deliver **carbon-free energy** to a mid-Atlantic power grid and offset **100%** of its electricity use. Plus, the yields of a **sustainable rooftop farm** and a partnership with a local fishing association that delivers **fresh fish** daily go directly to patients, while reducing the hospital's carbon footprint.

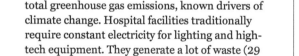

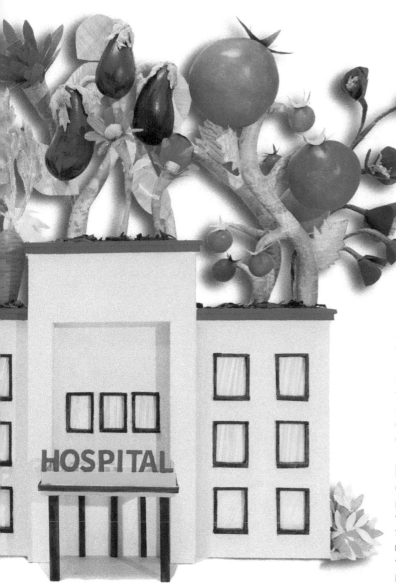

CALMING AND COOLING

Thomas Jefferson University Hospital in Philadelphia planted a **vegetative roof** to absorb rain water and heat. This, alongside other energy-conserving measures, has **saved the hospital over $132 million** since 2010. Other hospitals have similar sustainable roofs where patients benefit, too: The green space helps **reduce anxiety and blood pressure**, and speeds recovery after surgery.

HELLO, PAPER STRAWS

Bon Secours St. Francis Eastside Hospital in South Carolina has set out to reduce plastic waste by **replacing all plastic straws** with paper ones and swapping plastic utensils for reusable **stainless steel cutlery.** Such moves that curtail landfill waste help lessen the production of methane, a potent greenhouse gas with **25 times** the warming potential of carbon dioxide over a 100-year period.

REDUCING VEHICLE EMISSIONS

Children's Health in Dallas has installed a parking guidance system in its garage to help visitors find spots quickly, curbing emissions from cars circling the lot. Future projects: **replacing at least 30%** of the hospital's fleet with electric or **hybrid vehicles by 2022,** and partnering with rideshare programs to help transport patients and employees between campuses. Bike racks and 22 electric vehicle charging stations further encourage the use of green transportation.

A MOVE TO RENEWABLES

Chicago's Advocate Health Care has pledged to power all health care operations with **100% renewable electricity** by 2030 – an "impressive" aim for a Midwest grid largely powered by coal, says Gary Cohen, head of two organizations that help hospitals lessen their environmental impact. The initiative would cut annual carbon dioxide emissions by **over 392,000 metric tons,** equal to removing 84,000 cars from the road.

BEES AND GREENERY

At **Sibley Memorial Hospital in Washington, D.C.,** several buildings have **vegetative roofs** that help lower heating and cooling costs. One has **four beehives,** giving the imperiled bee population a home while helping with local pollination. And all that honey? It's given to employees, who can also use the large garden on hospital grounds to **grow their own vegetables or flowers.**

TOXIN TABOO

At **UPMC Magee-Womens Hospital in Pittsburgh,** the floors, walls and furniture are made with recycled materials **free of hazardous chemicals,** and nontoxic cleaning products are often used. The effort protects babies and moms from harsh toxins. The neonatal intensive care unit **banished plastic materials** containing DEHP, a chemical used in medical devices that may pose risks, especially to NICU infants. To slash waste, food containers are being upgraded to **biodegradable corn** and **paper products.**

Medical Marvels

These five patients have all survived big challenges

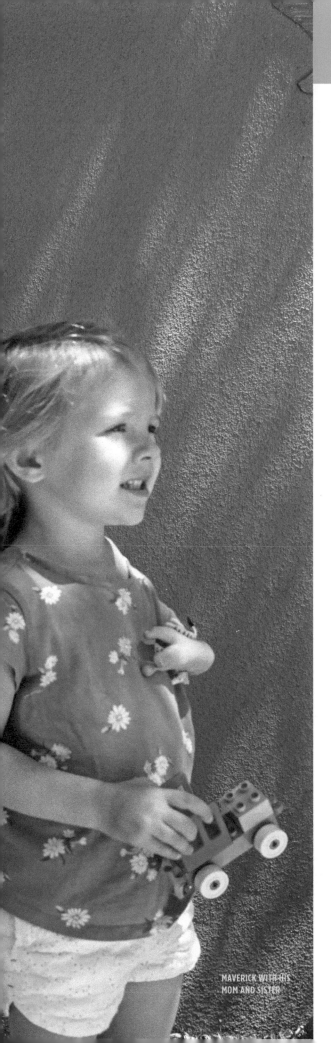

A LIFE-THREATENING MEDICAL mystery. Searing chronic pain. A ticking time bomb inside the body. Brain tumors that caused uncontrolled eating. A devastating leg injury in combat. The patients featured on the following pages were each given a chance at life – or got their lives back – with the help of pioneering treatments, procedures or technology, and quick-thinking medical teams who, in some cases, devised unconventional solutions to big problems, took risks and confirmed that medicine is equal parts science and art with a dash of luck mixed in. Prepare to be inspired.

MAVERICK COLTRIN • 2 years old

MAVERICK COLTRIN WAS SIX DAYS old and very, very sick. His parents were growing increasingly alarmed, first over his reluctance to eat, then jaundice and spasms. After Maverick stopped eating entirely, they raced him to the emergency room at Rady Children's Hospital in San Diego. There, he had another spasm, and started vomiting blood. A barrage of tests followed, and he was admitted to the neonatal intensive care unit. Brain monitoring revealed the spasms were actually seizures; doctors tried the usual medications in vain. "Nothing was working," recalls his mom, Kara. Meantime, the frequency of Maverick's seizures increased to as many as 30 per hour. And still, no one knew why he was sick.

Hometown:
Jamul, California

Hospital:
Rady Children's

His Challenge:
Pyridoxine-dependent epilepsy

Kara and Maverick's dad, Michael, were offered a chance to participate in a clinical trial for newborns admitted to the hospital with serious, unexplained disease. A new technology was being tested called rapid whole-genome sequencing, or rWGS, which analyzes the 3 billion-plus nucleotides that make up an individual's DNA sequence much more quickly than conventional whole-genome sequencing. "I told them I thought this was a very good option for us to see if we could get some answers as quickly as possible," says physician Kristen Wigby, then a clinical genetics fellow at Rady (and now on the faculty). The distinction between the two types of sequencing is like the difference "between a Ford Focus and a Formula One racing car," says Stephen Kingsmore, president and CEO of the Rady Children's Institute for Genomic Medicine, who conducted the trial.

Kara and Michael agreed to have Maverick participate, though they didn't pin their hopes on the trial; they also had their genomes sequenced so any changes in their son's DNA that he didn't inherit from them could be identified. Mean-

while, Maverick's organs were beginning to fail and his skin had turned a dusky blue. "We went from not knowing what was wrong to thinking he was going to die," Kara says.

Then, just 39 hours after blood was drawn, a diagnosis. Maverick had pyridoxine-dependent epilepsy, a rare condition caused by two mutations in his ALDH7A1 gene. Pyridoxine is also known as vitamin B6. The treatment for his frightening ordeal: simple supplementation. Maverick had already been given vitamin B6 as part of the protocol for unexplained seizures, but it hadn't started to work yet. In a textbook case, an infant with the disease responds within minutes, Wigby explains. But in real life, many don't respond for a few days. A diagnosis meant his medical team could keep giving him pyridoxine with confidence. Within 36 hours, the seizures completely stopped.

Kingsmore published a 2018 study showing that 18 of 42 infants who had rWGS to identify an illness or condition received a diagnosis, more than with standard genetic tests. For 13 of those infants, the diagnosis changed the treatment plan, altering outcomes for 11 of the babies. Even when the test reveals a genetic condition that is invariably fatal, getting an answer matters. Parents can start contemplating palliative care instead of leaving an infant on life support hoping for recovery, for example. And it can ease confusion and guilt. "Having a genetic diagnosis shows this wasn't a curse of God, or something that happened during pregnancy," Kingsmore says.

Mystery solved. Kara and Michael now know they are both carriers of the harmful mutation, and Kara can supplement with vitamin B6 if she is ever pregnant again, which could improve an affected baby's outcome. (Maverick has an unaffected older sister.) Rapid genomic screening, at more than $8,000 for the child only, is more expensive than conventional screening, which bottoms out at about $1,000 but often costs several times more. Kingsmore says getting quick answers can save on the costs of hospitalization and unnecessary tests and procedures. He'd like to see the technology made available in every NICU. So far it's not widely used, but some institutions are doing it as part of clinical trials or on a fee-for-service basis. Insurance coverage is still low, but increasing, Kingsmore explains.

As for Maverick, "he hasn't had a seizure since," Kara says. "He's a happy, healthy, chunky boy." He's only slightly behind developmentally and is learning to walk and talk. His treatment remains simple. He is on a special diet that restricts the amino acid lysine, and he gets regular vitamin B6 supplements. "I buy them at Target," she says. –Katherine Hobson

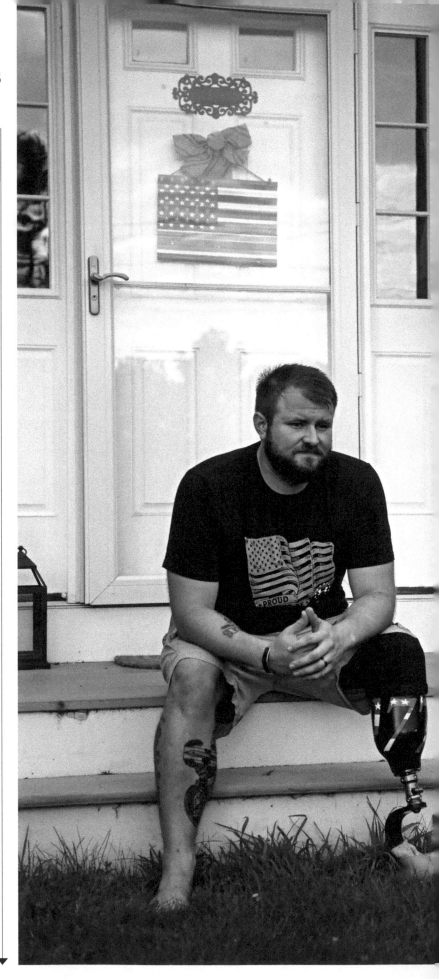

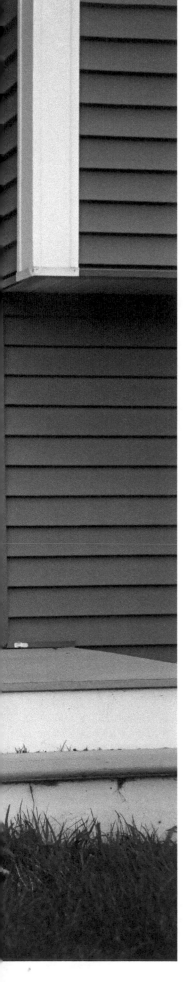

BRANDON KORONA • 28 years old

IN 2013, BRANDON Korona was serving as a U.S. Army combat engineer in Afghanistan when his left leg was severely damaged after an improvised explosive device detonated under his truck. His doctors performed multiple surgeries to try and save it, including an ankle fusion and heel reconstruction. But Brandon wasn't happy with the result. "I could walk and get around, but I had no quality of life. I was in constant pain," Brandon says. "I couldn't run or be active again."

So with the support of his wife, Chelsea, Brandon opted to have the leg removed below the knee in 2017. His doctors referred him to Brigham Health in Boston, where he became the second patient ever to undergo an experimental surgery called the Ewing Amputation. The goal of the procedure, developed by his Brigham surgeon, Matthew Carty, in collaboration with double-amputee Hugh Herr and his team of researchers at Massachusetts Institute of Technology's Center for Extreme Bionics, was to enable Brandon's stump to interact with his prosthetic limb as if it were a real leg. He would be able to perform complex actions – running, climbing stairs, effectively anything he could do before – just by thinking about it.

In a traditional amputation, the dynamic nerve connections between muscles and the brain are destroyed, leaving a stump that can house a prosthetic limb but that can't easily perform complex movements like climbing stairs, or offer amputees normal proprioception – the ability to know where a limb is in space without looking at it. During the Ewing Amputation – named for the first patient to undergo the procedure, rock climber Jim Ewing – surgeons preserve the ability of special fibers and receptors in the muscles of the affected stump so they can channel spatial details to the brain.

More natural. "We believe we're restoring the natural inputs to the brain, so it interprets the limb as being intact," says Carty, director of the Lower Extremity Transplant Program at Brigham and Women's Hospital and an associate professor of surgery at Harvard. "Patients have a precise perception of where

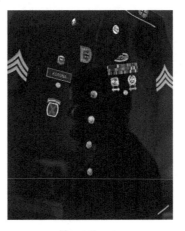

Hometown:
Dracut, Massachusetts
Hospital:
Brigham Health
His Challenge:
Severe leg injury

their limb is in space." There are other advantages, he adds. Patients are less likely to experience "phantom" pain in the missing limb or nerve pain in the stump, and they have less muscle loss than traditional amputees typically suffer over time.

Brandon's initial recovery took about three months. After the surgery, he worked with a physical therapist to train his modified limb to work with a prosthesis. Within a month of getting onto a prosthetic, he could walk as if the limb were his own. "I know where the foot is. I feel the sensation of the foot hitting the ground and stepping forward," he says.

"People don't realize I'm an amputee unless I'm wearing shorts."

It wasn't long before he could run. He has since completed five road races and is training for the 2020 Boston Marathon. The race will have special meaning for him: The initial research behind the development of the Ewing Amputation was funded by the Gillian Reny Stepping Strong Center for Trauma Innovation, named for a survivor of the 2013 Boston Marathon bombings, who was treated for life-threatening limb injuries at Brigham and Women's Hospital. Carty's team now has funding from the Department of Defense to develop a similar technique for people who need upper limb amputation. And Herr's team at MIT has developed a prototype of a "bionic" leg specifically designed to interact with the limbs of patients who have had the Ewing Amputation. It contains electrodes that link these individuals to this new technology so they can better perform complex "reflexive" behaviors – stretching the heel to climb stairs, say – more naturally than they can with standard prostheses.

The bionic leg isn't yet on the market, but Brandon has tested it out. "I was able to control it with my muscles," he says. "I look forward to seeing the potential of it to help me run even better than I can with my prosthetic limb." For now, he's thrilled by how much the Ewing Amputation has improved his life. "I don't have any pain. I have no limitations anymore," he says. "It's a complete 180 from where I was." *–Arlene Weintraub*

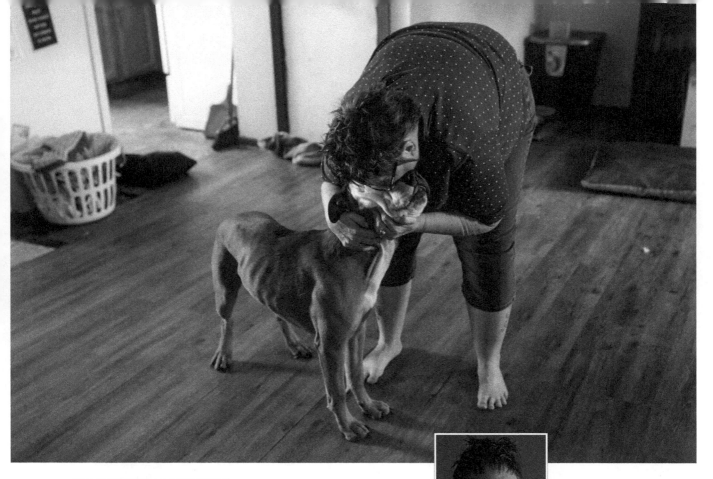

TAMMY DURFEE • 57 years old

Hometown:
Higginsville, Missouri
Hospital:
University of Maryland
Medical Center
Her Challenge:
Thalamocortical
dysrhythmia

IN 2008, Tammy Durfee awoke with a pain in her left hip and leg. Had she tweaked it the day before? Or slept on it wrong?

Ten years later, after having two spinal fusions (surgeons reinforced her spine using screws and bone grafts) and a device implanted to send electrical signals to her spinal cord in an attempt to override the now searing pain, Tammy had become "a hermit," she says. "I had timed exactly how long it took to get ready for work and didn't get out of bed until I absolutely had to. When I got home, I got back into bed as soon as possible."

Finally, a neurosurgeon diagnosed neuropathic pain associated with thalamocortical dysrhythmia, in which misfiring in the thalamus region of the brain sends pain signals out to the body. Roughly 8% of Americans suffer from neuropathic pain of some kind, a leading reason doctors prescribe opioids. Tammy had spent years trying the potent painkillers until finally telling her doctor, "I'm not taking them anymore."

Desperate for relief, she reached out to the University of Maryland School of Medicine, which was recruiting people for a clinical trial of MRI-guided focused ultrasound to the brain as a treatment for neuropathic pain. The technology, which relies on intense ultrasound beams to burn targeted tissue, is used to treat tremors, bone tumors and uterine fibroids. Building on Swiss research, Dheeraj Gandhi, a professor of diagnostic radiology and nuclear medicine, neurology and neurosurgery at the medical school, wanted to determine if it might be effective against neuropathic pain. On Sept. 13, 2018, Tammy became the first person in the U.S. to undergo MRI-guided focused ultrasound for that purpose, at the University of Maryland Medical Center.

Burning the pain away. Gandhi and his team affixed a metallic frame to her head to immobilize it within the MRI machine. They connected it to a helmet-like contraption that directed more than 1,000 ultrasound beams to tiny spots on her thalamus. Gradually, the energy output was increased, raising the temperature to between 55 and 60 degrees Celsius (131 to 140 degrees Fahrenheit), burning the precise area of tissue to disrupt the errant signals. With each increase, the team checked in with Tammy.

"My head started to feel hot, which made me anxious," she says. She focused on deep breathing. Patients may feel fleeting discomfort, dizziness and headaches during the treatment, Gandhi says.

"The beautiful thing about this is that patients tend to be completely awake during the procedure, meaning you can test them for improvement while they are still in the magnet," Gandhi says. "They go home the same day, and there's no incision apart from the steel frame that is secured to the skull. It's not like spinal cord stimulators or deep brain stimulation, which can have serious side effects like bleeding or stroke." After the four-hour treatment, Tammy says she literally danced out of the surgery room.

"I can do anything and everything I want now," she says. "I can walk my dogs, carry laundry, ride in the car, actually sit through an entire TV show. I have my life back."

Gandhi's hope is that the technique might help people cut their pain and disability by 40% and 30%, respectively, and that the trial will lead to more research and Food and Drug Administration approval. It's early, but results are promising. And Tammy's pain is gone: "I tell everyone about my success, but that it's not approved or available yet. I hope it will be soon, so that more people like me can get the help they need." *–K. Aleisha Fetters*

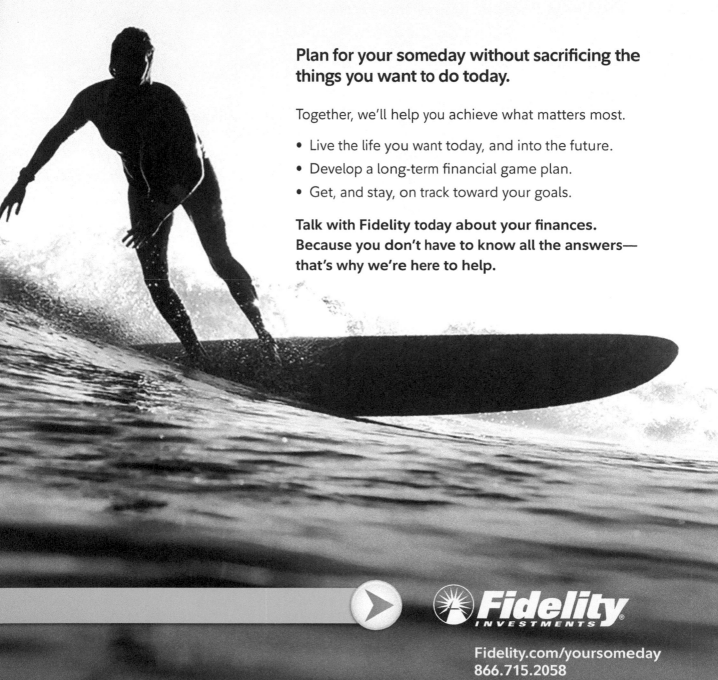

BECAUSE SOMEDAY

I'll spend every day making the morning rounds.

Plan for your someday without sacrificing the things you want to do today.

Together, we'll help you achieve what matters most.

- Live the life you want today, and into the future.
- Develop a long-term financial game plan.
- Get, and stay, on track toward your goals.

Talk with Fidelity today about your finances. Because you don't have to know all the answers— that's why we're here to help.

Fidelity INVESTMENTS

Fidelity.com/yoursomeday
866.715.2058

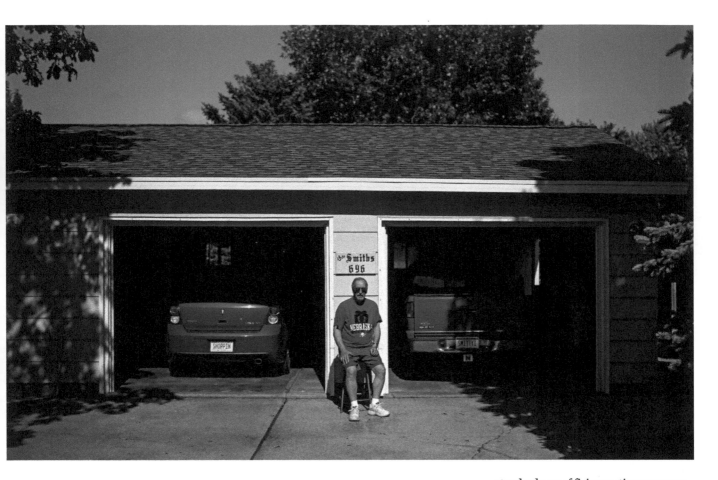

JIMMIE SMITH • 72 years old

JIMMIE SMITH THOUGHT he was healthy – until a routine checkup led to a deadly diagnosis. Doctors discovered a ticking time bomb inside his body that threatened to kill him within six months.

His nightmare began in 2018, when a blood test signaled that his kidney function was off, prompting a CT scan. The test revealed that Jimmie, who lives with his wife, Karen, in a small Nebraska town (population: just over 400), had a very large aortic aneurysm. And it could erupt at any time.

"That was very scary. I had no pain or any symptoms," he says. The aorta is the body's largest blood vessel. Shaped like a cane with shoots of feeder blood vessels to vital organs, it ferries blood from the heart to the rest of the body. When the aorta's wall weakens, an aneurysm can form – a balloon-like bulge that can burst, triggering internal bleeding and even death. Doctors don't know what causes aortic aneurysms, though hardening of the arteries, high blood pressure, genetic predisposition and smoking

might play a role – and Jimmie was a lifelong smoker who has since quit.

A subsequent scan detected multiple aneurysms in his aorta, making his perilous condition beyond the scope of what his doctors in Nebraska could handle. That's how he ended up at Mayo Clinic in Minnesota, nearly 500 miles from home. There he met with vascular surgeon Gustavo Oderich, an internationally recognized expert in aneurysm repair.

What made Jimmie's situation even more treacherous was the location of the aneurysms – in the curve of the aorta by his collarbone and in other tricky-to-fix spots. Basically, his whole aorta was affected. "He had a perfect storm; really the worst of the worst-case scenario," says Oderich, Mayo's chair of vascular and endovascular surgery. "He was lucky that he survived so many years."

Jimmie wasn't a good candidate for the

Hometown:
Giltner, Nebraska

Hospital:
Mayo Clinic

His Challenge:
Aortic aneurysms

standard way of fixing aortic aneurysms, whereby a large incision is made in the abdomen and chest to expose the aorta, the heart is stopped, and patients are placed on a heart-lung machine to keep blood circulating. The surgeon then repairs the aortic aneurysm by sewing a thin mesh sleeve to the blood vessel, strengthening the weak spot and preventing rupture. "Because of the position of his aneurysms, he would need two very large open surgeries," Oderich says; half of patients who need this sequence of procedures "never recover enough to tolerate a second operation," he explains.

Jimmie would require an out-of-the-box approach – and with every beat of his heart, every whoosh of his blood, his aneurysms threatened to burst. There was a 50-50 chance he could die before reaching the operating table.

So Oderich made a bold decision: His team would rebuild Jimmie's entire aorta – from the arch of his collarbone to his

(CONTINUED ON PAGE 60)

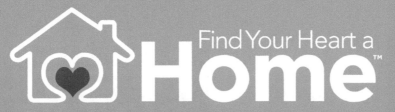

Find Your Heart a
Home™
Connecting heart patients with the right hospital

🔍 Do You Or a Loved One Need Cardiac Care?

- **Heart Attack** (Stent, Surgery)
- **Heart Rhythm Disorder** (AFib Ablation, Implantable Cardioverter-Defibrillator)
- **Heart Valve Disease** (TAVR, Surgery)

For these and other treatments, use the online tool to …

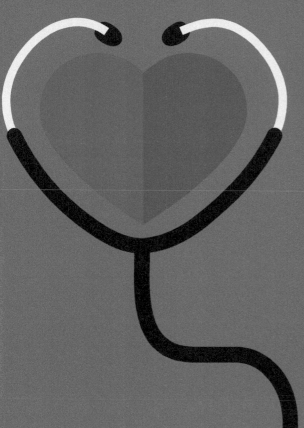

SEARCH
over **700 hospitals**

COMPARE
their **performance**

SELECT
the **right hospital**

Get Started at *FindYourHeartaHome.org*

Powered by ACC's NCDR® and CardioSmart®

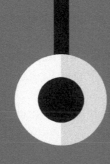

New and Improved Navigation!

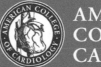

AMERICAN COLLEGE *of* **CARDIOLOGY**

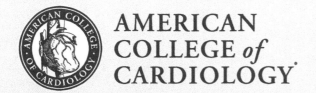

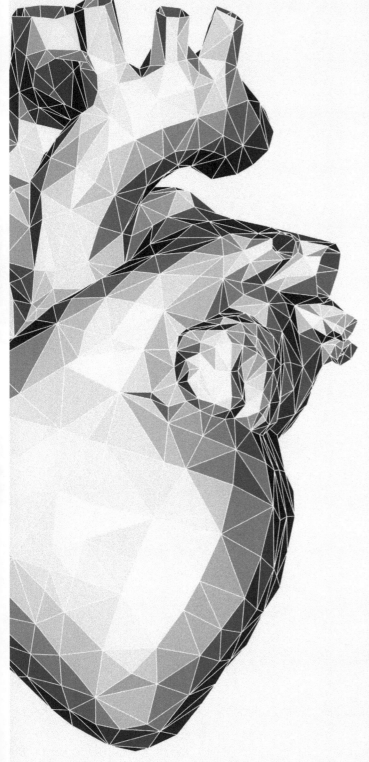

THE HEART OF QUALITY PATIENT CARE

As the global professional organization for the entire cardiovascular care team, the American College of Cardiology is committed to supporting patients, caregivers and health care providers by ensuring the highest quality care is delivered to every patient, every time.

ACC Accreditation Services

ACC's Accreditation Services links performance improvement to patient outcomes and promotes consistent processes across the care continuum. We work with hospitals and health systems to build communities of excellence by advancing the highest standards of quality patient care.

NCDR (National Cardiovascular Data Registry)

The NCDR is ACC's suite of data registries helping hospitals and health systems measure and improve the quality of cardiovascular care they provide. The NCDR utilizes real-world evidence to improve patient outcomes and achieve quality heart care.

The following pages list more than 2,000 hospitals and health systems who rely on ACC's NCDR and Accreditation Services. Patients and caregivers can trust hospitals and health systems who participate in the NCDR, receive the ACC's Accreditation seal of approval, and are recognized with the Chest Pain – MI Registry Performance Achievement Award and the HeartCARE Center Award for delivering the best in patient care.

FOR CARDIOVASCULAR PROFESSIONALS, please visit *CVQuality.ACC.org* to learn more about ACC's Quality Improvement for Institutions program.

FOR PATIENTS AND CAREGIVERS, please visit *CardioSmart.org* to learn more about ACC's provider-directed heart health education and resources.

ACC Accreditation Services

AF Atrial Fibrillation Accreditation
Incorporates evidence-based guidelines and clinical best practices to treat patients with atrial fibrillation.

CL Cardiac Cath Lab Accreditation
Merges the latest evidence-based science and process improvement methodologies, while addressing pre-procedure, peri-procedure and post-procedure care for patients undergoing treatment in the Cath Lab.

CP Chest Pain Center Accreditation
Integrates triage treatment protocols, risk stratification, and best practices for the emergency care of acute coronary syndrome patients.

EP Electrophysiology Accreditation
Links the latest science, process improvement methodologies and patient outcomes across the care continuum for patients undergoing treatment in the EP Lab.

HF Heart Failure Accreditation
Leverages guideline-directed medical therapies and best practices to ensure greater operational efficiency and a more consistent approach to treatment.

NCDR

A AFib Ablation Registry™
(Catheter-based atrial fibrillation ablation procedures) Assesses the prevalence, demographics, acute management and outcomes of patients undergoing atrial fibrillation (AFib) catheter ablation procedures.

C CathPCI Registry®
(Diagnostic cardiac catheterization and percutaneous coronary intervention) Measures adherence to the ACC/AHA clinical practice guideline recommendations, procedure performance standards and appropriate use criteria for coronary revascularization.

CP Chest Pain - MI Registry™
(Acute myocardial infarction treatment) Leverages national evidence-based standards for understanding and improving the quality, safety and outcomes of care provided for heart attack patients.

I ICD Registry™
(Implantable cardioverter defibrillator and leads procedures) Provides a national standard on the implant, revision, replacement or explant of ICD/CRT-D to understand treatment patterns, clinical outcomes, device safety and overall quality of care.

IM IMPACT Registry®
(Pediatric and adult congenital treatment procedures) Assesses the prevalence, demographics, management and outcomes of pediatric and adult congenital heart disease (CHD) patients who undergo diagnostic catheterizations and catheter-based interventions.

L LAAO Registry™
(Left atrial appendage occlusion procedures) Captures data on left atrial appendage occlusion (LAAO) procedures to assess real-world procedural outcomes, short and long-term safety, and comparative effectiveness.

P PVI Registry™
(Lower extremity peripheral vascular interventions, carotid artery revascularization, and endarterectomy procedures) Measures the prevalence, demographics, management and outcomes of patients undergoing lower extremity peripheral arterial catheter-based interventions.

T STS/ACC TVT Registry™
(Transcatheter valve therapy procedures) Monitors real-world outcomes on transcatheter valve therapies leading to improved patient outcomes, enhanced assessment of treatment options and results, and more informed decision making.

Chest Pain - MI Registry™ Performance Achievement Award
Recognizes hospitals participating in Chest Pain – MI Registry who have demonstrated sustained, top level performance in quality of care and adherence to guideline recommendations.

▲ Platinum
▲ Gold
▲ Silver

◆ HeartCARE Center™
Recognizes hospitals who have demonstrated a commitment to world-class cardiovascular care through comprehensive process improvement, disease and procedure-specific accreditation, professional excellence, and community engagement.

ALABAMA

Hospital	Accreditations
Andalusia Regional Hospital	I HF
Baptist Medical Center South	C CP I
Brookwood Baptist Medical Center	C L P T
Children's of Alabama	IM
Crestwood Medical Center	C CP I CP
Cullman Regional Medical Center	C CL CP HF
DCH Regional Medical Center	C I P
Dekalb Regional Medical Center	C I CP
East Alabama Medical Center - Opelika	C
Eliza Coffee Memorial Hospital	CP
Flowers Hospital	C CP I ▲
Gadsden Regional Medical Center	C I CP
Grandview Medical Center	C CP I L T CL CP
Helen Keller Hospital	I
Huntsville Hospital	C CP I L P T
Jackson Hospital	C
Marshall Medical Centers	C I
Medical Center Enterprise	CP
Mobile Infirmary	C L T
North Alabama Medical Center	C P
Princeton Baptist Medical Center	C I IM L T
Providence Hospital - Mobile	C I
Regional Medical Center - Anniston	C I
Regional Medical Center - Stringfellow	CP
Riverview Regional Medical Center	C I CP
Russell Medical Center	C
Shelby Baptist Medical Center	C L P T
Shoals Hospital	CP
South Baldwin Regional Medical Center	C I CP
Southeast Health	C L T CP
Springhill Medical Center	C T
St. Vincent's Birmingham	C L T
St. Vincent's East	C L T
Thomas Hospital	C CP I
UAB Hospital	A C I L T
University Hospital	C
Vaughan Regional Medical Center	C CP
Walker Baptist Medical Center	C

ALASKA

Hospital	Accreditations
Alaska Cardiovascular Surgery Center, LLC	I
Alaska Native Medical Center	C
Alaska Regional Hospital	C L AF CP HF
Central Peninsula Hospital	C
Fairbanks Memorial Hospital	C I
Mat-Su Regional Medical Center	C I CP
Providence Alaska Medical Center	A C CP T ▲

ARIZONA

Hospital	Accreditations
Abrazo Arizona Heart Hospital	C CP I L P T CL CP
Abrazo Arrowhead Campus	C CP I L P T CP
Abrazo Central Campus	C CP I CP
Abrazo Scottsdale Campus	C CP I
Abrazo West Campus	C CP I CP
Banner Baywood Medical Center	CP
Banner Boswell Medical Center	L T
Banner Desert Medical Center	T
Banner Heart Hospital	C L T
Banner Thunderbird Medical Center	L T
Banner University Medical Center South	C
Banner University Medical Center Tucson	C I IM L
Canyon Vista Medical Center	C I
Carondelet Health Network	C CP CP
Chandler Regional Medical Center	C CP L P T CP
Flagstaff Medical Center	C I L
Havasu Regional Medical Center	C I CL CP
HonorHealth Deer Valley Medical Center	C
HonorHealth John C. Lincoln Medical Center	C
HonorHealth Scottsdale - Osborn Medical Center	C
HonorHealth Scottsdale - Shea Medical Center	C L T
HonorHealth Scottsdale - Thompson Peak Medical Center	C
Kingman Regional Medical Center	C I P
La Paz Regional Hospital	I
Maricopa Medical Center	I
Mayo Clinic Hospital - Arizona	C L T
Mercy Gilbert Medical Center	C CP CP

Continues on next page

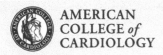

(Arizona, continued)

Hospital	Badges
Mountain Vista Medical Center	C CP CP
Northwest Medical Center	C I T CP
Oro Valley Hospital	C I CP
Phoenix Children's Hospital	IM
St. Joseph Hospital	
St. Joseph's Hospital and Medical Center	C CP L P T CP
St. Luke's Medical Center	CP
St. Mary Hospital	C CP I T CP
Summit Healthcare Regional Medical Center	C I
Tucson Medical Center	C CP I L T CP
University Medical Center Phoenix - Banner	C L T
Valley View Medical Center	C I CP
Verde Valley Medical Center	C I
Western Arizona Regional Medical Center	C CP I
Yavapai Regional Medical Center	I L T
Yuma Regional Medical Center	C I P T

ARKANSAS

Hospital	Badges
Arkansas Children's Hospital	IM
Arkansas Heart Hospital	C CP I L P T
Baptist Health - Fort Smith	C CP I P CP
Baptist Health Medical Center - Conway	CP
Baptist Health Medical Center - Little Rock	C CP I L T
Baptist Health Medical Center - North Little Rock	C CP I
Baxter Regional Medical Center	C CP I P ★
CHI St. Vincent Hot Springs	C CP I
CHI St. Vincent Infirmary	A C CP I L T
CHI St. Vincent North	C CP I
Conway Regional Medical Center	C CP I
Jefferson Regional Medical Center	CP I
Medical Center of South Arkansas	C CP I
Mercy Hospital Fort Smith	C CP CP
Mercy Hospital Northwest Arkansas	C CP L T CP ★
National Park Medical Center	CP I
NEA Baptist Memorial Hospital	C CP ★
Northwest Medical Center - Bentonville	C CP I
Northwest Medical Center - Springdale	C CP I
Saline Memorial Hospital	CP
Siloam Springs Regional Hospital	CP
St. Bernards Medical Center	CP L T ★
St. Mary's Regional Medical Center	C CP I
Unity Health - White County Medical Center	C CP I
University of Arkansas for Medical Sciences Medical Center	CP
Washington Regional Medical Center	C CP I L T CP
White River Medical Center	CP

CALIFORNIA

Hospital	Badges
Adventist Health and Rideout	C CP I
Adventist Health Bakersfield	C CP I CP HF ★
Adventist Health Glendale	C I T CP
Adventist Health Hanford	I
Adventist Health Lodi Memorial	I
Adventist Health Simi Valley	C I
Adventist Health Sonora	I
Adventist Health St. Helena	C I L P T
Adventist Health White Memorial	C I T AF CP
AHMC Anaheim Regional Medical Center	C I T
Alameda Health System	C
Alta Bates Summit Medical Center - Summit Campus	C I L P T
Alvarado Hospital Medical Center	C
Antelope Valley Hospital	C CP I CP ★
Arcadia Outpatient Surgery Center, LP	I
Arrowhead Regional Medical Center	C CP I
Bakersfield Heart Hospital	C CP I CP HF
Barstow Community Hospital	I CP
Beverly Hospital	I
California Hospital Medical Center	C
California Pacific Medical Center - Pacific Campus	C CP I L T ★
Cedars-Sinai Medical Center	C I IM L T
Centinela Hospital Medical Center	C I
CHA Hollywood Presbyterian Medical Center	C
Children's Hospital Los Angeles	I IM
Children's Hospital of Orange County (CHOC)	IM
Chino Valley Medical Center	C
Clovis Community Medical Center	C I
Community Hospital of the Monterey Peninsula	C L T CP
Community Memorial Hospital - San Buenaventura	C CP I L T
Community Regional Medical Center	C I P T
Corona Regional Medical Center	C I
Dameron Hospital	C I
Desert Regional Medical Center	C CP I L AF CP
Desert Valley Hospital	C CP I
Doctors Medical Center Modesto	C CP I L T CP ★
Dominican Hospital	C P T
Eisenhower Health	C I L T CP
El Camino Hospital System	A C CP L P T ★
El Centro Regional Medical Center	I CP
Emanate Health	C I T
Emanuel Medical Center	C CP CP
Enloe Medical Center	C I
Fountain Valley Regional Hospital & Medical Center	C
French Hospital Medical Center	C CP L T ★
Fresno Heart & Surgical Hospital	C I L P T
Garfield Medical Center	C CP I P T
Glendale Memorial Hospital	C I CP
Good Samaritan Health System - Regional Medical Center of San Jose	C
Good Samaritan Health System - Good Samaritan Hospital - San Jose	C L T
Good Samaritan Hospital - Los Angeles	C I L T
Hemet Valley Medical Center	I
Henry Mayo Newhall Memorial Hospital	C I
Hoag Hospital Irvine	A C I L T
Huntington Hospital	C I L T
JFK Memorial Hospital	C CP
John Muir Medical Center - Concord Campus	C CP I L T ★
John Muir Medical Center - Walnut Creek Campus	C CP I
Kaiser Permanente Fontana Medical Center	C I T
Kaiser Permanente Los Angeles Medical Center	C I
Kaiser Permanente Modesto Medical Center	C
Kaiser Permanente Oakland Medical Center	C IM
Kaiser Permanente Orange County - Anaheim Medical Center	I
Kaiser Permanente Orange County - Irvine Medical Center	C I
Kaiser Permanente Redwood City Medical Center	C
Kaiser Permanente Fremont Medical Center	C
Kaiser Permanente Orchard Medical Offices	I
Kaiser Permanente Roseville Medical Center	C
Kaiser Permanente Sacramento Medical Center	C
Kaiser Permanente San Francisco Medical Center	C T
Kaiser Permanente San Jose Medical Center	C
Kaiser Permanente San Rafael Medical Center	C
Kaiser Permanente Santa Clara Medical Center	C L
Kaiser Permanente South Sacramento Medical Center	C
Kaiser Permanente Vallejo Medical Center	C
Kaiser Permanente Walnut Creek Medical Center	C
Kaweah Delta Health Care District	C I T
Keck Medicine of USC	C I L T
Lakewood Regional Medical Center	C
Loma Linda University Medical Center	C I IM L T CP
Loma Linda University Medical Center Murrieta	C I T CP
Long Beach Medical Center	C I IM L T
Los Alamitos Medical Center	C
Los Robles Health System - Los Robles Regional Medical Center	A C L T CP
Lucile Packard Children's Hospital Stanford	I IM
Marian Regional Medical Center	C L
Marin General Hospital	C I L T CP
Marshall Medical Center	I
Memorial Hospital	C CP L T CP
Memorial Medical Center	C CP I T CP ★
Menifee Valley Medical Center	I
Mercy General Hospital	C L T
Mercy Medical Center Merced	C
Mercy Medical Center Redding	C
Mercy San Juan Medical Center	C
Methodist Hospital of Southern California	C I P
Mills - Peninsula Health Services	A C I L T
Mission Hospital Mission Viejo	C
NorthBay Medical Center	C CP I CP ★
Northridge Hospital Medical Center	C
O'Connor Hospital	C
Orange Coast Medical Center	C I
Orange County Global Medical Center	I
Palmdale Regional Medical Center	C I
Palomar Medical Center Escondido	C CP I P T ★
PIH Health - Whittier	C I
PIH Health Hospital - Downey	C I
Placentia-Linda Hospital	C
Pomona Valley Hospital Medical Center	C CP L T CP
Providence Holy Cross Medical Center	C
Providence Little Company of Mary Medical Center Torrance	A C T
Providence St. John's Health Center	A C L
Providence St. Joseph Medical Center	A C
Providence Tarzana Medical Center	A C
Queen of the Valley Medical Center	C I
Rady Children's Hospital San Diego	IM
Rancho Springs Medical Center	I
Ridgecrest Regional Hospital	I
Riverside Community Hospital	C CP I
Riverside University Health System Medical Center	I
Ronald Reagan UCLA Medical Center	C CP I IM L T
Sacramento Heart Ambulatory Surgery Center, Inc	CP I
Saddleback Medical Center	C I L T
Salinas Valley Memorial Hospital	CP I L P T ★
San Antonio Regional Hospital	I T CP
San Joaquin General Hospital	I
San Ramon Regional Medical Center	C
Santa Barbara Cottage Hospital	C I L T
Santa Rosa Memorial Hospital	C I T
Scripps Memorial Hospital La Jolla	C L T
Scripps Mercy Hospital San Diego	C
Sequoia Hospital	C
Sharp Chula Vista Medical Center	C L T
Sharp Grossmont Hospital	C L T
Sharp Memorial Hospital	C L T
Shasta Regional Medical Center	C I CP
Sierra View Medical Center	C
Skypark Surgery Center	I
St. Agnes Medical Center	C I L T
St. Bernardine Medical Center	C P T
St. Francis Medical Center	C CP I P
St. John's Regional Medical Center	C L T
St. Joseph Hospital - Eureka	C I
St. Joseph Hospital Orange	A C L T

Legend

Registries
- A — AFib Ablation Registry™
- C — CathPCI Registry®
- CP — Chest Pain - MI Registry™
- I — ICD Registry™
- IM — IMPACT Registry®
- L — LAAO Registry™
- P — PVI Registry™
- T — STS/ACC TVT Registry™

Accreditations
- AF — Atrial Fibrillation
- CL — Cardiac Cath Lab
- CP — Chest Pain Center
- EP — Electrophysiology
- HF — Heart Failure

Awards
- ★ Chest Pain - MI Registry™ Award Silver
- ★ Chest Pain - MI Registry™ Award Gold
- ★ Chest Pain - MI Registry™ Award Platinum
- ◆ HeartCARE Center™

St. Joseph's Medical Center .... C CP I L P T ★
St. Jude Medical Center .... A C
St. Mary Medical Center .... C CP
St. Mary Medical Center Long Beach C
St. Mary's Medical Center C
St. Rose Hospital .... C I
St. Vincent Medical Center I
Stanford Health Care .... C I T
Stanford Health Care - ValleyCare Medical Center .... C I
Sutter Amador Surgery Center I
Sutter Delta Medical Center .... C I
Sutter Medical Center -
Jose Adams Medical Pavilion .... C I L T
Sutter Roseville Medical Center .... C I
Sutter Santa Rosa Regional Hospital .... A C I
Sutter Solano Medical Center I
Temecula Valley Hospital .... C CP I P CP
Torrance Memorial Medical Center .... A C L T
Tri-City Medical Center .... C CP I
UC Irvine Medical Center .... C I T
UC San Diego Health -
La Jolla Sulpizio Cardiovascular Center .... C CP I L T
UCSF Benioff Children's Hospital Oakland .... IM
University Of California – Santa Monica .... C I
University of California
Davis Medical Center .... C CP I IM L P T
University of California
San Francisco Health System .... C I IM L T
USC Verdugo Hills Hospital I
Valley Children's Hospital .... IM
Valley Presbyterian Hospital .... C I
Washington Hospital .... C I
Watsonville Community Hospital I
West Anaheim Medical Center .... C CP
West Hills Hospital & Medical Center I

COLORADO

Avista Adventist Hospital .... C CP
Boulder Community Health .... C I L T
Castle Rock Adventist Hospital .... C CP
Children's Hospital Colorado System .... I IM CP
Colorado Plains Medical Center .... CP
Denver Health .... C CP I
Good Samaritan Medical Center .... C CP P CP ★
Littleton Adventist Hospital .... C CP CP ★
Longmont United Hospital .... C CP
Lutheran Medical Center .... C CP P CP ★
McKee Medical Center .... C CP ★
Mercy Regional Medical Center .... C CP ★
North Colorado Medical Center .... C CP L T ★
North Suburban Medical Center .... C CP
Parker Adventist Hospital .... C CP CP
Parkview Medical Center .... C CP I L C CP ★
Penrose-St. Francis Health Services .... C CP L T ★
Platte Valley Medical Center .... C CP CP
Porter Adventist Hospital .... A C CP L AF CP HF
Poudre Valley Hospital .... C CP I
Presbyterian/St. Luke's Medical Center .... C CP IM ★
Rose Medical Center .... A C CP I L AF CL CP ★ ◆
Sky Ridge Medical Center .... C CP CP ★
St. Anthony Hospital .... A C CP L T CP ★
St. Anthony North Health Campus .... C CP
St. Francis Medical Center .... C CP ★
St. Joseph Hospital .... C CP L T CP ★
St. Mary's Medical Center .... C CP T CP ★
Swedish Medical Center .... C CP I IM P T ★
The Medical Center of Aurora -
Main Campus .... C CP I L T AF CP ★
UCHealth Medical Center
of the Rockies .... A C CP I L P T ★

UCHealth Memorial
Hospital Central .... C CP I L T AF CP ★ ◆
UCHealth Memorial Hospital North .... CP
UCHealth University of Colorado Hospital .... CP
University Of Colorado
Hospital Authority .... A C CP I L T ★
Vail Health .... C I
Valley View Hospital .... A C CP I

CONNECTICUT

Bridgeport Hospital .... A C L T
Connecticut Children's Medical Center .... I IM
Danbury Hospital .... C I T CP
Greenwich Hospital C
Hartford Hospital .... A C I T
Lawrence & Memorial Hospital I
MidState Medical Center I
Norwalk Hospital .... C I CP
St. Francis Hospital and Medical Center .... A C I T
St. Mary's Hospital .... A C CP I CP
St. Vincent's Medical Center .... C CP I L T ★
Stamford Hospital .... C I L T
The Hospital of Central Connecticut -
New Britain General Campus .... C I
The William W. Backus Hospital I
UConn John Dempsey Hospital .... C CP I
Waterbury Hospital .... C I
Yale New Haven Hospital .... A C IM L T

DISTRICT OF COLUMBIA

Children's National Medical Center .... IM
George Washington University Hospital .... A C CP I L T
MedStar Washington Hospital Center .... A C CP I L T

DELAWARE

Bayhealth .... C I T
Beebe Healthcare .... C I L
Christiana Care Health System .... C CP I L T ★
Nanticoke Memorial Hospital .... C P
Nemours Alfred duPont Hospital for Children .... IM
St. Francis Healthcare .... C CP I

FLORIDA

AdventHealth Altamonte Springs .... C I
Adventhealth Apopka I
AdventHealth Carrollwood .... C I
AdventHealth Celebration .... C CP I
AdventHealth Dade City .... C I AF CP
AdventHealth Daytona Beach .... C I L T
AdventHealth DeLand .... C I
AdventHealth East Orlando .... C I
AdventHealth Fish Memorial .... C I
AdventHealth New Smyrna Beach .... C I
AdventHealth North Pinellas .... C CP I CP
AdventHealth Ocala .... C I L P T AF
AdventHealth Orlando .... A C I IM L T
AdventHealth Palm Coast C
AdventHealth Pepin Heart Institute .... C CP I L T CP
AdventHealth Sebring .... C I P
AdventHealth Tampa .... CP
AdventHealth Waterman .... A C CP I T
AdventHealth Wesley Chapel .... C I
AdventHealth Zephyrhills .... C CP I CP
Ascension - St. Vincent's Medical Center Clay County C
Ascension - St. Vincent's
Medical Center Riverside .... A C I L T
Ascension - St. Vincent's Medical Center Southside .... C I
Aventura Hospital & Medical Center .... A C I L T
Baptist Health - Jacksonville FL .... A C I L T
Baptist Hospital - Miami .... A C I L P T
Baptist Hospital - Pensacola .... C CP I L T
Bartow Regional Medical Center .... C I

Bay Medical Center Sacred Heart .... C I P T
Bayfront Health - Brooksville .... C I
Bayfront Health - Port Charlotte .... C I L CP
Bayfront Health - Punta Gorda .... CP
Bayfront Health - Seven Rivers .... C CP
Bayfront Health - St. Petersburg .... C CP I
Bethesda Heart Hospital .... C I L T
Blake Medical Center .... C I T
Boca Raton Regional Hospital .... C I T
Brandon Regional Hospital .... C L T
Broward Health Imperial Point .... C I
Broward Health Medical Center .... C I L T
Broward Health North .... C I
Cape Canaveral Hospital C
Cape Coral Hospital .... HF
Capital Regional Medical Center .... C CP
Central Florida Regional Hospital .... C CP L T CP
Citrus Memorial Hospital .... C T
Clearwater Cardiovascular
& Interventional Consultants MD PA C
Cleveland Clinic Florida .... C I L
Cleveland Clinic Indian River Hospital .... C CP I T CP
Cleveland Clinic Tradition Hospital C
Delray Medical Center .... C I L T
Doctors Hospital .... I P
Doctors Hospital of Sarasota C
Dr. P. Phillips Hospital .... C CP HF
Englewood Community Hospital .... C CP
Fawcett Memorial Hospital .... C L
Flagler Hospital .... C I
Florida Medical Center .... C I L T
Fort Walton Beach Medical Center .... C L P CP
Golisano Children's Hospital of Southwest Florida .... C I T
Good Samaritan Medical Center .... C CP
Gulf Breeze Hospital I
Gulf Coast Medical Center .... C I HF
Gulf Coast Regional Medical Center .... C CP
Halifax Health Medical Center
of Daytona Beach .... C I L T
HCA North Florida Division -
Ocala Health System .... C T AF CP HF
Health Central Hospital .... C CP HF
Heart and Rhythm Institute of Trinity .... CP I
Heart of Florida Regional Medical Center .... C CP I CP
Highlands Regional Medical Center C
Holmes Regional Medical Center .... A C L T
Holy Cross Hospital .... C I L T
Homestead Hospital .... I P
Jackson Memorial Hospital .... C I IM P T
Jackson North Medical Center .... C I
Jackson South Medical Center .... C I
JFK Medical Center .... A C L T CP
Joe Dimaggio Children's Hospital
at Memorial Regional Hospital .... IM
Johns Hopkins All Children's Hospital .... IM
Jupiter Medical Center .... C I
Kendall Regional Medical Center C
Lake City Medical Center .... C I CP
Lake Wales Medical Center .... I CP
Lakeland Regional Health
Medical Center .... C I L P T CP
Lakewood Ranch Medical Center .... C CP
Largo Medical Center .... A C L
Lawnwood Regional Medical Center
& Heart Institute .... C L T
Lee Memorial Hospital .... HF
Leesburg Regional Medical Center .... C CP I T CP
Lower Keys Medical Center .... C I CP
Manatee Memorial Hospital .... C CP I L T ★
Martin Health System .... C I T

Continues on next page

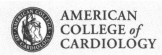

- Mayo Clinic Hospital - Florida — C L T
- Mease Countryside Hospital — C CP I P
- Medical Center of Trinity — C
- Melbourne Regional Medical Center — C I
- Memorial Hospital Jacksonville — A C L P T CP
- Memorial Hospital of Tampa — C
- Memorial Hospital West — C
- Memorial Regional Hospital — C L T
- Mercy Hospital — C CP
- Morton Plant Hospital — A C CP I L P T
- Morton Plant North Bay Hospital — C CP I P
- Mount Sinai Medical Center — C CP P T CP ★
- NCH Baker Hospital — C L T
- Nemours Children's Hospital — IM
- Nicklaus Children's Hospital — IM
- North Florida Regional Medical Center — C L T CP
- North Okaloosa Medical Center — C CP I P CP
- North Shore Medical Center — C I
- Northside Hospital — A C L T CP
- Northwest Medical Center — C CP
- Oak Hill Hospital — C
- Ocala Regional Medical Center — CP
- Orange Park Medical Center — C L T CP
- Orlando Health — C IM L T CP HF
- Osceola Regional Medical Center — A C CP L T CP
- Oviedo Medical Center — C CP
- Palm Bay Hospital — C
- Palm Beach Gardens Medical Center — C L T
- Palmetto General Hospital — C T
- Palms of Pasadena Hospital — C
- Palms West Hospital — C
- Parrish Medical Center — C I P
- Physicians Regional Medical Center - Collier Boulevard — CP
- Physicians Regional Medical Center - Pine Ridge — A C CP I CP
- Poinciana Medical Center — C
- Putnam Community Medical Center — C
- Regional Medical Center Bayonet Point — C L P T
- Rockledge Regional Medical Center — C CP L
- Sacred Heart Hospital on the Emerald Coast — C I
- Sacred Heart Hospital Pensacola — C I L T
- Santa Rosa Medical Center — CP
- Sarasota Memorial Hospital — A C CP I L T CP
- Sebastian River Medical Center — C
- Shands Live Oak Regional Medical Center — CP
- Shands Starke Regional Medical Center — CP
- South Bay Hospital — C
- South Florida Baptist Hospital — C CP I P
- South Lake Hospital — C CP HF
- South Miami Hospital — A C I L P
- South Seminole Hospital — C CP HF
- St. Anthony's Hospital — C CP I
- St. Cloud Regional Medical Center — C I CP
- St. Joseph's Children's Hospital — A C CP I IM L P T
- St. Joseph's Hospital - North — C CP I P
- St. Joseph's Hospital - South — C CP I P
- St. Lucie Medical Center — C CP
- Tallahassee Memorial HealthCare — C I L T AF CP
- Tampa General Hospital — C CP I L T AF CP HF
- The Villages Regional Hospital — C CP I CP

Registries	Accreditations	Awards
A AFib Ablation Registry™	AF Atrial Fibrillation	★ Chest Pain - MI Registry™ Award Silver
C CathPCI Registry®	CL Cardiac Cath Lab	★ Chest Pain - MI Registry™ Award Gold
CP Chest Pain - MI Registry™	CP Chest Pain Center	★ Chest Pain - MI Registry™ Award Platinum
I ICD Registry™	EP Electrophysiology	◆ HeartCARE Center™
IM IMPACT Registry®	HF Heart Failure	
L LAAO Registry™		
P PVI Registry™		
T STS/ACC TVT Registry™		

- UF Health Jacksonville — A C CP I L P T ★
- UF Health Shands Hospital — C I IM T CP
- University of Miami Health System — C I L T
- Venice Regional Bayfront Health — C I L T
- Wellington Regional Medical Center — C CP I CP
- West Florida Hospital — C CP P AF CP
- West Kendall Baptist Hospital — I P
- West Marion Community Hospital — CP
- Westside Regional Medical Center — C CP
- Winter Haven Hospital — A C CP I L P
- Wolfson Children's Hospital — I IM

GEORGIA

- Archbold Medical Center — C I
- Augusta University Medical Center — A C I L T CL CP
- Cartersville Medical Center — C CP
- Children's Healthcare of Atlanta - Egleston Hospital — I IM
- Coffee Regional Medical Center — C CP CP
- Coliseum Medical Centers — C L
- Doctors Hospital of Augusta — C CP
- East Georgia Regional Medical Center — C I
- Eastside Medical Center — C CP
- Emory Decatur Hospital — C
- Emory Johns Creek Hospital — C
- Emory St. Joseph's Hospital — C L T
- Emory University Hospital — C T CP
- Emory University Hospital Midtown — C L T
- Fairview Limited Partnership — C
- Fairview Park Hospital — CP
- Floyd Medical Center — C I CP
- Grady Hospital — C I
- Gwinnett Health System — C CP L T
- Hamilton Medical Center — C CP I CP
- Houston Medical Center — C I
- Meadows Health — C CP
- Medical Center Navicent Health — C I L T AF CP HF
- Memorial Health University Medical Center — C CP L T CP
- Memorial Satilla Health — C CP
- Northeast Georgia Medical Center — C L T
- Northeast Georgia Medical Center Braselton — C
- Northside Hospital Atlanta — C
- Northside Hospital Cherokee — C
- Northside Hospital Forsyth — C
- Phoebe Putney Memorial Hospital — C I L T
- Piedmont Athens Regional Medical Center — C CP L T CP ★
- Piedmont Atlanta Hospital — C CP L T CP
- Piedmont Columbus Regional - Midtown — C
- Piedmont Fayette Hospital — C CP CP ★
- Piedmont Henry Hospital — C CP CP HF
- Piedmont Mountainside Hospital — CP
- Piedmont Newnan Hospital — C CP CP ★
- Piedmont Rockdale Hospital — C CP CP
- Polk Medical Center — CP
- Redmond Regional Medical Center — C CP T CP ★
- South Georgia Medical Center — C CP I P
- Southeast Georgia Health System — C I
- Southern Regional Medical Center — C CP I CP ★
- St. Francis Hospital — C I CP
- St. Joseph's Hospital — C CP I L T CP
- St. Mary's Health Care System - GA — C CP I CP ★
- Tanner Medical Center - Carrollton — C I CP
- Tanner Medical Center - Villa Rica — C CP
- Tift Regional Medical Center — C I
- Union General Hospital — CP
- University Health Care System — C CP I L T CP
- WellStar Atlanta Medical Center — C I
- WellStar Atlanta Medical Center South — C I
- WellStar Cobb Hospital — C I
- WellStar Douglas Hospital — C
- WellStar Kennestone Hospital — C I L T

- WellStar North Fulton Hospital — C I
- WellStar Paulding Hospital — C I
- WellStar Spalding Regional Hospital — C I
- WellStar West Georgia Medical Center — C I

HAWAII

- Hilo Medical Center — C I
- Kaiser Permanente Moanalua Medical Center — C I
- Maui Memorial Medical Center — C I
- Pali Momi Medical Center — C
- Straub Medical Center — C IM L T
- The Queen's Medical Center — C I L T

IDAHO

- Eastern Idaho Regional Medical Center — C CP L T AF CP ★
- Kootenai Health — A C CP I L T
- Portneuf Medical Center — C CP T CP
- St. Alphonsus Medical Center - Nampa — C CP CP
- St. Alphonsus Regional Medical Center - Boise — A C CP I T CP ★
- St. Joseph Regional Medical Center — C I
- St. Luke's Health System - Boise — C CP I L T
- St. Luke's Magic Valley Medical Center — C
- West Valley Medical Center — C CP CP

ILLINOIS

- Advocate BroMenn Medical Center — C CP I CP ★
- Advocate Children's Hospital - Oak Lawn — IM
- Advocate Christ Medical Center — C CP I L P T
- Advocate Condell Medical Center — C I L
- Advocate Dreyer Vascular Center — P
- Advocate Good Samaritan Hospital — C I L P T
- Advocate Good Shepherd Hospital — C I
- Advocate Illinois Masonic Medical Center — C I L
- Advocate Lutheran General Hospital — C I L T
- Advocate Sherman Hospital — C CP I L CP ★
- Advocate South Suburban Hospital — C I
- Advocate Trinity Hospital — C I
- Alton Memorial Hospital — C
- AMITA Health Adventist Medical Center Bolingbrook — C CP I
- AMITA Health Adventist Medical Center GlenOaks — C CP I
- AMITA Health Adventist Medical Center Hinsdale — C CP I ★
- AMITA Health Adventist Medical Center La Grange — C CP I ★
- AMITA Health Alexian Brothers Medical Center Elk Grove Village — C I L T
- AMITA Health St. Alexius Medical Center Hoffman Estates — C I
- Anderson Hospital — C CP
- Ann & Robert H. Lurie Childrens Hospital of Chicago — IM
- Blessing Hospital — C I CP
- Carle Foundation Hospital — C CP I L T CP ★
- CGH Medical Center — C I CP
- Community First Medical Center — C CP I
- Edward Hospital — C CP I L P T ★
- Elmhurst Hospital — C CP I P ★
- Evanston Hospital — A C I L T
- FHN Memorial Hospital — C I
- Franciscan Health Olympia Fields — C CP I CP ★
- Galesburg Cottage Hospital — CP CP
- Gateway Regional Medical Center — C I
- Genesis Medical Center - Silvis — C I
- Glenbrook Hospital — C I
- Gottlieb Memorial Hospital — C
- Heartland Regional Medical Center — C I CP
- Herrin Hospital — CP
- Highland Park Hospital — A C I
- HSHS St. Anthony's Memorial Hospital — C

HSHS St. Elizabeth's Hospital ... C CP I L T CP ★
HSHS St. John's Hospital ... C CP L P T ★
HSHS St. Mary's Hospital ... C CP I
Iroquois Memorial Hospital ... I
Jersey Community Hospital ... I
Katherine Shaw Bethea Hospital ... C
Loyola University Medical Center ... A C CP I L T ★
MacNeal Hospital ... C CP I
Memorial Hospital Belleville ... C CP CP ★
Memorial Hospital East ... C CP
Memorial Hospital of Carbondale ... C CP I L P T ★
Memorial Medical Center ... C CP L T
Mercy Hospital and Medical Center ... C CP I
Mercyhealth Javon Bea Hospital - Rockton ... C I CP
Metrosouth Medical Center ... C CP I
Morris Hospital & Healthcare Centers ... I
Mt. Sinai Hospital Medical Center ... C I CP
Northwest Community Hospital ... C I L T
Northwestern Medicine Central
DuPage Hospital ... C CP I T
Northwestern Medicine Delnor Hospital ... C CP I ★
Northwestern Medicine Huntley Hospital ... C CP I CP ★
Northwestern Medicine Kishwaukee Hospital ... C I
Northwestern Medicine Lake Forest Hospital ... C CP I ★
Northwestern Medicine McHenry Hospital ... C CP I T CP ★
Northwestern Memorial Hospital ... C I L T
Norwegian American Hospital ... C I
OSF Heart of Mary Medical Center ... I CP
OSF St. Anthony Medical Center ... C CP I L T ★
OSF St. Francis Medical Center ... A C CP I IM L T ★
OSF St. Joseph Medical Center ... C CP I ★
Palos Hospital ... C L
Presence Mercy Medical Center ... C I CP
Presence Resurrection Medical Center ... C CP I CP
Presence Saint Mary and Elizabeth Medical Center -
St. Mary Campus ... C CP I CP
Presence St. Francis Hospital ... C CP I CP
Presence St. Joseph Hospital - Chicago ... C CP I CP

Presence St. Joseph Hospital - Elgin ... C I
Presence St. Joseph Medical Center ... C CP I L P CP
Presence St. Mary's Hospital ... C CP I CP
Red Bud Regional Hospital ... CP
Riverside Medical Center ... C CP I P CP HF ★
Rush Copley Medical Center ... A C CP I P CP ★
Rush Oak Park Hospital ... C CP ★
Rush University Medical Center ... A C CP IM L P T ★
Sarah Bush Lincoln Health Center ... C I
Silver Cross Hospital ... C I
Skokie Hospital ... C I
SSM Health Good Samaritan Hospital - Mt. Vernon ... C I
Swedish Covenant Hospital ... C I
SwedishAmerican Hospital ... I
The University of Chicago Medical Center ... C CP I L T
Trinity Rock Island ... A C CP I P T
UChicago Medicine Ingalls Memorial Hospital ... C CP I CP
Union County Hospital ... CP
UnityPoint Health - Methodist ... C CP I P ★
UnityPoint Health - Proctor Hospital ... C CP I P
University of Illinois Hospital ... C I L T
Vista Medical Center - East ... C I
Weiss Memorial Hospital ... C I
West Suburban Medical Center ... C CP I CP
Westlake Hospital ... C I

INDIANA

Baptist Health Floyd ... C L P
Bluffton Regional Medical Center ... CP
Clark Memorial Hospital ... C CP I CP
Columbus Regional Hospital ... C CP I CP ★
Community Heart and Vascular Hospital ... C I L T
Community Hospital ... C CP I L T
Community Hospital Anderson ... C I
Community Hospital East ... C I
Community Hospital South ... C I
Community Howard Regional Health ... C I
Deaconess Midtown Hospital ... C CP I P ★

Dukes Memorial Hospital ... CP
Dupont Hospital ... CP
Elkhart General Hospital ... C T
Eskenazi Health ... C I
Franciscan Health Crown Point ... C I CP
Franciscan Health Dyer ... C I CP
Franciscan Health Hammond ... C I CP
Franciscan Health Indianapolis ... C CP I L T CP ★
Franciscan Health Lafayette East ... C CP I CP
Franciscan Health Michigan City ... C I CP
Franciscan Health Munster ... C I
Good Samaritan Hospital ... C
Goshen Health Hospital ... C CP I ★
Hancock Regional Hospital ... C CP
Hendricks Regional Health ... C
Hendricks Regional Health - Danville Hospital ... CP
Highpoint Health ... I
Indiana University Health Methodist Hospital ... AF
IU Health Arnett Hospital ... C CP I CP ★
IU Health Ball Memorial Hospital ... C CP I ★
IU Health Bloomington Hospital ... C CP I L ★
IU Health
Methodist Hospital ... A C CP I L T AF CL CP ★ ◆
IU Health Saxony Hospital ... C CP I ★
IU Health West Hospital ... C CP I ★
Johnson Memorial Hospital ... C
Kosciusko Community Hospital ... CP
La Porte Hospital ... A C CP I CP
Lutheran Hospital ... A C CP I L P T AF CL CP HF ◆
Marion General Hospital ... C I CP
Memorial Hospital and Health Care Center ... C
Memorial Hospital of South Bend ... C L T
Methodist Hospitals ... C CP CL CP
Methodist Hospitals - Southlake ... C CP I CL CP
Mishawaka Medical Center ... A C I L
Parkview Heart Institute ... A C I L P T HF ◆
Pinnacle Hospital ... C I P

Continues on next page

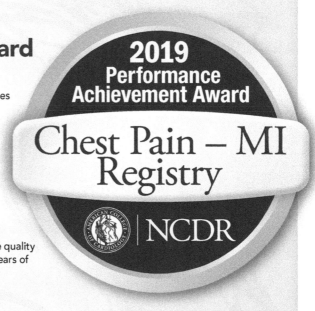

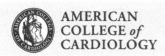

THE HEART OF QUALITY PATIENT

Porter Regional Hospital .... C I L T AF CP
Reid Health .... C I L P
Riley Hospital for Children at IU Health .... I IM
Riley Hospital for Children
at IU Health North Hospital .... C CP I
Riverview Health .... C CP I CP ★
St. Catherine Hospital .... C I
St. Joseph Hospital .... C I CL
St. Mary Medical Center .... C I L CP
St. Vincent Anderson Hospital .... C I T
St. Vincent Evansville Hospital .... C CP I T ★
St. Vincent Heart Center of Indiana .... C CP I L T ★
St. Vincent Indianapolis Hospital .... C CP I IM ★
Terre Haute Regional Hospital .... C CP
The Heart Hospital
at Deaconess Gateway .... C CP I L T ★
Union Hospital .... C I L T CP
Union Hospital Clinton .... CP
Witham Health Services C

IOWA

CHI Health Mercy Council Bluffs .... C I
Covenant Medical Center .... C CP I CP
Genesis Medical Center - East Rusholme Street ... C I T
Iowa Lutheran Hospital .... C CP CP
Iowa Methodist Medical Center .... C CP L T CP
Mary Greeley Medical Center I
Mercy Hospital - Iowa City .... C CP I CP
Mercy Medical Center - Cedar Rapids .... C I
Mercy Medical Center - Clinton .... C CP
Mercy Medical Center -
Des Moines .... A C CP I L T CP ★
Mercy Medical Center - Dubuque .... C I
Mercy Medical Center - North Iowa .... C CP I
Mercy Medical Center - Sioux City .... C CP I ★
Ottumwa Regional Health Center C
Trinity Bettendorf .... C CP I P
UnityPoint - Allen Hospital .... C CP P CP ★
UnityPoint Health -
Trinity Regional Medical Center .... C CP ★
UnityPoint Health Cedar Rapids -
St. Luke's Hospital .... A C CP I L T CP ★
UnityPoint Health Dubuque - Finley Hospital ...... C CP ★
UnityPoint Health Sioux City -
St. Luke's Regional Medical Center .... C CP I P ★
University of Iowa Hospitals & Clinics .... C IM L T

KANSAS

AdventHealth Shawnee Mission .... C CP I T CP ★
Ascension Via Christi Health .... C L T
Ascension Via Christi Hospital in Manhattan .... C I
Ascension Via Christi Hospital in Pittsburg I
Hays Medical Center .... C CP I CP ★
Kansas Medical Center .... C I T
Lawrence Memorial Hospital C
Menorah Medical Center .... C CP I ★
Newman Regional Health .... C I
Olathe Medical Center .... C CP L T ★
Overland Park Regional Medical Center ...... A C CP I L
Providence Medical Center .... C CP I CP
Salina Regional Health Center .... C I L P CP

Registries / Accreditations / Awards

Registries:
A AFib Ablation Registry™
C CathPCI Registry®
CP Chest Pain - MI Registry™
I ICD Registry™
IM IMPACT Registry®
L LAAO Registry™
P PVI Registry™
T STS/ACC TVT Registry™

Accreditations:
AF Atrial Fibrillation
CL Cardiac Cath Lab
CP Chest Pain Center
EP Electrophysiology
HF Heart Failure

Awards:
★ Chest Pain - MI Registry™ Award Silver
★ Chest Pain - MI Registry™ Award Gold
★ Chest Pain - MI Registry™ Award Platinum
◆ HeartCARE Center™

St. Catherine Hospital .... C CP
St. Luke's South Hospital .... C CP I ★
Stormont Vail Regional Health Center .... C CP L T ★
University of Kansas Health System
St. Francis Campus .... C CP I CP ★
University of Kansas Hospital ...... A C CP I L T CL CP ★
Wesley Medical Center .... C CP I L T
Wesley Woodlawn Hospital & ER .... C CP I
Western Plains Medical Complex .... C I CP

KENTUCKY

Baptist Health Corbin .... C CP CP
Baptist Health Lexington .... C I L P T AF CL CP
Baptist Health Louisville .... C CP T HF
Baptist Health Madisonville .... C I
Baptist Health Paducah .... C CP I L CP ★
Baptist Health Richmond .... C I
Bluegrass Community Hospital .... CP
Bourbon Community Hospital .... CP
Clark Regional Medical Center .... CP
Ephraim McDowell Regional Medical Center ..... C CP I
Fleming County Hospital .... CP
Frankfort Regional Medical Center .... C CP
Georgetown Community Hospital .... CP HF
Hardin Memorial Hospital .... C CP
Harrison Memorial Hospital .... C I CP
Hazard ARH Regional Medical Center .... C CP I
Highlands Regional Medical Center .... C I CP
Jackson Purchase Medical Center .... CP
Jewish Hospital .... C CP I L T
King's Daughters Medical Center .... C I T AF CP
Lake Cumberland Regional Hospital .... C I CP
Logan Memorial Hospital .... CP
Meadowview Regional Medical Center .... C I CP
Mercy Health - Lourdes Hospital .... C I
Mercy Health - Marcum and Wallace Hospital ..... CP
Norton Audubon Hospital .... C I T AF
Norton Brownsboro Hospital .... C CP
Norton Children's Hospital .... IM
Norton Hospital .... C L AF CP
Our Lady of Bellefonte Hospital .... C I
Owensboro Health Regional Hospital .... C I P
Paul B. Hall Regional Medical Center .... CP
Pikeville Medical Center .... C CP I L T AF CP ★
Spring View Hospital .... CP
St. Claire Regional Medical Center .... C CP I
St. Elizabeth - Edgewood .... C CP I L T CP ★
St. Joseph Berea .... CP
St. Joseph East .... C CP I CP
St. Joseph Hospital .... A C CP I T CP
St. Joseph London .... C I
Sts. Mary & Elizabeth Hospital C
The Medical Center at Bowling Green .... C I L T CP
Three Rivers Medical Center .... CP
TJ Samson Community Hospital .... C I CP
TriStar Greenview Regional Hospital .... C CP
UK Albert B Chandler Hospital .... C CP I IM L T
University of Louisville Hospital C

LOUISIANA

Acadian Medical Center .... CP
Baton Rouge General Medical Center -
Bluebonnet Campus .... C L
Beauregard Health System I
Childrens Hospital - Main Campus .... IM
CHRISTUS Ochsner
St. Patrick Hospital .... C CP I L P T HF ★
CHRISTUS Shreveport-Bossier Health System -
Highland .... C I L T
CHRISTUS St. Frances Cabrini Hospital .... C CP I
Cypress Pointe Hospital I

East Jefferson General Hospital .... C I HF
Glenwood Regional Medical Center .... C I T
Heart Hospital of Lafayette .... C CP I T
Lafayette General Medical Center .... C CP T
Lake Charles Memorial Hospital .... T
Lakeview Regional Medical Center .... C I
Lane Regional Medical Center .... I CP
Mercy Regional Medical Center .... I CP
Minden Medical Center I
North Oaks Medical Center .... C I P
Northern Louisiana Medical Center C
Ochsner Baptist Medical Center C
Ochsner LSU Hospital Monroe I
Ochsner LSU Hospital Shreveport I
Ochsner Medical Center - Baton Rouge C
Ochsner Medical Center - Kenner C
Ochsner Medical Center -
Main Campus .... A C I IM L P T
Ochsner Medical Center - West Bank Campus .....
Our Lady of Lourdes Regional Medical Center ..... C CP I
Our Lady of the Lake Regional
Medical Center .... C I T AF CP
Rapides Regional Medical Center .... C CP I T
Slidell Memorial Hospital .... C CP
St. Bernard Parish Hospital C
St. Charles Parish Hospital C
St. Francis Medical Center .... C CP I CP
St. Francis P&S Surgery & Heart Center .... C I
St. Tammany Parish Hospital .... CP I CP
Teche Regional Medical Center .... CP
Terrebonne General Medical Center .... C CP I P T CP
Touro Infirmary .... CP I
Tulane Lakeside Hospital for Women and Children .. C CP L
University Medical Center New Orleans .... C I T
West Calcasieu Cameron Hospital C
West Feliciana Parish Hospital .... CP
Willis-Knighton Medical Center .... A C I L T CP
Willis-Knighton Pierremont Health Center C
WK Bossier Health Center C

MAINE

Central Maine Medical Center .... C I T CP
Maine Medical Center .... C CP I IM L T
MaineGeneral Medical Center - Alfond Center for Health .. I
Northern Light Eastern Maine Medical Center ..... C I L T
York Hospital .... C I

MARYLAND

Adventist HealthCare
Shady Grove Medical Center .... C CP I P CL CP
Adventist HealthCare Washington
Adventist Hospital .... C CP I P T CP ★
Anne Arundel Medical Center .... C CP I CP ★
Carroll Hospital C
Frederick Memorial Hospital .... C CP I CP ★
Holy Cross Germantown Hospital I
Holy Cross Hospital .... C I
Howard County General Hospital .... C I
Johns Hopkins Bayview Medical Center .... C CP ★
MedStar Franklin Square Medical Center .... C I
MedStar Southern Maryland Hospital Center ... C CP I
MedStar Union Memorial Hospital .... C I L T
Mercy Medical Center .... C I
Meritus Medical Center .... C CP I
Northwest Hospital I
Peninsula Regional Medical Center .... A C I L T
Sinai Hospital of Baltimore .... C I L T
St. Agnes Hospital .... C CP I CP ★
Suburban Hospital .... C CP I T ★
The Johns Hopkins Hospital .... C CP I IM L T
UM Baltimore Washington Medical Center .... C I

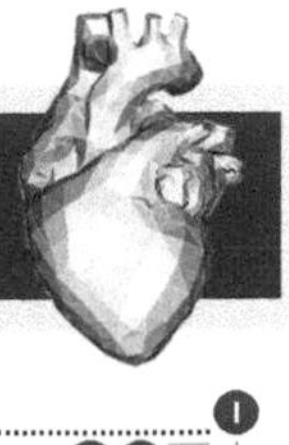

- UM Prince George's Hospital Center — C CP I
- UM St. Joseph Medical Center — C L T
- UM Upper Chesapeake Medical Center — C P
- University of Maryland Capital Region Health — CP
- University of Maryland Medical Center — C IM L T
- University of Maryland Shore Regional Health — C I
- Western Maryland Regional Medical Center — C CP I ★

MASSACHUSETTS

- Anna Jaques Hospital — C I
- Baystate Medical Center — A C I L T
- Berkshire Medical Center — C I
- Beth Israel Deaconess Hospital - Plymouth — C I
- Beth Israel Deaconess Medical Center — C I L T
- Beverly Hospital — C I
- Boston Children's Hospital — I IM
- Boston Medical Center — C I L T
- Brigham and Women's Hospital — C I L T
- Cape Cod Hospital — C I L T
- Charlton Memorial Hospital — C I L T
- Cooley Dickinson Hospital — C I
- Good Samaritan Medical Center — C CP
- Holy Family Hospital - Methuen — C
- Lahey Hospital & Medical Center - Burlington — A C I L T
- Lawrence General Hospital — C I CL CP HF ♦
- Lowell General Hospital - Main Campus — C I
- Massachusetts General Hospital — C I IM L P T
- MelroseWakefield Hospital — C I
- Mercy Medical Center — C I
- MetroWest Medical Center — C
- Milford Regional Medical Center — C I
- Mount Auburn Hospital — C I T
- North Shore Medical Center - Salem Hospital — C I
- Norwood Hospital — C
- Signature Healthcare Brockton Hospital — C I
- South Shore Hospital — C
- St. Anne's Hospital — C
- St. Elizabeth's Medical Center — C L P T
- St. Luke's Hospital — C I
- St. Vincent Hospital — C I L T
- Tufts Medical Center — C I L T
- UMass Memorial Medical Center — C I L T

MICHIGAN

- Ascension Borgess Health — C I L P T CP
- Ascension Genesys Hospital — C I T
- Ascension Macomb-Oakland Hospital - Warren Campus — C I
- Ascension Providence Hospital - Novi Campus — C I
- Ascension Providence Hospital - Southfield Campus — C I L T
- Ascension Providence Rochester Hospital — C I
- Ascension St. John Hospital — C I L T
- Ascension St. Mary's Hospital — C I L P T
- Beaumont Hospital - Dearborn — C L T
- Beaumont Hospital - Farmington Hills — C
- Beaumont Hospital - Grosse Pointe — C
- Beaumont Hospital - Royal Oak — C L T
- Beaumont Hospital - Trenton — C
- Beaumont Hospital - Troy — C
- Beaumont Hospital - Wayne — C
- Bronson Methodist Hospital — C CP I L T
- Children's Hospital of Michigan — IM
- Covenant Medical Center - Harrison — C L T
- DMC Harper University Hospital — C I L T
- DMC Huron Valley - Sinai Hospital — C I
- DMC Sinai - Grace Hospital — C I
- Garden City Hospital — C I
- Henry Ford Allegiance Health — C I T
- Henry Ford Hospital — C I L T
- Henry Ford Macomb Hospital - Clinton Township — C I T CP
- Henry Ford West Bloomfield Hospital — C I
- Henry Ford Wyandotte Hospital — C I
- Holland Hospital — C CP I ★
- Hurley Medical Center — C
- Lakeland Community Hospital Niles — CP
- Lakeland Regional Medical Center St Joseph — CP
- McLaren Bay Region — C CP I T
- McLaren Central Michigan — I
- McLaren Flint — C I L T
- McLaren Greater Lansing — C I
- McLaren Lapeer Region — I
- McLaren Macomb — C I T AF CP
- McLaren Northern Michigan — C CP I L T
- McLaren Oakland — C I CP
- McLaren Port Huron Hospital — C I P
- McLaren Thumb Region — I
- Mercy Health Mercy Campus — A C I T
- Mercy Health St. Mary's — C I
- Metro Health Hospital — C CP I CP ★
- Michigan Medicine — C IM L T
- MidMichigan Medical Center - Midland — C CP I L T
- Munson Medical Center — C I L T
- ProMedica Monroe Regional Hospital — C CL
- Sparrow Hospital — C CP L T ★
- Spectrum Health — A C CP I IM L T
- Spectrum Health Lakeland — A C I P CP
- St. Joseph Mercy Ann Arbor — A C I L T
- St. Joseph Mercy Oakland — C I T
- St. Mary Mercy Livonia — C I P
- UP Health System - Bell — CP
- UP Health System - Marquette — C CP I L T CL CP
- UP Health System - Portage Main Campus — CP

MINNESOTA

- Abbott Northwestern Hospital — C I L T
- CentraCare Health System — A C CP I L T ★
- Children's Hospitals & Clinics of Minnesota - Minneapolis — IM
- Essentia Health - St. Joseph's Medical Center — C
- Essentia Health - St. Mary's Medical Center — C CP L T CP ★
- Fairview Ridges Hospital — C
- Fairview Southdale Hospital — A C L T
- HealthEast St. Joseph's Hospital — A C L T
- Hennepin County Medical Center — C I
- Mayo Clinic Health System — C IM L T
- Mercy Hospital — C I L T
- North Memorial Health Hospital — HF
- North Memorial Health — C I L T
- Olmsted Medical Center — I
- Park Nicollet Methodist Hospital — C L T
- Prairie Ridge Hospital and Health Services — I
- Regions Hospital — C L T
- Ridgeview Medical Center — C
- Sanford Bemidji Medical Center — C CP
- St. Luke's Hospital — C CP I ★
- United Hospital — C I L T
- University of Minnesota Medical Center West Bank Hospital — A C IM T

MISSISSIPPI

- Anderson Regional Medical Center — C CP I CP ★
- Baptist Medical Center — C CP T
- Baptist Memorial Hospital - Golden Triangle — C CP L CP ★
- Baptist Memorial Hospital - Desoto — C CP AF CP HF ★
- Baptist Memorial Hospital - North Mississippi — C CP CP ★
- Bolivar Medical Center — CP
- Delta Regional Medical Center — CP ★
- Forrest General Hospital — C CP I L T ★
- Garden Park Medical Center — I
- Magnolia Regional Health Center — C CP CP ★
- Memorial Hospital at Gulfport — C CP I
- Merit Health Biloxi — C I
- Merit Health Central — C CP I
- Merit Health Natchez — I CP
- Merit Health River Oaks — C I
- Merit Health River Region — C CP I CP
- Merit Health Wesley — C CP I AF CP HF ★
- Methodist Olive Branch Hospital — C CP CP ★
- North Mississippi Medical Center - Tupelo — C CP I L P T ★
- Northwest Mississippi Regional Medical Center — CP
- Ocean Springs Hospital — C CP I T ★
- Rush Foundation Hospital — CP
- Singing River Hospital — C CP I
- Southwest Mississippi Regional Medical Center — C CP I ★
- St. Dominic-Jackson Memorial Hospital — A C CP T ★
- The University of Mississippi Medical Center — CP I L T

MISSOURI

- Barnes-Jewish Hospital — C CP L T ★
- Barnes-Jewish St. Peter's Hospital — C
- Belton Regional Medical Center — CP
- Boone Hospital Center — C T
- Bothwell Regional Health Center — I
- Capital Region Medical Center — C CP ★
- Centerpoint Medical Center — C CP I ★
- Children's Mercy Hospital and Clinics — I IM
- Christian Hospital — C CP T
- Citizens Memorial Hospital — CP
- Cox Medical Center - Branson — C CP I ★
- Cox Medical Center - South — C CP I L T ★
- Freeman Health System — C CP I P T ★
- Hannibal Regional Hospital — C CP I
- HHC ASC, LLC — CP I
- Lake Regional Health System — C
- Lee's Summit Medical Center — C CP I ★
- Liberty Hospital — C CP I CP ★
- Mercy Hospital Jefferson — C CP
- Mercy Hospital Joplin — C CP
- Mercy Hospital South — C CP L T
- Mercy Hospital Springfield — C CP T ★
- Mercy Hospital St. Louis — C CP L T
- Mercy Hospital Washington — C CP
- Merit Health Wesley — AF
- Missouri Baptist Medical Center — C T
- Moberly Regional Medical Center — C I
- Mosaic Life Care — C CP I P T CP
- Mosaic Life Care at St. Joseph - Medical Center — CP
- North Kansas City Hospital — C CP I L T CP HF ★
- Northeast Regional Medical Center — C I CP
- Ozarks Medical Center — C CP I CP
- Phelps County Regional Medical Center — C I
- Poplar Bluff Regional Medical Center - Oak Grove — C CP I CP
- Progress West Hospital — C
- Research Medical Center — A C CP I L T ★
- Southeast Hospital — C CP I T ★
- SSM Health Cardinal Glennon Children's Hospital — I IM
- SSM Health DePaul Hospital - St. Louis — C CP I L T
- SSM Health St. Clare Hospital - Fenton — C CP I
- SSM Health St. Joseph Hospital - Lake St. Louis — C CP
- SSM Health St. Joseph Hospital - St. Charles — C CP I
- SSM Health St. Louis University Hospital — C CP I L T
- SSM Health St. Mary's Hospital - Audrain — C CP I
- SSM Health St. Mary's Hospital - Jefferson City — C CP I ★
- SSM Health St. Mary's Hospital - St. Louis — C CP I
- St. Francis Medical Center — C CP I L T CP ★

Continues on next page

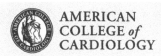

St. Joseph Medical Center .... C CP I CP
St. Louis Children's Hospital .... IM
St. Luke's Des Peres Hospital .... C I
St. Luke's East Hospital .... C CP I ★
St. Luke's Hospital .... C I L T
St. Luke's Hospital of Kansas City .... A C CP I L T ★
St. Luke's North Hospital - Barry Road ... C CP I ★
St. Mary's Medical Center .... C CP I
Truman Medical Centers .... C CP I
University Hospital .... A C I L T

MONTANA

Benefis Health System C
Billings Clinic Hospital .... C CP I L T CP ★
Bozeman Health Deaconess Hospital .... C CP I
Community Medical Center .... C CP I
Great Falls Clinic Hospital I
Kalispell Regional Medical Center .... C CP I L T ★
Providence St. Patrick Hospital .... A C CP I L T
St. James Healthcare .... C CP
St. Vincent Healthcare .... A C CP I L T ★

NEBRASKA

Bryan Health .... C I L T
CHI Health Creighton University Medical Center -
Bergan Mercy .... A C I L T
CHI Health Good Samaritan .... C I
CHI Health Immanuel .... C I
CHI Health Lakeside .... C I
CHI Health Midlands I
CHI Health Nebraska Heart .... A C I L T
CHI Health St. Francis .... C I
Children's Hospital & Medical Center .... I IM
Faith Regional Health Services .... C CP I CP ★
Great Plains Health .... C I P
Kearney Regional Medical Center .... C I P
Mary Lanning Memorial Hospital .... C CP I
Methodist Fremont Health .... C I
Nebraska Medicine .... CP
Nebraska Medicine - Bellevue .... C CP
Nebraska Medicine -
Nebraska Medical Center .... C CP I L T CP ★
Nebraska Methodist Hospital .... C I L T

NEVADA

Carson Tahoe Regional Medical Center .... C I
Centennial Hills Hospital Medical Center .... CP I CP
Coronado Surgery Center I
Desert Springs Hospital Medical Center ...... CP I CP
Dignity Health St. Rose Dominican -
San Martin Campus .... C CP CP
Dignity Health St. Rose Dominican -
Siena Campus .... C CP T CP
Henderson Hospital .... CP CP
Mesa View Regional Hospital .... CP
MountainView Hospital .... C CP L T
North Vista Hospital .... C CP CP
Northeastern Nevada Regional Hospital .... C CP I CL CP
Northern Nevada Medical Center .... C CP I CP
Renown Regional Medical Center ...... C CP L T CP HF
Renown South Meadows Medical Center .... CP

Southern Hills Hospital & Medical Center C
Spring Valley Hospital Medical Center .... CP I T CP
St. Mary's Regional Medical Center .... C CP I T CP ★
Summerlin Hospital Medical Center .... CP I T CP
Sunrise Hospital & Medical Center .... C L T
University Medical Center of Southern Nevada ...... C CP I CP
Valley Hospital Medical Center .... CP I CP

NEW HAMPSHIRE

Catholic Medical Center .... C I L T
Cheshire Medical Center/Dartmouth -
Hitchcock Keene I
Children's Hospital at Dartmouth - Hitchcock .... C I L T
Concord Hospital .... C I L T
Elliot Hospital .... C I
Exeter Hospital .... C I
Parkland Medical Center .... C C I
Portsmouth Regional Hospital .... A C T
Southern New Hampshire Medical Center .... C I
St. Joseph Hospital .... C I
Wentworth-Douglass Hospital C

NEW JERSEY

AtlantiCare Regional Medical Center -
Mainland Campus .... C I L T
Bayshore Medical Center .... C CP CP
Capital Health Medical Center - Hopewell .... CP CP
CentraState Medical Center .... CP
Chilton Medical Center C
Clara Maass Medical Center .... CP
Community Medical Center .... CP
Cooper University Hospital .... C I L T
Deborah Heart and Lung Center .... L T
Englewood Hospital and Medical Center ..... C CP L T
Hackensack University Medical Center ... C CP I L P T CP
Hackettstown Medical Center .... CP
Hunterdon Healthcare System C
Inspira Medical Center Elmer Hospital .... CP
Inspira Medical Center Vineland .... CP CP
Inspira Medical Center Woodbury .... C CP CP
Jersey Shore University
Medical Center .... C CP I L P T CP HF ★
JFK Medical Center .... C CP CL CP HF ★
Monmouth Medical Center C
Morristown Medical Center .... C I L T
Newark Beth Israel Medical Center ..... C I IM L T
Newton Medical Center C
Ocean Medical Center .... C CP P CP HF ★
Our Lady of Lourdes Medical Center .... I L T
Overlook Medical Center C
Raritan Bay Medical Center Perth Amboy .... CP
Riverview Medical Center .... C CP P CP HF ★
RWJ University Hospital New Brunswick ..... C I L T
RWJ University Hospital Somerset .... CP
Southern Ocean Medical Center .... C CP CP HF ★
St. Barnabas Medical Center .... I L T
St. Clare's Health C
St. Francis Medical Center .... I L
St. Joseph's Regional Medical Center .... T
St. Mary's General Hospital .... CP
St. Michael's Medical Center I
The University Hospital I
The Valley Hospital .... C CP I L T

NEW MEXICO

Carlsbad Medical Center .... C I CP
CHRISTUS St. Vincent Regional Medical Center C
Eastern New Mexico Medical Center .... C I CP
Gerald Champion Regional Medical Center ..... C CP I
Lea Regional Medical Center .... C I CP HF
Los Alamos Medical Center .... CP

Lovelace Medical Center .... C CP L T ★
Memorial Medical Center .... C I HF
Mimbres Memorial Hospital I
MountainView Regional Medical Center ..... C CP I ★
Presbyterian Hospital .... A C CP I IM L T ★
San Juan Regional Medical Center .... C CP I P CP
University of New Mexico Hospital .... I L

NEW YORK

Albany Medical Center .... C I L T
Albany Memorial Hospital .... CP CP
Arnot Ogden Medical Center .... C CP I
Bassett Medical Center .... C I
BronxCare Hospital Center -
Grand Concourse Campus .... CP I ★
Brookdale Hospital Medical Center I
Brooklyn Hospital Center at Downtown Campus ... C CP
Buffalo General Medical Center .... C I L T
Cayuga Medical Center at Ithaca .... C CP CP
Champlain Valley Physicians Hospital .... C I
Cohen Children's Medical Center .... I IM
Crouse Hospital .... CP I L
Ellis Hospital .... C CP L T
Fairview Southdale Hospital .... C CP L T
Glens Falls Hospital .... C I
Good Samaritan Hospital .... C I
Good Samaritan Hospital Medical Center ..... C I P T
Huntington Hospital .... C I
Jamaica Hospital Medical Center .... C CP I
Lenox Hill Hospital .... C I L T
Long Island Community Hospital .... C I
Long Island Jewish Medical Center .... C I L
Maimonides Medical Center .... C L T
Mercy Hospital of Buffalo .... C CP I L T ★
Montefiore Health System .... C I IM L T
Mount Sinai Beth Israel .... C I
Mount Sinai Medical Center .... C CP I IM L T ★
Mount Sinai St. Luke's .... C CP I L T
Mount Sinai West .... CP
NewYork-Presbyterian
Brooklyn Methodist Hospital .... C CP L T
NewYork-Presbyterian Lawrence Hospital .... C CP
NewYork-Presbyterian
Morgan Stanley Children's Hospital .... IM
NewYork-Presbyterian Queens .... A C CP I L
NewYork-Presbyterian/Weill
Cornell Medical Center .... C CP IM L T
Niagara Falls Memorial Medical Center C
North Shore University Hospital .... C I L T
NYC Health and Hospitals - Bellevue ...... A C CP L
NYU Langone Health Tisch Hospital ..... C I IM L T
NYU Langone Hospital - Brooklyn C
NYU Langone Hospital - Brooklyn C
NYU Winthrop Hospital .... C CP L T
Olean General Hospital .... C CP I CP
Orange Regional Medical Center .... C I
Peconic Bay Medical Center .... C I
Richmond University Medical Center .... C CP I
Rochester General Hospital .... L T
Samaritan Hospital .... C CP I CP
Saratoga Hospital C
South Nassau Communities Hospital .... C I
Southside Hospital .... C I L T
St. Barnabas Hospital .... C I
St. Catherine of Siena Medical Center .... C I
St. Elizabeth Campus .... C CP I L T
St. Francis Hospital - The Heart Center ..... C L P T
St. Joseph's Hospital
Health Center .... A C I L P T CP HF
St. Luke's Cornwall Hospital - Newburgh Campus .... C I
St. Peter's Hospital .... C CP I L T AF C HF

Legend

Registries
- A AFib Ablation Registry™
- C CathPCI Registry®
- CP Chest Pain - MI Registry™
- I ICD Registry™
- IM IMPACT Registry®
- L LAAO Registry™
- P PVI Registry™
- T STS/ACC TVT Registry™

Accreditations
- AF Atrial Fibrillation
- CL Cardiac Cath Lab
- CP Chest Pain Center
- EP Electrophysiology
- HF Heart Failure

Awards
- ★ Chest Pain - MI Registry™ Award Silver
- ★ Chest Pain - MI Registry™ Award Gold
- ★ Chest Pain - MI Registry™ Award Platinum
- ◆ HeartCARE Center™

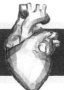

Staten Island University Hospital - North Campus — C I L T
Stony Brook Southampton Hospital — C I
Stony Brook University Hospital — A C CP L P T CP
Strong Memorial Hospital — A C CP I IM L T ★
SUNY Upstate Medical University — C I L
UHS Wilson Medical Center — CP HF
United Health Services — L T
UPMC Chautauqua — I
Vassar Brothers Medical Center — C C I L T
Westchester Medical Center — C CP I IM L T
White Plains Hospital — C
Wyckoff Heights Medical Center — I

NORTH CAROLINA

Atrium Health Pineville — C CP ★
Atrium Health Union — C
Betsy Johnson Hospital — CP
Cape Fear Valley Health System — C C CP I T CP ☆
Cape Fear Valley Medical Center — CP
CarolinaEast Medical Center — C CP I L CL CP HF ★
Carolinas HealthCare System NorthEast — C CP ★
Carolinas Medical Center — C CP I IM L T ★
CaroMont Regional Medical Center — C CP I P T CP
Carteret General Hospital — C
Catawba Valley Medical Center — C CP I CP HF ★
Central Carolina Hospital — C CP HF
Central Harnett Hospital —
Cone Health Alamance Regional Medical Center — C C CP I P ☆
Cone Health Moses Cone Hospital — C CP I L P T ★
Davis Regional Medical Center — C I CP
DLP Cardiac Partners LLC — C
DLP Cardiac Partners LLC — C
DLP Maria Parham Medical Center LLC — C
Duke Raleigh Hospital — C CP I
Duke Regional Hospital — C CP I
Duke University Hospital — C CP I IM L T ★
FirstHealth - Moore Regional Hospital — C T
Forsyth Medical Center — C CP I L T ★
Frye Regional Medical Center — C CP I CL CP ★
Halifax Regional Medical Center — C
Harris Regional Hospital — CP
Haywood Regional Medical Center — C I CP
Huntersville Medical Center — C CP I
Iredell Memorial Hospital — C I CP
Johnston Health — C I
Johnston Health Clayton — C I
Lake Norman Regional Medical Center — C CP
Margaret R. Pardee Memorial Hospital — CP ☆
Maria Parham Medical Center — CP
Matthew's Medical Center — C CP I
Mission Hospital - Asheville — C CP L T CP ★
Nash UNC Health Care - Nash General Hospital — C CP CP ★
New Hanover Regional Medical Center — A C CP I L T CL CP ★
Pardee Hospital — C CP
Person Memorial Hospital — CP
Presbyterian Medical Center — C CP I L T ★
Rowan Medical Center — C CP I ★
Rutherford Regional Medical Center — CP
Scotland Memorial Hospital — C
Sentara Albemarle Medical Center — C CP I
Southeastern Health — A C CP I P
Swain Community Hospital — CP
UNC Lenoir Health Care — CP
UNC Medical Center — A C CP I IM L T CP ★
UNC Rex Hospital — C CP I L P T CP ☆ ◆
Vidant Health — CP
Vidant Medical Center — C CP I IM L T CP ★

Wake Forest Baptist Health - High Point Medical Center — C CP CP ☆
Wake Forest Baptist Health - Wilkes Medical Center — CP
Wake Forest Baptist Medical Center — C CP IM L T ★
WakeMed Cary Hospital — C CP CP
WakeMed Raleigh Campus — C C CP L P T CP HF ★
Watauga Medical Center — C CP I
Wayne UNC Health Care — C CP P
Wilson Medical Center — C I

NORTH DAKOTA

Altru Health System — C CP I L T
CHI St. Alexius Health — A C I P
Essentia Health - Fargo — C CP CP
Sanford Medical Center Bismarck — C CP T ★
Sanford Medical Center Fargo — C CP L T CP ★
Trinity Hospital — C CP I

OHIO

Adena Regional Medical Center — C CP I
Affinity Medical Center - Massillon — CP
Akron Children's Hospital — IM
Ashtabula County Medical Center — I
Atrium Medical Center — C I L CP
Aultman Hospital — A C I L T CP ★
Bethesda North Hospital — C I CP
Blanchard Valley Hospital — C I CP
Cincinnati Children's Hospital Medical Center - Burnet Campus — I IM
Cleveland Clinic Akron General — C I L T CP
Cleveland Clinic Main Campus — C I IM L T
Clinton Memorial Hospital — C
Community Hospitals and Wellness Centers — C I
Coshocton Regional Medical Center — CP
East Liverpool City Hospital — CP
Fairfield Medical Center — A C CP I P T ★
Fairview Hospital — C CP I CP ★
Firelands Regional Medical Center — C CP I CP ★
Fisher-Titus Medical Center — C I
Fort Hamilton Hospital — C I
Galion Hospital — C P
Genesis Hospital — C T CL CP
Good Samaritan Hospital — A C I L T
Good Samaritan Hospital & Health Center — L
Grandview Medical Center — A C I L P
Grant Medical Center — C L T
Hillcrest Hospital — C CP I CP ★
Holzer Medical Center - Gallipolis — C I
Kettering Medical Center — A C I L P T
Knox Community Hospital — C CP CP
Licking Memorial Hospital — C CP ★
Lima Memorial Health System — C I CP
Marietta Memorial Hospital — C I
Mary Rutan Hospital — I
Memorial Hospital of Union County — C I
Mercy Health - Anderson Hospital — C CP I CL CP
Mercy Health - Fairfield Hospital — C CP I P T CL CP ★
Mercy Health - Lorain Hospital — C I P
Mercy Health - Springfield Regional Medical Center — C CP I
Mercy Health - St. Anne Hospital — C I
Mercy Health - St. Elizabeth Youngstown Hospital — A C CP I L T
Mercy Health - St. Rita's Medical Center — C CP I L P T
Mercy Health - St. Vincent Medical Center — C I T
Mercy Health - Tiffin Hospital — C
Mercy Health - West Hospital — C CP I L P CL CP
Mercy Medical Center — C I T CL HF
Miami Valley Hospital — C I L T
Miami Valley Hospital North — C

Miami Valley Hospital South — C
Mount Carmel East — C C CP I L T EP
Mount Carmel St. Ann's — C CP I EP
Mount Carmel West — C CP I EP
Nationwide Children's Hospital — I IM
Ohio State University Hospital East — C
Ohio State University Wexner Medical Center — C I L T
OhioHealth Doctors Hospital — C
OhioHealth Mansfield Hospital — C
OhioHealth Marion General Hospital — C
OhioHealth Riverside Methodist Hospital — C L T
Ontario Hospital — C
ProMedica Toledo Hospital — A C CP I L T CL CP
Soin Medical Center — C I
Southern Ohio Medical Center — C I
Southview Medical Center — C I
Southwest General Health Center — A C C I P ★
St. Luke's Hospital — C I CP
St. Vincent Charity Medical Center — I
Summa Health System - Akron Campus — A C CP I L T CP HF ◆
Summa Health System - Barberton Campus — C CP CP
Taylor Station Surgical Center — CP I
The Christ Hospital — C CP L T ★
The Jewish Hospital - Mercy Health — C CP I L P CL CP
The MetroHealth System — C CP L ★
Trinity Medical Center West — A C I CP
Trumbull Regional Medical Center — C I CP
UH Cleveland Medical Center — C I L T
UH Rainbow Babies & Children's Hospital — IM
University Hospitals Ahuja Medical Center — C I CP
University Hospitals Bedford Medical Center — CP
University Hospitals Conneaut Medical Center — CP
University Hospitals Elyria Medical Center — C CP I P CP ★
University Hospitals Geauga Medical Center — C I CP
University Hospitals Geneva Medical Center — C I CP
University Hospitals Parma Medical Center — C I CP
University Hospitals Portage Medical Center — C I CP
University Hospitals Richmond Medical Center — I CP
University Hospitals Samaritan Medical Center — CP
University Hospitals St. John Medical Center — C CP I CP ★
University of Cincinnati Medical Center — C I L T
University of Toledo Medical Center — C CP I L ★
Upper Valley Medical Center — C I
West Chester Hospital — C I L CP
West Medical Center — CP
Western Reserve Hospital — CP
Wooster Community Hospital — C I CP

OKLAHOMA

AllianceHealth Clinton — CP
AllianceHealth Durant — C I CP
AllianceHealth Madill — CP
AllianceHealth Midwest — C CP I CP
AllianceHealth Ponca City — I CP
AllianceHealth Seminole — I CP
AllianceHealth Woodward — CP
Comanche County Memorial Hospital — C
Hillcrest Hospital South — C CP I P CL CP ◆
Hillcrest Medical Center — C CP I L P T
INTEGRIS Baptist Medical Center — C CP I L P T
INTEGRIS Deaconess — C CP I CL CP ★
INTEGRIS Grove Hospital — C I
INTEGRIS Southwest Medical Center — C I P
Jane Phillips Medical Center — C I P
McAlester Regional Health Center — C
Mercy Hospital Ardmore — C
Norman Regional Health System — CP I CP ★
Norman Regional Hospital — CP

Continues on next page

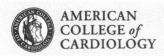
Northeastern Health System Tahlequah .... (I)
Oklahoma Heart Hospital Health System .... (C)(I)(T)
Oklahoma Heart Hospital South Campus .... (C)(I)(T)
Oklahoma State University Medical Center .... (I)
Oklahoma Surgical Hospital .... (I)
OU Medicine .... (C)(CP)(I)(IM)(P)(T)
SSM Health St. Anthony Hospital - Oklahoma City ..... (C)(I)(T)
SSM Health St. Anthony Hospital - Shawnee .... (C)(I)
St. Francis Hospital - The Heart Center .... (C)(I)(L)(T)
St. Francis Hospital Muskogee .... (I)
St. Francis Hospital South .... (C)(I)
St. John Medical Center .... (C)(CP)(I)(L)(P)(T)★
St. Mary's Regional Medical Center .... (CP)(I)
Stillwater Medical Center .... (C)

OREGON

Adventist Health Portland .... (CP)(I)
Asante Rogue Regional Medical Center .... (C)(CP)(L)(T)★
Bay Area Hospital .... (C)(CP)(I)
CHI Mercy Health Mercy Medical Center .... (C)(I)(P)
Good Samaritan Regional Medical Center .... (C)(I)(T)
Kaiser Sunnyside Medical Center .... (C)(I)(L)(T)
Legacy Emanuel Medical Center .... (C)(CP)(I)(L)(T)★
Legacy Good Samaritan Medical Center .... (C)(CP)(I)
Legacy Meridian Park Medical Center .... (C)(CP)(I)★
Legacy Mount Hood Medical Center .... (C)
McKenzie-Willamette Medical Center .... (C)(CP)(P)
Oregon Health and Science University ..... (A)(C)(CP)(IM)(L)(T)
PeaceHealth Sacred Heart
Medical Center at RiverBend .... (C)(I)(T)
Providence Medford Medical Center .... (C)(CP)(CP)★
Providence Milwaukie Hospital .... (CP)
Providence Newberg Medical Center .... (CP)
Providence Portland Medical Center .... (C)(CP)(I)★
Providence St. Vincent Medical Center .... (C)(CP)(L)(T)★
Salem Hospital (Regional Health Services) ...... (C)(L)(T)
St. Charles Health System .... (C)(CP)(I)(P)(T)
Tuality Community Hospital .... (C)

PENNSYLVANIA

Abington Hospital - Jefferson Health .... (C)(I)(L)(T)(CP)
ACMH Hospital .... (C)(CP)
Allegheny General Hospital .... (C)(CP)(I)(L)(T)
Brandywine Hospital .... (C)(I)(CP)
Bryn Mawr Hospital .... (C)(L)
Butler Memorial Hospital .... (C)(CP)(I)(L)(P)(T)(CP)★
Chambersburg Hospital .... (C)(CP)(I)★
Chan Soon-Shiong Medical Center at Windber .... (C)
Chester County Hospital .... (C)(CP)(I)(CL)(CP)◆
Chestnut Hill Hospital .... (CP)
Children's Hospital of Philadelphia .... (I)(IM)
Conemaugh Memorial Medical Center -
Main Campus .... (C)(CP)(I)(P)(T)(CL)(CP)(HF)◆
Conemaugh Meyersdale Medical Center .... (CP)
Conemaugh Miners Medical Center .... (CP)
Conemaugh Nason Medical Center .... (C)(I)(CP)
Crozer-Chester Medical Center .... (C)(CP)(I)
Doylestown Hospital .... (A)(C)(CP)(I)(L)(T)(CP)★
Easton Hospital .... (C)(CP)(L)(CP)
Einstein Medical Center - Montgomery .... (C)(I)(T)(CP)

Einstein Medical Center -
Philadelphia .... (C)(CP)(I)(L)(P)(T)(CP)
Evangelical Community Hospital .... (C)
Excela Health Frick Hospital .... (CP)
Excela Health Latrobe Hospital .... (CP)
Excela Health Westmoreland
Regional Hospital .... (A)(C)(CP)(I)
Forbes Hospital .... (C)(CP)(I)
Geisinger Community Medical Center .... (C)
Geisinger Holy Spirit .... (C)(L)(T)
Geisinger Medical Center .... (C)(IM)(L)(T)
Geisinger Wyoming Valley Medical Center .... (C)(L)(T)
Grand View Hospital .... (C)
Guthrie Healthcare .... (C)(I)(L)(T)
Hahnemann University Hospital .... (C)(I)(L)
Heritage Valley Beaver .... (I)(P)(T)
Holy Redeemer Hospital and Medical Center .... (C)
Hospital of the University
of Pennsylvania .... (C)(CP)(I)(L)(T)★
Indiana Regional Medical Center .... (C)(I)
JC Blair Memorial Hospital .... (C)(I)
Jeanes Hospital .... (C)(CP)(I)
Jefferson Bucks Hospital .... (C)
Jefferson Hospital .... (C)(CP)(I)
Jefferson Torresdale Hospital .... (C)(L)
Lancaster General Hospital .... (C)(I)(T)
Lankenau Medical Center .... (C)(L)(T)
Lehigh Valley Hospital - Muhlenberg .... (C)(I)(L)
Lehigh Valley Hospital - Cedar Crest ..... (C)(I)(L)(P)(T)
Lehigh Valley Hospital - Pocono .... (C)(I)
Lower Bucks Hospital .... (C)
Meadville Medical Center .... (C)(CP)★
Mercy Fitzgerald Hospital .... (C)(CP)(I)(CP)★
Monongahela Valley Hospital .... (C)(I)
Moses Taylor Hospital .... (CP)
Mount Nittany Medical Center .... (C)(I)
Nazareth Hospital .... (C)(CP)
Paoli Hospital .... (C)
Penn Highlands Dubois .... (C)
Penn Presbyterian Medical Center .... (C)(CP)(I)(L)(T)
Penn State Health Milton S. Hershey
Medical Center .... (C)(I)(IM)(L)(T)
Penn State Health St. Joseph Medical Center -
Main Campus .... (C)(CP)(I)(L)(P)(T)
Pennsylvania Hospital .... (C)(CP)(I)
Phoenixville Hospital .... (C)(I)(L)(C)
Pottstown Hospital .... (CP)(HF)
Reading Hospital .... (A)(C)(CP)(I)(L)(T)
Regional Hospital of Scranton ...... (C)(CP)(I)(L)(T)(AF)(CL)(CP)◆
Riddle Hospital .... (C)
Sharon Regional Medical Center .... (C)(CP)(CP)★
St. Christopher's Hospital For Children .... (IM)
St. Clair Memorial Hospital .... (C)(I)
St. Luke's Hospital - Allentown Campus .... (C)(CP)
St. Luke's Hospital - Anderson Campus .... (C)
St. Luke's Hospital - Miners Campus .... (CP)
St. Luke's Hospital - Monroe Campus .... (C)
St. Luke's University Health Network .... (C)(I)(L)(T)(CP)
St. Luke's University Hospital - Bethlehem .... (C)
St. Mary Medical Center .... (C)(CP)(I)(L)(T)(CP)
St. Vincent Hospital .... (C)(CP)(I)(L)(T)(CP)
Temple University Hospital .... (C)(CP)(I)(L)(P)(T)
Thomas Jefferson University Hospital .... (C)(I)(L)(T)
Tyler Memorial Hospital .... (CP)
Uniontown Hospital .... (C)
UPMC Altoona .... (C)(CP)(I)(L)(T)(CL)(CP)
UPMC Children's Hospital of Pittsburgh .... (IM)
UPMC East .... (C)(CP)(I)
UPMC Hamot .... (C)(CP)(I)(L)(T)
UPMC Jameson .... (C)
UPMC McKeesport .... (C)(I)

UPMC Mercy .... (C)(CP)(I)
UPMC Passavant - McCandless .... (C)(CP)(I)(P)
UPMC Pinnacle Carlisle .... (CP)
UPMC Pinnacle Hanover .... (C)(CP)(I)(P)★
UPMC Pinnacle Harrisburg .... (C)(CP)(I)(L)(P)(T)★
UPMC Pinnacle Lititz .... (C)
UPMC Pinnacle Memorial .... (C)(CP)(I)(CP)
UPMC Pinnacle West Shore .... (C)(CP)(I)(P)★
UPMC Presbyterian .... (C)(CP)(I)(L)
UPMC Shadyside .... (C)(I)(T)
UPMC Somerset .... (C)(CP)(P)
UPMC Susquehanna .... (C)(CP)(I)(T)
Washington Health System .... (C)(CP)(I)
Wayne Memorial Hospital .... (C)(I)
WellSpan Ephrata Community Hospital .... (C)(I)
Wellspan Gettysburg Hospital .... (C)(I)
WellSpan Good Samaritan Hospital .... (C)(I)(P)
WellSpan York Hospital .... (C)(I)(L)(T)(CP)
West Penn Hospital .... (C)(CP)(I)
Wilkes-Barre General Hospital ..... (C)(CP)(I)(P)(CL)(CP)

PUERTO RICO

Auxilio Mutuo Hospital .... (CP)
Cayey Mennonite Medical Center .... (C)(L)(T)
Centro Cardiovascular of Puerto Rico
and the Caribbean .... (I)(L)(P)(T)(CP)
HIMA San Pablo - Bayamon .... (I)
Hospital Episcopal San Lucas Ponce .... (I)(L)
Hospital Pavia Santurce .... (I)(L)(T)

RHODE ISLAND

Kent Hospital .... (C)(I)
Landmark Medical Center .... (C)(I)
Miriam Hospital .... (C)
Rhode Island Hospital .... (C)(I)(L)(T)
Roger Williams Medical Center .... (I)
South County Hospital .... (I)

SOUTH CAROLINA

Aiken Regional Medical Center .... (P)
AnMed Health Medical Center .... (CP)
AnMed Health System .... (C)(CP)(L)(T)(CP)★
Beaufort Memorial Hospital .... (C)(CP)(I)★
Carolina Pines Regional Medical Center .... (I)(CP)
Carolinas Hospital System .... (C)(CP)(I)(CP)
Cherokee Medical Center .... (CP)
Colleton Medical Center .... (CP)
Conway Medical Center .... (C)(CP)(I)
East Cooper Medical Center .... (C)
Grand Strand Medical Center .... (C)(L)(T)
Greenville Memorial Hospital .... (C)(L)(P)(T)(CP)
Hilton Head Regional Medical Center .... (C)(CP)
KershawHealth Medical Center .... (I)
Lexington Medical Center .... (C)(CP)(I)(L)(T)(CP)★
Mary Black Campus of Spartanburg Medical Center .... (I)(CP)
McLeod Regional Medical Center .... (C)(CP)(I)(L)(T)★
Medical University of South Carolina -
Ashley River Tower .... (C)(IM)(L)(T)
MUSC Health Marion Center .... (CP)
Piedmont Medical Center .... (C)(CP)(I)(L)(P)(CP)
Prisma Health Richland Hospital .... (C)(CP)(L)(T)(CP)★
Providence Health .... (C)(CP)(I)(L)(T)(CP)★
Roper St. Francis Healthcare - Roper Hospital .... (C)(L)(T)
Self Regional Healthcare .... (C)(CP)(I)(T)(CP)★
Spartanburg Medical Center .... (CP)
Spartanburg Regional
Healthcare System .... (A)(C)(CP)(I)(L)(T)(CP)★
Springs Memorial Hospital .... (I)(CP)
St. Francis Downtown .... (C)(CP)(I)(L)(T)★
Tidelands Georgetown Memorial Hospital .... (C)(CP)
Trident Medical Center .... (A)(C)(CP)(L)(T)(CP)★

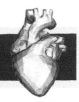

CARE — Participants in ACC's NCDR Registries, Accreditation Services and Awardees

SOUTH DAKOTA

Avera - Sacred Heart Hospital .... (I) (P)
Avera - St. Luke's Hospital.. (C) (CP)
Avera Heart Hospital .... (C) (CP) (L) (T) (CP) ★
Avera McKennan Hospital & University Health Center .... (CP)
Prairie Lakes Healthcare System........................ (C) (CP) ☆
Regional Health Rapid City Hospital ..... (C) (CP) (I) (L) (P) (T) ★
Sanford Aberdeen Medical Center.................................. (CP)
Sanford USD Medical Center .... (C) (CP) (IM) (L) (T) (AF) (CP) ★

TENNESSEE

Baptist Memorial Hospital - Memphis ... (C) (CP) (L) (P) (T) (CP) ★
Baptist Memorial Hospital Carroll County............................... (CP)
Blount Memorial Hospital... (CP) ★
Bristol Regional Medical Center........................ (C) (CP) (P) ★
CHI Memorial.......................... (A) (C) (CP) (I) (L) (P) (T) (CP)
CHI Memorial Hospital Hixson .... (CP)
Cookeville Regional Medical Center..................... (C) (T) (CP)
Erlanger Baroness Hospital........................ (C) (CP) (I) (L) (T)
Erlanger East Hospital... (C)
Fort Sanders Regional Medical Center .... (I)
Hardin Medical Center .... (CP)
Holston Valley Medical Center .... (C) (CP) (P) (T) ★
Jackson-Madison County
General Hospital........................ (C) (C) (P) (I) (T) (CP) ★
Jefferson Memorial Hospital... (CP)
Johnson City Medical Center .... (C) (CP) (I) (L) (T)
Laughlin Memorial Hospital .... (C)
Le Bonheur Children's Hospital................................... (IM)
Livingston Regional Hospital.. (CP)
Maury Regional Medical Center........................ (C) (CP) (I) (CP)
Methodist Le Bonheur
Germantown Hospital .... (C) (I) (L) (T) (CP)
Methodist Medical Center of Oak Ridge .... (C) (I)
Methodist North Hospital........................... (C) (I) (CP)
Methodist South Hospital... (C)
Methodist University Hospital .... (C) (CP) (I) (CP)
Morristown-Hamblen Healthcare System .... (I)

North Knoxville Medical Center .... (C) (CP) (I) (CP)
NorthCrest Medical Center .... (C) (CP) (I) ☆
Parkridge East Hospital.. (CP)
Parkridge Medical Center .... (A) (C) (L) (CP)
Parkwest Medical Center.. (I) (T)
Riverview Regional Medical Center.............................. (CP)
Roane Medical Center.. (I)
Southern Tennessee Regional Health System.......... (C) (I) (CP) (HF)
Southern Tennessee Regional Health System -
Lawrenceburg.. (CP)
Southern Tennessee Regional Health System - Sewanee ...... (CP)
Southern Tennessee Regional Health System -
Winchester .... (CP) (HF)
St. Francis Hospital Bartlett........................ (C) (CP) (I) (CP)
St. Francis Hospital Memphis .... (C) (CP) (I) (CP) ☆
St. Thomas Midtown Hospital........................ (C) (I) (L)
St. Thomas Rutherford Hospital .... (C) (I)
St. Thomas West Hospital........................ (C) (I) (L) (T)
Starr Regional Medical Center - Athens Campus.................. (CP)
Sumner Regional Medical Center........................ (C) (I) (CP)
Tennova - Lakeway Regional Hospital........................... (CP)
Tennova Healthcare - Clarksville........................ (C) (I) (CP)
Tennova Healthcare - Cleveland .... (C) (CP)
Tennova Healthcare - Harton........................ (C) (CP) (I) (CP)
Tennova Healthcare - Lebanon........................ (C) (CP)
Tennova Healthcare - Shelbyville..................................... (CP)
TriStar Centennial Medical Center .... (A) (C) (L) (T) (CP)
TriStar Hendersonville Medical Center .... (C) (CP)
TriStar Horizon Medical Center .... (C) (CP)
TriStar Skyline Medical Center........................ (C) (CP)
TriStar Southern Hills Medical Center .... (C) (CP)
TriStar StoneCrest Medical Center .... (C) (CP)
TriStar Summit Medical Center........................ (C) (CP)
Trousdale Medical Center .... (CP)
Turkey Creek Medical Center..... (A) (C) (CP) (I) (L) (P) (T) (CP) ☆
University of Tennessee Medical Center..... (C) (CP) (I) (L) (T) ★
Vanderbilt University Medical Center................ (C) (CP) (L) (T) (CP)
Vanderbilt University Medical Center System................ (IM) (CP)

West Tennessee Healthcare Dyersburg Hospital.......... (C) (I) (CP)
West Tennessee Healthcare Volunteer Hospital................ (CP)
Williamson Medical Center .... (CP)

TEXAS

Abilene Regional Medical Center................ (C) (I) (CL) (CP)
AdventHealth Central Texas.................... (C) (CP) (I)
Ascension Dell Children's
Medical Center of Central Texas................................. (IM)
Ascension Dell Seton Medical Center
at the University of Texas................ (C) (CP) (I) (P)
Ascension Providence................ (CP) (I) (T) ★
Ascension Seton Medical Center Austin..... (C) (CP) (I) (L) (T) ★
Ascension Seton Medical Center Hays................ (C) (CP) (I) ★
Ascension Seton Medical Center Williamson .... (C) (CP) (I) ★
Baptist Hospitals of Southeast Texas - Beaumont .... (I) (T)
Baptist Medical Center................ (C) (CP) (I) (T) (CP)
Bay Area Regional Medical Center .... (CP)
Baylor Jack and Jane Hamilton Heart
and Vascular Hospital at Dallas................ (C) (CP) (I) (L) (T) ☆
Baylor Scott & White -
Fort Worth's Andrews Women's Hospital .... (C) (I) (L)
Baylor Scott & White All Saints Medical Center -
Fort Worth .... (CP) (T) ☆
Baylor Scott & White Medical Center - Carrollton .... (C) (CP) (I)
Baylor Scott & White Medical Center - Centennial...... (C) (CP) (I)
Baylor Scott & White Medical Center -
College Station................ (C) (CP) (I)
Baylor Scott & White Medical Center -
Grapevine .... (C) (CP) (I) ☆
Baylor Scott & White Medical Center -
Hillcrest................ (C) (CP) (I) (L) ★
Baylor Scott & White Medical Center - Irving............. (C) (CP) (I)
Baylor Scott & White Medical Center - Lake Pointe ..... (C) (CP) (I)
Baylor Scott & White Medical Center - Lakeway............. (C) (CP)
Baylor Scott & White Medical Center - Marble Falls .... (C)

Continues on next page

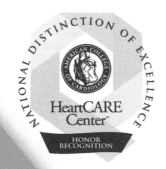

Congratulations
To Our Inaugural Year HeartCARE Center Awardees

THE AMERICAN COLLEGE OF CARDIOLOGY CELEBRATES THE GREAT ACHIEVEMENT OF THOSE HOSPITALS THAT HAVE EARNED THIS PRESTIGIOUS AWARD.

CHI ST. LUKE'S HEALTH MEMORIAL LUFKIN, LUFKIN, TX
CHRISTUS MOTHER FRANCES HOSPITAL-TYLER, TYLER, TX
CONEMAUGH MEMORIAL MEDICAL CENTER, JOHNSTOWN, PA
INDIANA UNIVERSITY HEALTH METHODIST HOSPITAL, INDIANAPOLIS, IN
LAWRENCE GENERAL HOSPITAL, LAWRENCE, MA
LUTHERAN HOSPITAL, FORT WAYNE, IN
METHODIST TEXSAN HOSPITAL, SAN ANTONIO, TX
PARKVIEW HEART INSTITUTE, FORT WAYNE, IN
PENN MEDICINE CHESTER COUNTY HOSPITAL, WEST CHESTER, PA
REGIONAL HOSPITAL OF SCRANTON, SCRANTON, PA
SUMMA HEALTH SYSTEM – AKRON CAMPUS, AKRON, OH
THE HOSPITALS OF PROVIDENCE - SIERRA CAMPUS, EL PASO, TX
UCHEALTH MEMORIAL HOSPITAL, COLORADO SPRINGS, CO
UNC REX HEALTHCARE, RALEIGH, NC
ROSE MEDICAL CENTER, DENVER, CO
HILLCREST HOSPITAL SOUTH, TULSA, OK

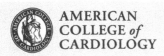
Baylor Scott & White Medical Center - McKinney.................... C CP I CP
Baylor Scott & White Medical Center - Round Rock.. C CP I ★
Baylor Scott & White Medical Center - Sunnyvale ...... C CP I
Baylor Scott & White Medical Center - Waxahachie .... CP
Bayshore Medical Center........................ C CP L P CP
Ben Taub Hospital .... CP I CP ★
Brownwood Regional Medical Center................ C C P I
BSA Hospital .... C I
Cardiology Center of Amarillo........................ I
Cedar Park Regional Medical Center .... C CP I
Central Texas Medical Center .... CP
CHI St. Joseph Regional Health Care Center........ C I
CHI St. Luke's Health - Baylor St. Luke's Medical Center .... A C CP I L P T CL
CHI St. Luke's Health - Lakeside Hospital .... C I
CHI St. Luke's Health - Memorial Lufkin .... C CP I L CP HF ◆
CHI St. Luke's Health - Patients Medical Center .... C CP I
CHI St. Luke's Health - Sugar Land Hospital .... C CP I CP
CHI St. Luke's Health - The Vintage Hospital .... C CP I CP
CHI St. Luke's Health - The Woodlands Hospital .... C CP I P ★
Children's Medical Center of Dallas...................... IM
CHRISTUS Good Shepherd Medical Center - Longview.............. C CP I L ★
CHRISTUS Mother Frances Hospital - Tyler......... C CP I L T CL CP HF ★ ★ ◆
CHRISTUS Santa Rosa - New Braunfels .... A C CP I L
CHRISTUS Santa Rosa - The Children's Hospital of San Antonio............. IM
CHRISTUS Santa Rosa - Westover Hills .... C CP I L CP
CHRISTUS Santa Rosa Hospital - Medical Center.............. C
CHRISTUS Southeast Texas - St. Elizabeth.............. C CP I
CHRISTUS Southeast Texas St. Mary.............. C
CHRISTUS Spohn Hospital Alice .... C I
CHRISTUS Spohn Hospital Corpus Christi - Shoreline............ CP I L T CP
CHRISTUS St. Michael Atlanta...................... CP
CHRISTUS St. Michael Health System........... C CP I CP
Citizens Medical Center .... CP CP ★
City Hospital at White Rock........................ C CP I
Clear Lake Regional Medical Center........... C CP L P T CP
College Station Medical Center.................... C I CP
Conroe Regional Medical Center .... C CP L CP
Cook Children's Medical Center.................... IM
Corpus Christi Medical Center - Bay Area........ C CP L T CP
Corpus Christi Medical Center - Doctors Regional............ CP
Covenant Medical Center.......................... A C I T
Dallas Regional Medical Center.................... CP I CP
Del Sol Medical Center............................ C CP CP
DeTar Hospital Navarro .... C CP I CP
Doctors Hospital at Renaissance........... CP I IM P T CP HF
Doctors Hospital of Laredo .... I CP
Driscoll Children's Hospital .... IM
Ennis Regional Medical Center .... CP
Guadalupe Regional Medical Center C
Harlingen Medical Center.......................... C I
HCA Houston Healthcare - West.................. AF
Heart Hospital of Austin .... A C L T
Hendrick Medical Center.......................... C I
Houston Methodist Baytown Hospital .... C CP I

Houston Methodist Clear Lake Hospital .... C CP I CP
Houston Methodist Hospital....................... C CP I L P T
Houston Methodist Sugar Land Hospital ...... C CP I L P
Houston Methodist the Woodlands Hospital.. C CP I L P ★
Houston Methodist West Hospital................ C CP I CP
Houston Methodist Willowbrook Hospital...... C CP I CP
Houston Northwest Medical Center............... C CP CP
Hunt Regional Medical Center C
Huntsville Memorial Hospital .... C I
John Peter Smith Hospital .... C CP I
Kingwood Medical Center .... C CP L CP
Lake Granbury Medical Center .... C CP I
Laredo Medical Center............................ C I
Las Palmas Medical Center .... C CP L
Longview Regional Medical Center .... C I L P T
Lubbock Heart & Surgical Hospital .... C I
Mainland Medical Center .... C CP P CP
Matagorda Regional Medical Center C
McAllen Heart Hospital .... CP I CP
Medical Center Hospital.......................... C CP I
Medical City Alliance C
Medical City Arlington .... C CP CP
Medical City Dallas............................... A C L T CP
Medical City Denton.............................. C CP CP
Medical City Fort Worth .... C L T
Medical City Frisco............................... C
Medical City Las Colinas......................... C
Medical City Lewisville........................... C CP
Medical City McKinney........................... C
Medical City North Hills.......................... C CP
Medical City Plano............................... C CP
Medical City Weatherford........................ C CP
Memorial Hermann Cypress Hospital .... CP
Memorial Hermann Greater Heights Hospital........ CP
Memorial Hermann Heart & Vascular Institute - Southwest............ CP L T
Memorial Hermann Katy Hospital................ CP
Memorial Hermann Memorial City Medical Center .... CP L
Memorial Hermann Northeast Hospital.......... CP
Memorial Hermann Pearland Hospital........... CP
Memorial Hermann Southeast Hospital.......... CP
Memorial Hermann Sugar Land Hospital......... CP
Memorial Hermann Texas Medical Center....... CP IM L T
Memorial Hermann the Woodlands .... CP L T ★
Methodist Charlton Medical Center............... C CP ★
Methodist Dallas Medical Center................. C CP L T
Methodist Hospital .... A C CP I IM L T CL CP ★
Methodist Mansfield Medical Center............. C CP
Methodist Richardson Medical Center........... C CP L T
Methodist Specialty and Transplant Hospital .... C I
Methodist Stone Oak Hospital .... C CP I
Methodist Texsan Hospital....................... C CP I L ★ ◆
Metropolitan Methodist Hospital................. A C CP HF
Midland Memorial Hospital....................... C I
Mission Trail Baptist Hospital.................... C CP I CP
Nacogdoches Medical Center..................... C I
Nacogdoches Memorial Hospital................. I
Navarro Regional Hospital........................ CP
North Central Baptist Hospital .... C CP I CP ★
North Cypress Medical Center.................... C I CP
Northeast Baptist Hospital........................ C CP I L CP
Northeast Methodist Hospital................... A C CP I L CP ★
Northwest Children's Hospital of Northwest Texas Healthcare System............... C I
Northwest Texas Healthcare System............ CP
OakBend Medical Center Health System .... CP
Odessa Regional Medical Center................. C CP CP
Palestine Regional Medical Center .... C I CP
Paris Regional Medical Center.................... I P CP
Park Plaza Hospital .... C CP
Parkland Health and Hospital System .... C I L

Parkview Regional Hospital....................... CP
Pearland Medical Center.......................... C CP CP
Peterson Regional Medical Center................ C
Resolute Health Hospital......................... C CP I CP
Rio Grande Regional Hospital.................... C CP CP
San Angelo Community Medical Center........... C CP I CP HF
Scott & White Medical Center - Temple...... C CP I L T ★
Seton Medical Center Harker Heights .... C CP I CL ★
Shannon Medical Center........................ C CP T ★
Southwest General Hospital...................... CP
St. David's Georgetown Hospital .... CP
St. David's Medical Center........................ A C I L
St. David's North Austin Medical Center C
St. David's Round Rock Medical Center .... A C
St. David's South Austin Medical Center .... A C CP I L
St. Joseph Medical Center........................ C CP I
St. Luke's Baptist Hospital........................ C CP I CP
Texas Children's Hospital......................... IM
Texas Health Azle................................. CP
Texas Health Harris Methodist Hospital - Fort Worth................ C CP I T
Texas Health Harris Methodist Hospital Alliance C
Texas Health Harris Methodist Hospital Hurst-Euless-Bedford................ C CP I ★
Texas Health Harris Methodist Hospital Southwest Fort Worth................ C
Texas Health Heart and Vascular Hospital Arlington................ C CP I T
Texas Health Huguley Hospital Fort Worth South................ C CP I
Texas Health Presbyterian Hospital Allen C
Texas Health Presbyterian Hospital Dallas .... C CP I L P T ★
Texas Health Presbyterian Hospital Denton......... C CP I
Texas Health Presbyterian Hospital Plano .... C CP I
Texoma Medical Center.......................... C I T CP
The Heart Hospital at Providence .... CP
The Heart Hospital Baylor - Denton.............. C CP I CP ★
The Heart Hospital Baylor - Plano.............. C CP I L T CP ★
The Hospitals of Providence - East Campus .... C CP
The Hospitals of Providence - Memorial Campus...... C CP I P
The Hospitals of Providence - Sierra Campus............. C CP I L T CL CP HF ★ ◆
The Hospitals of Providence - Transmountain Campus ..... C CP
The Medical Center of Southeast Texas .... C CP CP
The University of Texas Medical Branch Clear Lake................ C I L
Tomball Regional Medical Center .... C CP CP
United Regional Medical Center.................. CP I CP HF
University Hospital................ C CP I L T CP ★
University Medical Center........................ C I L T
University Medical Center of El Paso............. C CP P CP
University of Texas MD Anderson Cancer Center......... I
University of Texas Medical Branch Health .... C I L T
UT Health Tyler.................................. C CP I T CP
Valley Baptist Medical Center - Brownsville ...... C CP I
Valley Baptist Medical Center - Harlingen .... C I
Valley Regional Medical Center................... C CP L CP
Wadley Regional Medical Center .... C CP I
West Houston Medical Center.................... C CP L AF CP
William P. Clements Jr. University Hospital .... C CP I L T ★
Wise Health Surgical Hospital - Parkway .... C I
Wise Health System............................. C CP I CP
Woodland Heights Medical Center............... C I L CL CP

UTAH

Ashley Regional Medical Center .... CP
Brigham City Community Hospital................ CP
Castleview Hospital.............................. CP
Davis Hospital and Medical Center............... C P CP

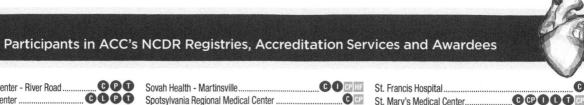

Dixie Regional Medical Center - River Road ... C P T
Intermountain Medical Center ... C L P T
Jordan Valley Medical Center ... C
Jordan Valley Medical Center - West Valley Campus ... C I
Lakeview Hospital ... C CP CP
Lone Peak Hospital ... CP
McKay-Dee Hospital ... L P T
Mountain Point Medical Center ...
Mountain View Hospital ... C CP CP
Mountain West Medical Center ...
Ogden Regional Medical Center ... C CP AF CP HF
Primary Children's Hospital ... I IM
Salt Lake Regional Medical Center ... C L
St. Mark's Hospital ... C CP I L T CP ★
Timpanogos Regional Hospital ... C CP L CP
University of Utah Health Care ... A C CP I L T ★
Utah Valley Hospital ... C L P

VERMONT

Central Vermont Medical Center ... I
Rutland Regional Medical Center ... I
The University of Vermont Medical Center ... A C I L T

VIRGINIA

Augusta Health ... C CP I CP
Bon Secours DePaul Medical Center ... C I P
Bon Secours Mary Immaculate Hospital ... C I
Bon Secours Maryview Medical Center ... C I P
Carilion New River Valley Medical Center ... C I
Carilion Roanoke Memorial Hospital ... C CP I L T CP
Centra Lynchburg General Hospital ... C CP I P T AF CP ★
Centra Southside Community Hospital ... C
Chesapeake Regional Medical Center ... C CP I CP
Children's Hospital of the King's Daughters ... I IM
Chippenham Hospital ... A C CP L T
Clinch Valley Medical Center ... C
Fauquier Health ... C
Fauquier Hospital ... CP
Henrico Doctors Hospital ... C CP T
Inova Alexandria Hospital ... C CP I ★
Inova Fairfax Hospital ... A C CP I IM L T ★
Inova Loudoun Hospital ... C CP I ★
John Randolph Medical Center ... CP
Johnston Memorial Hospital ... C CP I ★
LewisGale Hospital Alleghany ... CP
LewisGale Hospital Montgomery ... C CP CP
LewisGale Hospital Pulaski ... CP
LewisGale Medical Center ... C CP CP
Mary Washington Hospital ... C I L T
Memorial Regional Medical Center ... C I L
Naval Medical Center Portsmouth ... CP
Novant Health UVA Health System
Prince William Medical Center ... C CP I ★
Reston Hospital Center ... C CP CP
Riverside Regional Medical Center ... C CP I L CP
Riverside Walter Reed Hospital ... CP
Sentara Careplex Hospital ... C CP I ★
Sentara Halifax Regional Hospital ... C CP I
Sentara Leigh Hospital ... C CP I ★
Sentara Martha Jefferson Hospital ... C CP I CP ★
Sentara Norfolk General Hospital ... C CP I L T ★
Sentara Northern Virginia Medical Center ... C CP I ★
Sentara Obici Hospital ... C CP I
Sentara Princess Anne Hospital ... C CP ★
Sentara RMH Medical Center ... C CP I L T ★
Sentara Virginia Beach General Hospital ... C CP I CP ★
Sentara Williamsburg Regional Medical Center ... C CP I CP ★
Southern Virginia Regional Medical Center ... CP
Southside Regional Medical Center ... C CP I P CL CP
Sovah Health - Danville ... C CP I CP HF

Sovah Health - Martinsville ... C I CP HF
Spotsylvania Regional Medical Center ... C I
St. Francis Medical Center ... C I
St. Mary's Hospital ... C I P T
Stafford Hospital Center ... C CP
StoneSprings Hospital Center ... C CP
Twin County Regional Hospital ... CP
University of Virginia
Children's Hospital ... A C CP I L T ★
VCU Health ... C C I IM L T
VCU Medical Center Main Hospital ...
Virginia Hospital Center - Arlington ... C CP I L T
Warren Memorial Hospital ... C CP
Winchester Medical Center ... C CP I L T AF CL CP HF ★
Wythe County Community Hospital ... CP

WASHINGTON

Astria Regional Medical Center ... CP
Astria Sunnyside Hospital ... C
Capital Medical Center ... I
Central Washington Hospital ... C CP I
EvergreenHealth ... C I
Harrison Medical Center - Bremerton ... A C CP I L T ★
Highline Medical Center ... C CP I ★
Kadlec Regional Medical Center ... C
Legacy Salmon Creek Medical Center ... C I
MultiCare Auburn Medical Center ... C CP
MultiCare Deaconess Hospital ... A C CP I CP
MultiCare Good Samaritan ... C CP
MultiCare Tacoma General Hospital ... C CP I L T
MultiCare Valley Hospital ... CP
Northwest Hospital & Medical Center ... C
Overlake Hospital Medical Center ... C I T
PeaceHealth Southwest Medical Center ... C I L T
PeaceHealth St. John Medical Center ... C I
PeaceHealth St. Joseph Medical Center ... C I L T
Providence Regional Medical Center Everett ... A C L T
Providence Sacred Heart Medical Center & Children's Hospital ... C CP IM L T
Providence St. Mary Medical Center ... C
Providence St. Peter Hospital ... C CP T
Seattle Children's Hospital ... IM
Skagit Valley Hospital ... C
St. Anthony Hospital ... I
St. Francis Hospital ... C CP
St. Joseph Medical Center ... A C CP I L P T ★
Swedish Medical Center - Cherry Hill Campus ... A C L T
Swedish Medical Center - Edmonds Campus ... C
Trios Women's & Children's Hospital ... C
University of Washington Medicine ... C L T
Valley Medical Center ... C
Virginia Mason Memorial ... C I
Virginia Mason Seattle Medical Center ... C CP I L T ★
Winchester Medical Center ... AF

WEST VIRGINIA

Beckley ARH Hospital ... C
Berkeley Medical Center ... C I
Bluefield Regional Medical Center ... C CP
Cabell Huntington Hospital ... CP
Camden Clark Medical Center - Memorial Campus ... C CP I T
Charleston Area Medical Center Health System ... C CP I T
Greenbrier Valley Medical Center ... C CP
Logan Regional Medical Center ... CP
Mon Health ... C CP I L T ★
Princeton Community Hospital ... C
Raleigh General Hospital ... C CP I CP
Reynolds Memorial Hospital ... C

St. Francis Hospital ... C I
St. Mary's Medical Center ... C CP I L T CP ★
Thomas Memorial Hospital ... C I
United Hospital Center ... C I
Weirton Medical Center ... C I
Wheeling Hospital ... A C CP I L T CP ★
WVU Medicine Childrens Hospital ... C I L T

WISCONSIN

Ascension All Saints Hospital Spring Street Campus ... C I
Ascension Columbia St. Mary's Hospital Ozaukee ... C I
Ascension Columbia St. Mary's Women's Hospital ... C I T
Ascension SE Wisconsin Hospital - Elmbrook Campus ... C I
Ascension SE Wisconsin Hospital - Franklin Campus ... C I
Ascension SE Wisconsin Hospital - St. Joseph Campus ... C I
Ascension St. Clare's Hospital ... C CP I T ★
Ascension St. Francis Hospital ... C I
Aspirus Wausau Hospital ... C CP L P T ★
Aurora BayCare Medical Center ... A C CP I ★
Aurora Lakeland Medical Center ... CP
Aurora Medical Center in Burlington ... C I
Aurora Medical Center in Grafton ... A C CP I CP ★
Aurora Medical Center in Kenosha ... C I CP
Aurora Medical Center in Oshkosh ... C I
Aurora Medical Center In Summit ... C CP I CP
Aurora Sheboygan Memorial Medical Center ... C I
Aurora St. Luke's Medical Center ... A C CP I L T CP ★
Bellin Health ... C T
Beloit Hospital ... I
Children's Hospital of Wisconsin ... IM
Community Memorial Hospital ... C I CP
Froedtert Hospital ... C I L T CP
Gundersen Lutheran Medical Center ... C CP I T
Holy Family Memorial Medical Center ... C CP ★
HSHS Sacred Heart Hospital ... C CP I P
HSHS St. Mary's Hospital Medical Center ... C
HSHS St. Vincent Hospital ... C T
Kenosha Medical Center ... C
Marshfield Clinic - Wausau Center ... C CP I
Marshfield Medical Center - Eau Claire ... C CP
Marshfield Medical Center - Marshfield ... A C CP I L T
Mayo Clinic Hospital - Eau Claire ... C T
Mayo Clinic Hospital - Franciscan La Crosse Hospital ... C
Mercyhealth Hospital and Medical Center - Walworth ... CP
Mercyhealth Hospital and Trauma Center - Janesville ... C CP I CP
ProHealth Oconomowoc Memorial Hospital ... C I
ProHealth Waukesha Memorial Hospital ... C I L T CL CP
SSM Health St. Mary's Hospital - Madison ... C CP I L T ★
St. Agnes Hospital ... C I L
St. Joseph's Hospital ... CP
The Monroe Clinic ... C I
ThedaCare Regional Medical Center - Appleton ... C CP I T CL CP
UnityPoint Health - Meriter ... C CP I
University of Wisconsin Health ... C CP I IM L P T ★
Watertown Regional Medical Center ... C I CP

WYOMING

Campbell County Memorial Hospital ... C CP I ★
Cheyenne Regional Medical Center - West Campus ... C CP ★
Evanston Regional Hospital ... CP
SageWest Health Care - Lander ... CP
SageWest Health Care - Riverton ... CP
Sheridan Memorial Hospital ... C I
Wyoming Medical Center ... C CP I ★

(JIMMIE SMITH CONTINUED FROM 44)

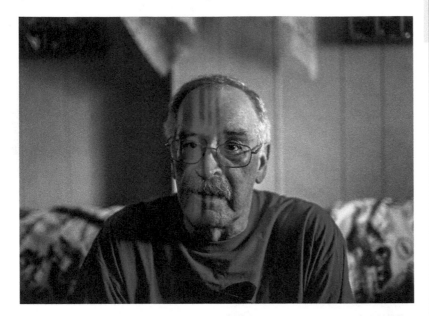

JIMMIE SMITH WAS DIAGNOSED WITH DANGEROUS ANEURYSMS IN HIS AORTA. HIS WIFE SHOWS OFF A DIAGRAM (RIGHT) OF THE 12 STENTS PLACED TO PREVENT THE BULGES FROM BURSTING.

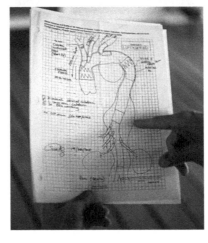

kidneys – using special, experimental stents that aren't yet commercially available in the U.S. (Stents are thin mesh tubes that help reinforce weak areas.) A repair this extensive would be a first for Mayo Clinic and is believed to be only the third full aorta reconstruction in the nation.

The surgery would be done using a minimally invasive approach that wouldn't require large incisions. Ongoing studies show that minimally invasive aortic aneurysm repair can greatly reduce the risk of death and life-threatening complications, and get patients home sooner than traditional open surgery.

First, the experts did 3D modeling of Jimmie's anatomy, and took precise measurements of his aorta to ensure the stents would fit securely. Oderich then worked closely with companies overseas to customize special stents for Jimmie, and with the Food and Drug Administration to quickly get approval to use them. To permanently maintain blood flow to the kidneys, intestines and the brain, Oderich needed stents that would enable him to create a sort of tree trunk; smaller branch stents could then split off and keep blood circulating to these vital organs.

Moment of truth. Jimmie underwent three separate operations – the first in July 2018 and the last in April 2019 – done through a small incision in each leg, at the groin. The stents were inserted inside the artery, using a thin plastic tube to guide each one to the precise place. The second procedure was the trickiest – the aneurysm was bulging like a pouch and hard to reach – but the third was the most dangerous because it was right near his heart, and it rebuilt the vessels to Jimmie's neck, head and arms.

"Between surgeries, I knew the aneurysms were there, waiting to get repaired, which was nerve-wracking because I never knew if they would burst," says Jimmie, who has completely recovered and is enjoying "the good life" with his family and new puppy, Boo. "I owe these doctors my life." *–Linda Marsa*

STELLA CROWLEY
17 years old

TO DESCRIBE HER as resilient? Understatement of the century. For nearly 18 years, Stella Crowley has lived with three benign brain tumors that – another understatement – have played havoc with her life.

Because of their consistency, akin to stretched-out cotton balls with fibers invading surrounding tissue, the tumors couldn't simply be removed. So "watchful waiting" was prescribed. But because of their location, in brain regions vital to hormone control, Stella faced the prospect of early puberty and of having her first period at age 5. Panic jolted through her mom, Christine, when doctors delivered that news. "Thankfully, there are medications to stave that off," she says.

It didn't end there. The tumors were interfering with Stella's brain-gut communication, meaning she never – ever – felt full. Around fourth grade, thanks to insatiable cravings and the beginnings of a pattern of uncontrolled eating, Stella started to rapidly gain weight.

The problem had a name – hypothalamic obesity – but no easy solution. Nothing worked. Not wellness camps. Not cognitive behavioral therapy. Not special diets, or appetite-suppressant medications or diligent exercise with a personal trainer. "There wasn't a way to block this urge," Christine says. Stella vividly remembers sneaking sacks of bagels and potato chips to her room and "eating bags and bags and bags of them in the darkness," she says. "It was nothing I could physically control."

Desperation. By high school, Stella was gaining about 25 pounds a year. Liposuction and a tummy tuck proved agonizingly ineffective: The cravings always won out. At 16, she weighed 237 pounds, nearly twice the average for a teen girl her age. Kids had been pelting her with "fat waste of space" insults forever, but Stella's self-confidence hit a new low when a boy rejected her with a glib, "Sorry, I only date girls who are 125 pounds or less."

Eventually, one expert warned that if she didn't lose weight, she risked having a heart attack by age 20. "I cried for a couple of hours," says Stella, mourning her goals of becoming a high school chemistry teacher and starting a family. Given that it was still too dangerous to

remove the tumors or risk the side effects of radiation, and that six rounds of chemo had accomplished nothing, her doctor proposed one last idea: gastric bypass surgery performed by Thomas Inge, director of adolescent bariatric surgery at Children's Hospital Colorado.

Inge and a growing body of evidence had been showing that the surgery – in which the stomach, typically the size of a football, is stapled off to about the size of an egg – could halt the extreme food cravings hijacking patients with hypothalamic obesity for reasons not entirely understood. "You wouldn't predict that an operation on the stomach would trump what's going on in the brain, and yet it happens," he says. That's because the brain and the gut talk to each other. A lot. And that conversation, it seems, can be dramatically redirected.

Hometown:
Carlsbad, California

Hospital:
Children's Hospital Colorado

Her Challenge:
Hypothalamic obesity

"We think the operation is working on two levels," Inge notes. "It's toning down the appetite signaling from gut to brain and amplifying messaging around being full." Since 2007, Inge has operated on about a dozen such patients with encouraging results. Because of their complex biology, he tells patients with hypothalamic obesity that there will be unknowns; they may not lose as much weight as those without the condition, but that in most cases, a loss of 10% to 25% is possible.

Severe obesity is rising in U.S. youth. And so are its health complications. Regardless of its cause – hypothalamic or otherwise – Inge wants families to know that his team's most recent data suggest that it may be more beneficial to consider weight loss surgery when patients are teenagers versus waiting

until they are adults. While the procedure yields similar weight loss results in adults and teenagers, adolescents with severe obesity saw greater reversal of Type 2 diabetes and high blood pressure than adults who had gastric bypass, per a study Inge recently published in the New England Journal of Medicine.

Inge and his team performed Stella's surgery through tiny incisions in October 2018. She has since lost nearly 80 pounds, and has overhauled her closet three times. She no longer gets winded when talking at length. She can chase her two Rottweiler puppies and even ski. What seemed like an inevitable life sentence of weight gain has been reversed. "We thought she was going to be homebound," Christine says. And those cravings? They're on mute. "It's been completely life-changing," Stella says. "It's allowed me to open so many doors to the future that I didn't even know were there." *–Lindsay Lyon*

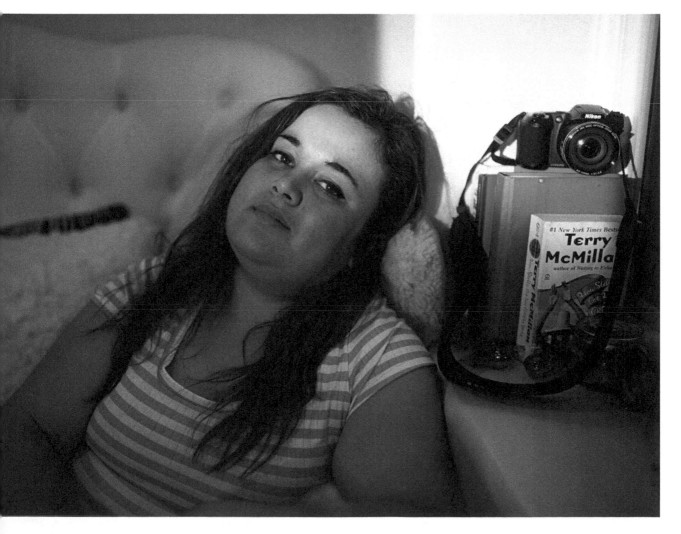

You bring out the Better in us.

It's amazing what you can achieve when you never settle.

From conquering heart disease to beating cancer to defeating joint pain, your fighting spirit is what drives us to get Better. After all, our greatest achievement is seeing you thrive.

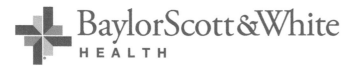

BaylorScott&White
HEALTH

Changing Healthcare For The Better

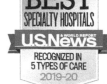
BSW The Heart Hospital Plano*
BEST SPECIALTY HOSPITALS
U.S.News & WORLD REPORT
RECOGNIZED IN 5 TYPES OF CARE
2019-20

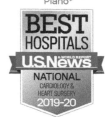
BSW The Heart Hospital Plano*
BEST HOSPITALS
U.S.News & WORLD REPORT
NATIONAL
CARDIOLOGY & HEART SURGERY
2019-20

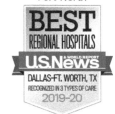
Fort Worth
BEST REGIONAL HOSPITALS
U.S.News & WORLD REPORT
DALLAS-FT. WORTH, TX
RECOGNIZED IN 3 TYPES OF CARE
2019-20

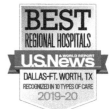
Dallas
BEST REGIONAL HOSPITALS
U.S.News & WORLD REPORT
DALLAS-FT. WORTH, TX
RECOGNIZED IN 10 TYPES OF CARE
2019-20

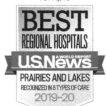
Temple
BEST REGIONAL HOSPITALS
U.S.News & WORLD REPORT
PRAIRIES AND LAKES
RECOGNIZED IN 8 TYPES OF CARE
2019-20

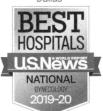
Dallas
BEST HOSPITALS
U.S.News & WORLD REPORT
NATIONAL
GYNECOLOGY
2019-20

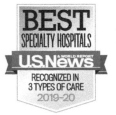
BSW The Heart Hospital Denton*
BEST SPECIALTY HOSPITALS
U.S.News & WORLD REPORT
RECOGNIZED IN 3 TYPES OF CARE
2019-20

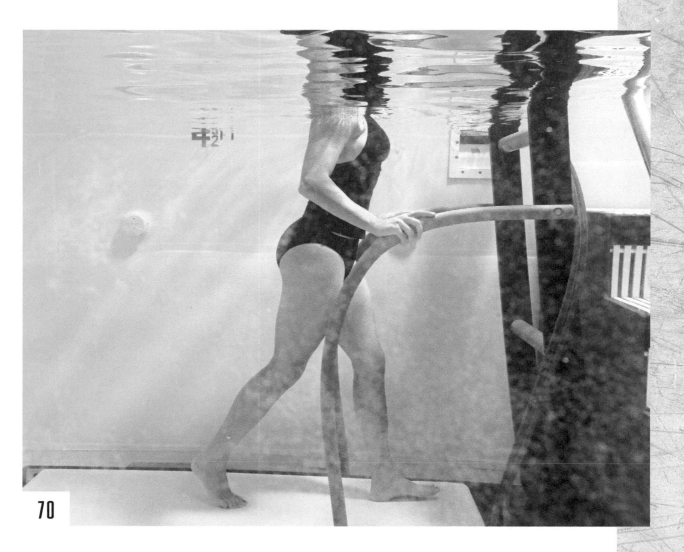

70

Patient Power

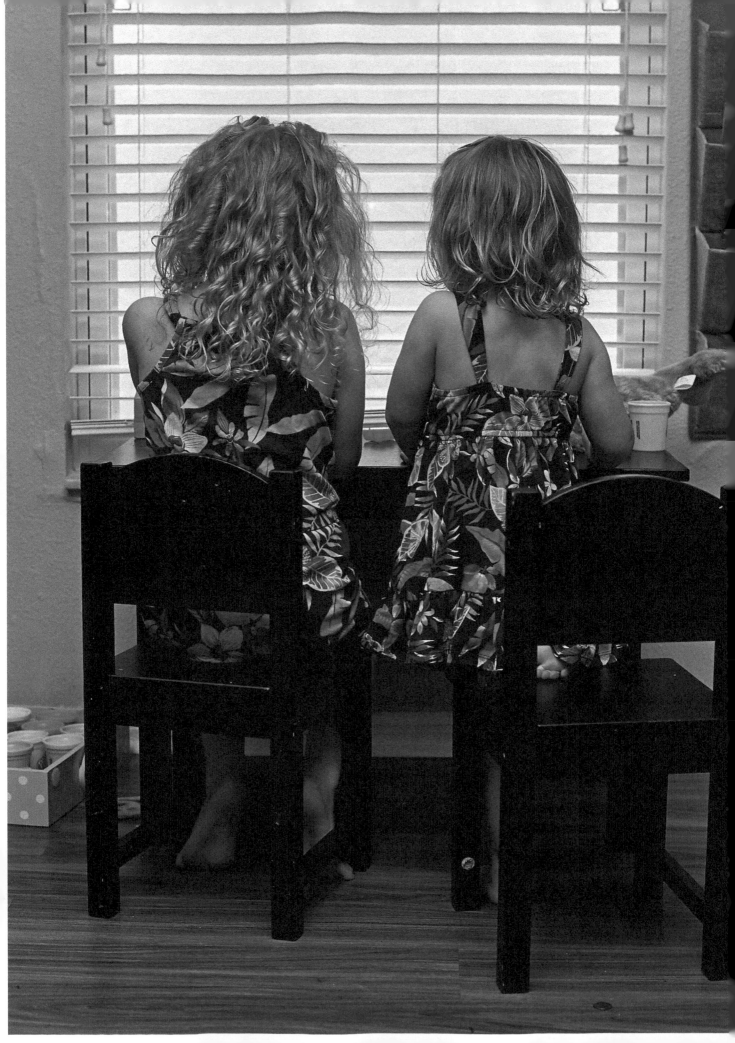

Hope for a Fertile Future

More patients are being offered the chance to conceive after cancer

by **Beth Howard**

WHEN LILY WEINBACH, 19, started having gastrointestinal problems last fall, her doctor suspected Crohn's disease. But the diagnosis turned out to be much worse: colon cancer.

The University of Michigan freshman needed treatment right away. But in the two-week sliver of time before starting chemotherapy – which could potentially leave her infertile – Weinbach not only had surgery to remove her tumor but also opted to have 17 eggs extracted from her ovary and frozen for when she's ready to start a family. "This was a priority for me," she says. "I have always known I wanted to have children."

While chemotherapy, radiation and other therapies effectively kill cancer cells in the body, they can also harm healthy tissue, including the reproductive organs. But over the last decade or so, experts in the burgeoning field of oncofertility have been fine-tuning processes that allow patients of reproductive age to store their eggs, sperm, or ovarian and testicular tissue, offering the chance to conceive after cancer. And scientists are tantalizingly close to being able to preserve fertility in young children – even infants – facing cancer.

One of the driving forces behind these technologies is the spectacular rise in survival rates. Since 1991, the U.S. cancer death rate has dropped 27 percent. Many of the millions of Americans conquering their cancers expect to live a full and normal life, including raising kids. "The success of cancer treatments is so much better than it used to be that we can think about patients' quality of life long term," says Christos Coutifaris, professor of obstetrics and gynecology at the University of Pennsylvania Perelman School of Medicine and immediate past president of the American Society for Reproductive Medicine.

The right to reproduce. Preserving fertility hasn't historically been a priority in the cancer-treatment equation. The message from oncologists has traditionally been: "Focus on the disease first and fertility

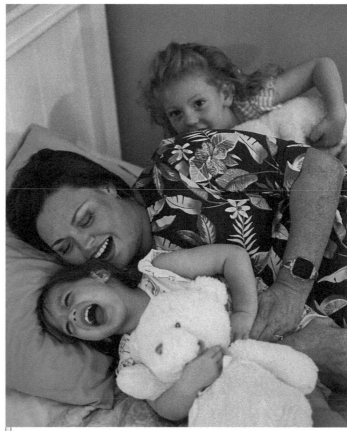

RACHELL MOODIE, 34, IS NOW CANCER-FREE. ONE OF HER DAUGHTERS WAS CONCEIVED FROM A FROZEN EMBRYO; THE OTHER, SPONTANEOUSLY.

later," says Teresa Woodruff, professor of obstetrics and gynecology at the Northwestern University Feinberg School of Medicine and founder of the 12-year-old Oncofertility Consortium, which partners with some 230 institutions to make fertility preservation options available.

Yet often, "patients who have been through this kind of life-altering experience come out on the other side and want to share all that life has to offer with

a child," says Leslie Appiah, co-director of the Fertility Preservation and Reproductive Health Program at the Ohio State University Comprehensive Cancer Center's James Cancer Hospital. "For those who can't," she says, "it really is devastating." Appiah often hears grief and frustration from patients in survivorship who weren't offered fertility preservation procedures or were unable to undergo them.

The issue is particularly fraught for women, because preserving eggs is much more complicated than preserving sperm. After puberty, most males can produce a sperm sample, and freezing and banking sperm prior to cancer treatment has been common for years, even among adolescents.

When Jordan Johnson, 18, was diagnosed with a rare head and neck cancer a year ago, he faced a grueling regimen of chemotherapy and radiation. So his team at the Aflac Cancer and Blood Disorders Center at Children's Healthcare of Atlanta offered to freeze his sperm, and it's now in storage, ready should he choose to become a biological dad. "Honestly, that was the last thing on my mind," says his mother, Shannon. "Just knowing that one day my son can still have a child is very exciting."

Since reproductive-age women and girls release only a single egg a month, preserving their fertility requires taking hormones that allow multiple eggs to mature and then suctioning the eggs through a tiny tube so that they can later be used for in vitro fertilization. Traditionally, the process has taken up to eight weeks – time that many cancer patients don't have. Consequently, until recently, "young women were very often not told by their doctors" that cancer treatments might cause infertility, Woodruff says.

'3D-printed ovaries may be on the horizon.'

Fertility breakthroughs. Doctors have discovered ways to speed up the egg-harvesting process to reduce delays in cancer treatment. "We figured out that we can get patients through a lot faster than what we traditionally thought," says Clarisa Gracia, chief of reproductive endocrinology and infertility and director of Fertility Preservation at the University of Pennsylvania's Perelman School of Medicine. "Now you can meet with my nurse, learn how to give yourself the shots, start the injections that day and boom! We'll be done within two weeks."

That's how it went for Rachell Moodie, 34, of Wesley Chapel, Florida, after a 2009 breast cancer diagnosis. "You have a couple weeks of testing, like heart and chest scans, and I did fertility preservation simultaneously with that," says Moodie, who got care at Moffitt Cancer Center in Tampa. "I started a hormone pill, my husband gave me injections twice a day, and I went in every day for them to check my blood and measure my eggs to see what was happening." Moodie is now cancer-free and has two daughters, ages 3 and 4 – the first from a frozen embryo; the other conceived spontaneously.

While putting sperm and embryos on ice has been done for decades, freezing the eggs themselves, when patients don't have a sperm source they wish to use, has been a tougher challenge. Eggs have a high water content; when they are frozen, ice crystals form that can destroy the eggs when they're later thawed.

The game changer is a freezing method called vitrification, which rapidly

cools and flash freezes the eggs using a high concentration of cryoprotectant to prevent those ice crystals from forming. The technology has worked so well that the American Society for Reproductive Medicine removed the experimental label from egg freezing in 2012, Woodruff says.

Doctors are also preserving parts of the ovary itself, surgically removing small strips of the organ tissue and freezing them before cancer treatment begins. After treatment, when a woman is ready

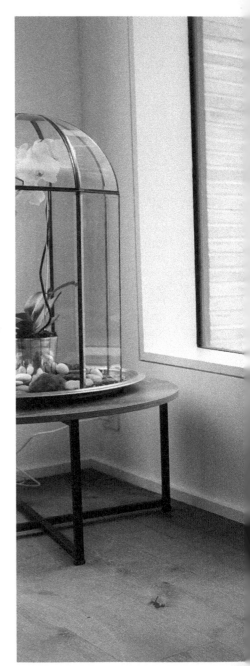

to become pregnant, the tissue is thawed and sewn back into the ovary to stimulate ovulation. This method allows doctors to preserve fertility without taking time to stimulate the ovaries for egg freezing – important when cancer treatment needs to start immediately. So far, about 130 births have resulted from the technique worldwide, Gracia says. The challenge yet to be fully worked out is making sure that no cancer resides in the tissue before it is reimplanted. (That is not a worry with eggs and sperm.) Thus far, she says, "it is generally performed in patients who are at low risk for having malignancy in the ovary."

Male adolescent or adult cancer patients who aren't able to produce a semen sample may benefit from a more routinely done procedure, testicular sperm extraction, through which sperm are retrieved from a biopsy of the testicles. And for males and females undergoing radiation only, the placement of a protective shield over the reproductive organs may reduce the collateral damage.

Pioneering options for children. Such advances are increasingly becoming the standard of care. Now, doctors and scientists are homing in on the next big challenge: Safeguarding fertility in young kids with cancer, for whom overall survival has increased from 10% to nearly 90% in the last 40 years.

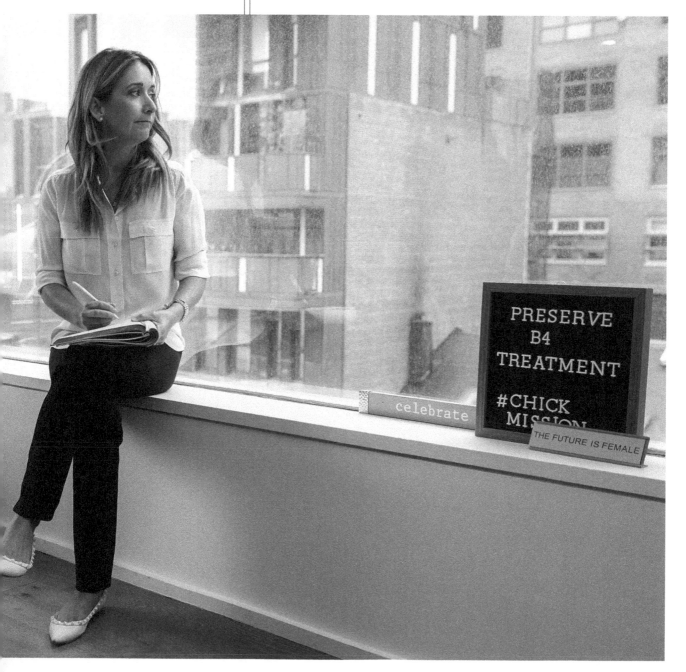

CANCER SURVIVOR AND ADVOCATE AMANDA RICE, 42, IN HER HOME OFFICE

After puberty, cancer patients as young as 12 or 13 may be able to undergo sperm and egg banking. But it's a different story for kids who have not undergone pubertal development, since they do not have mature sperm or eggs, says Courtney A. Finlayson, pediatric endocrinologist at Ann and Robert H. Lurie Children's Hospital of Chicago and assistant professor of pediatrics at Northwestern's Feinberg School of Medicine. "Ovarian tissue or testicular tissue is surgically removed and then frozen in hopes that someday we will be able to use it" to help kids have a biologically related child. Pediatric patients as young as five months have had their ovarian tissue banked in these experimental protocols.

Scientists are also exploring "bio-prosthetic ovaries" made with 3D printers out of gelatin ink. Doctors may be able to seed these artificial ovaries with a child's ovarian follicles (immature egg cells), potentially restoring functions that allow eggs to mature. The process works in a mouse model, though human studies are still years away, says principal investigator Monica Laronda, a researcher with Lurie Children's and an assistant professor of pediatrics at Northwestern.

There's also hope for young boys, using their testicular tissue, which contains sperm stem cells, the precursors to sperm. "We believe we can mature that tissue so that it could allow a cancer survivor to have a biological child," says Kyle Orwig, professor of obstetrics, gynecology and reproductive sciences at the University of Pittsburgh School of Medicine. In March of 2019 his team proved the concept in monkeys, stimulating sperm production after the frozen tissue was transplanted back to the animals – and eventually producing a live birth. Orwig expects to start human trials in the next few years.

Overcoming obstacles. Despite the breakthroughs, barriers remain. "It's a shame how infrequently women in their fertile years are made aware of reproductive risks and fertility potential and pathways to preserve," says Matthew Zachary, 45, a Brooklyn-based survivor who founded Stupid Cancer, an advocacy and support organization for young adults with cancer. Some oncologists aren't up to date on the options or they don't recognize the need to coordinate with reproductive spe-

'Science is edging closer to preserving fertility in babies facing cancer.'

cialists, he says. Or: "They don't want to deliver another blow after they've already said, 'You have cancer,'" notes Amanda Rice, 42, a breast cancer and melanoma survivor in New York City, who had several of her eggs frozen and stored before chemotherapy. And patients and families may not think to ask about the effects of treatment on reproductive organs.

Of course, some patients aren't eligible for oncofertility procedures – for instance, their diagnosis requires cancer treatment to start immediately. However, "patients have a right to make a decision about their reproductive health," says Barbara Lockart, a pediatric nurse practitioner at Lurie Children's who counsels patients about their options.

And then there's cost. The process to retrieve a woman's eggs alone can have a price tag of $10,000-plus, though many hospitals offer help to defray the expense, says James Klosky, psychologist for the Fertility Preservation Program at Children's Healthcare of Atlanta's Aflac Cancer and Blood Disorders Center. Some national pharmacy programs will provide fertility-related medications for free to cancer patients. On the other hand, negotiated storage fees at sperm banks can be as low as $60 a year. "Some offer reduced rates for cancer patients," Klosky says. Help can also come from foundations like Livestrong and organizations such as Chick Mission, founded by survivor Amanda Rice, which raises money to fund fertility preservation options for female cancer patients.

There's encouraging progress on the insurance front, too. Since 2017, 21 states have introduced legislation that would mandate coverage of medically necessary fertility preservation for cancer patients or others who are at risk. Six states – Connecticut, Rhode Island, Maryland, Delaware, Illinois and New York – have enacted this legislation, and several have bills pending, according to the Alliance for Fertility Preservation. More are expected to follow suit, opening the door for greater numbers of cancer patients to preserve their fertility. Says Woodruff: "The outlook has never been better for cancer patients who want to have their own biological children." •

Top 10 New Osteopathic Physicians Across America

Voted By State Peers

SUMEET GOEL, DO

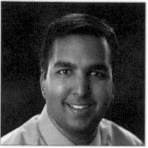

Family Medicine
Wisconsin

JENNIFER BELSKY, DO

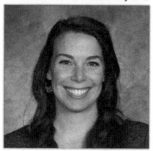

Pediatric Oncology
Ohio

ADAM C. HUNT, DO

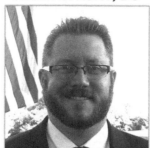

Emergency Medicine
and Family Medicine
Michigan

ANDREW LEVIN, DO

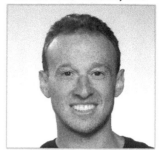

Physical Medicine
and Rehabilitation
Pennsylvania

COLE ZANETTI, DO

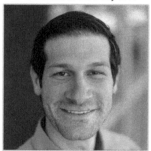

Family Medicine/
Preventative Medicine
Colorado

JASON SNEED, DO

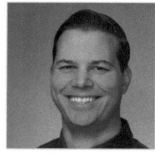

Osteopathic
Manipulative Medicine
Virginia

**DANIELLE
BARNETT-TRAPP, DO**

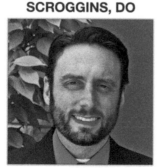

Family Medicine
Arizona

**BRADLEY
SCROGGINS, DO**

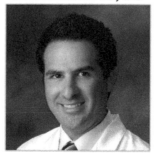

Pediatrics
New Mexico

SEGER MORRIS, DO

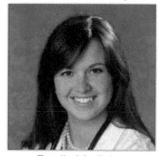

Internal Medicine
Mississippi

ERRIN WEISMAN, DO

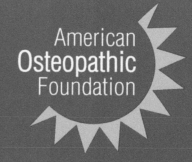

Family Medicine
Indiana

Congratulations

The American Osteopathic Foundation is proud to celebrate
2019's TOP EMERGING LEADERS in their first 5 years of practice
within the osteopathic profession.

We salute your commitment to osteopathic principles
and your tireless efforts to enhance patient-centered care.

American
Osteopathic
Foundation

Getting in Shape for

**Patients are boosting
their results with
targeted prep regimens**

by **Stacey Colino**

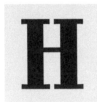

HAVING MAJOR SURGERY is like running a marathon – both challenges require training, physical conditioning and stamina, experts say. That's why doctors and hospitals are prescribing prehabilitation – basically rehabilitation performed before a surgical procedure, be it joint replacement, cardiac, transplant, colorectal or cancer surgery.

The goal? To help patients get stronger, fitter and more functional ahead of treatment – chemotherapy and radiation included, says Julie Silver, a physician and researcher at Harvard Medical School and Spaulding Rehabilitation Hospital. Prehab can encompass exercise or physical therapy (on land or in water), dietary changes and smoking cessation. It can also include fortifying mental strength through psychological interventions, she explains.

While research hasn't definitively proven the perks of prehab, "that in no way implies that it isn't of tremendous value," says Jonathan Whiteson, vice chair for clinical operations and medical director of cardiac and pulmonary rehabilitation at Rusk Rehabilitation at NYU Langone Health. In Europe and Canada, where there are often lengthy waitlists for surgery, research shows prehab may lower the risk of complications, shorten hospital stays and boost outcomes. "The window of opportunity to conduct research is smaller in the U.S. because we don't have long waitlists" for surgery, he adds.

Nothing cookie cutter about it. There isn't a one-size-fits-all approach to prehab. It's tailored to individual needs and accounts for the specific challenges a particular patient might face after a given procedure, says Silver, author of "Before and After Cancer Treatment: Heal Faster, Better, Stronger." "It's not general wellness – everybody knows to eat right and exercise. These are specific, targeted approaches to facilitate certain outcomes," like averting bleeding or infection after surgery.

Indeed, a Spanish study published in 2018 showed that pa-

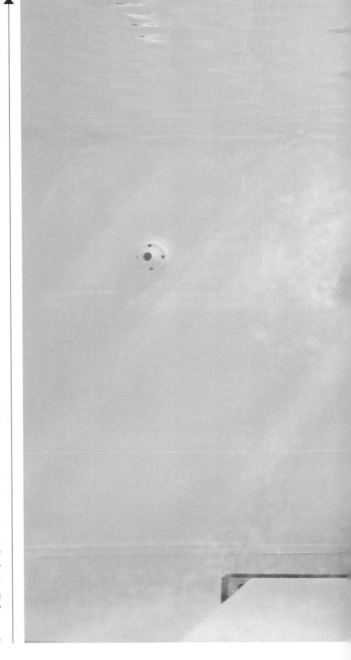

Surgery

tients who did a personalized prehab program involving high-intensity endurance exercise training before undergoing elective major abdominal surgery had fewer post-op complications compared to those who received standard care, because of their increased aerobic capacity. In a review of nine studies, Canadian researchers found that patients undergoing colorectal surgery who did nutritional prehabilitation (with oral nutritional supplements) alone or combined with exercise decreased their hospital stay by two days.

Prehab comes in different formats, from group classes to one-on-one training to self-directed at-home exercises. Duration? Often two to six weeks. "We want patients to quit smoking at

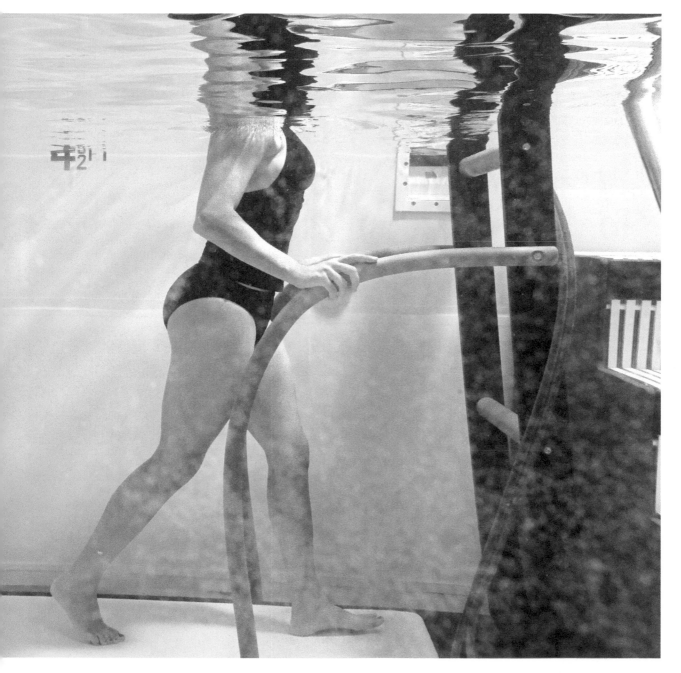

least four to six weeks before surgery because smoking can lead to lung infections and wound infections after surgery," says R. Matthew Walsh, Cleveland Clinic's chair of general surgery. "It takes a while for the effects of smoking to wear off." Prehab can also involve efforts to get diabetes, hypertension or other chronic conditions under control before surgery.

Sometimes, prehab means the difference between being cleared – or not – for a given treatment. For example, with lung cancer, the surgical-eligibility bar is set fairly high and some patients may be too sick or weak to qualify initially, Silver says. "If they get stronger with prehab, they might be transformed into surgical candidates," which may thereby improve their odds of survival. For those patients, says Silver, "That would be a really big game-changer."

Patients needing an organ transplant are often weak and frail. Prehabilitation can help them get strong enough to tolerate the surgery, Whiteson says. Depending on how frail they are, the prehab Rx may be dietary. "If patients are underweight and have lost muscle, we'll increase their protein and calorie intake and encourage them to have small, frequent meals and take a vitamin and mineral supplement,"

'Prehab paves the way for better outcomes.'

says Jeanette Hasse, transplant nutrition manager at Baylor University Medical Center in Dallas.

Joanna King, 66, was diagnosed with idiopathic pulmonary fibrosis in 2018 after developing severe shortness of breath. She was put on oxygen therapy and told she wouldn't survive without a lung transplant. But to even be considered for surgery, she had to get stronger. While on oxygen therapy, King began prehab at NYU Langone Health. It involved doing physical therapy, working with a psychologist and learning specific breathing techniques to boost oxygen levels and promote calmness.

Better outcomes. "The physical therapy built my strength, which made me feel good, and the psychologist helped me feel calm and confident," says King, a retired headhunter in New York City. "I went from being terrified to really looking forward to the surgery." In October 2018, King had a left lung transplant and no longer needs oxygen therapy. "I came out of the surgery really well."

With most sports medicine operations, prehab can set the stage for better outcomes, too. If someone is scheduled to have an ACL (the anterior cruciate ligament) reconstruction, a prehab regimen can improve range of motion, swelling and muscle activation in the knee before surgery, says Rachel M. Frank, assistant professor of orthopaedic surgery and director of the joint preservation program at the University of Colorado School of Medicine. "If you go in for surgery with an angry

knee, your chances of having stiffness in the knee after surgery are greater, as are your chances of having a decreased functional outcome and a slower return to sport." A 2018 study found that patients with knee osteoarthritis who did a six-week home-based prehabilitation exercise program before undergoing total knee arthroplasty had greater improvements in pain and functionality up to six months after surgery, compared to those in a control group.

After Ellie Venafro, 45, tore her ACL while skiing in January 2019, her knee was so swollen she couldn't straighten her leg. She needed surgery, but "Dr. Frank didn't want to do [it] until I had almost full range of motion," says Venafro, a health care finance director. So she went to physical therapy once weekly and did twice-daily exercises at home to strengthen her leg muscles. "I'm a very avid exerciser, and I wanted to get back to it as soon as I could."

She had surgery in February and was thrilled with the results. "I'd heard horror stories about how long recovery could take and how much pain I might be in," she says. "My recovery was pretty remarkable: I immediately had more range of motion than is typical, and by the second week, I was already on the bike, which is where someone would usually be by the seventh week." Venafro is now hiking and running on the treadmill again.

Sometimes patients end up in better shape than before surgery, Silver says. "The earlier people get in for prehab, the better they function on the other side," adds physical therapist Melanie Gaeta, orthopedic program manager at the Center for Restorative Therapies at Mercy Medical Center in Baltimore. The ideal scenario: prehab plus traditional postoperative rehabilitation, Whiteson says.

Interest in prehab is growing. "It's a field, a trend, a movement that makes tremendous sense," Whiteson says. "There's no doubt that there's a benefit to getting stronger before elective surgery." Walsh agrees: "We're so geared up to enhance recovery after surgery. What we do before surgery can enhance recovery after surgery even more." ●

A Very Delicate Balance

The secret life of the microbes that call the human body home

by **Elizabeth Gardner**

SPOILER ALERT: This story about the miraculous medical potential of the human microbiome is going to end with some big unknowns, and be served up with a side of guidance to eat more fermentable fiber.

New discoveries about the microbiome – the trillions of microorganisms that inhabit the body and interact with its cells – are piling up rapidly and may impact every aspect of medical practice in the coming decades. However, they have so far resulted in only one reliable cure, for a stubborn bacterial infection, despite a proliferation of over-the-counter "probiotics" promising

smoother digestion, a stronger immune system – even a better mood. Experts say that while there are many encouraging research avenues, most microbiome-related product claims should, for now, be taken with a grain of salt (or maybe a bowl of chili).

Each person's microbiome is a unique collection of mostly bacteria, along with some fungi, viruses and other microorganisms. Estimates of the microbiome's size vary wildly, but conservatively, it equals the number of cells in the body (some 38 trillion in a 155-pound person, though all those microbes weigh only about half a pound).

Off-kilter. A healthy microbiome is required for the body to function properly. Research associates microbiome disruptions with diseases and chronic ailments that plague millions: celiac disease, asthma, allergies and even colon cancer. Many people experience temporary digestive chaos from antibiotics that attack good gut bacteria along with their intended targets, and some studies show that just one course of antibiotics can change the gut microbiome for months.

"We have good evidence that these microcolonies are essential to our biology," says Jens Walter, professor of agricultural, food and nutritional science at the University of Alberta. "We exist in a state of symbiosis with these communities, and what we do in modern life disrupts this symbiosis." Walter has been studying the microbiome since 1999 and has recently been exploring how it might be implicated in multiple sclerosis. Studies have shown differences in the gut microbiome of people with and without MS. The federal website

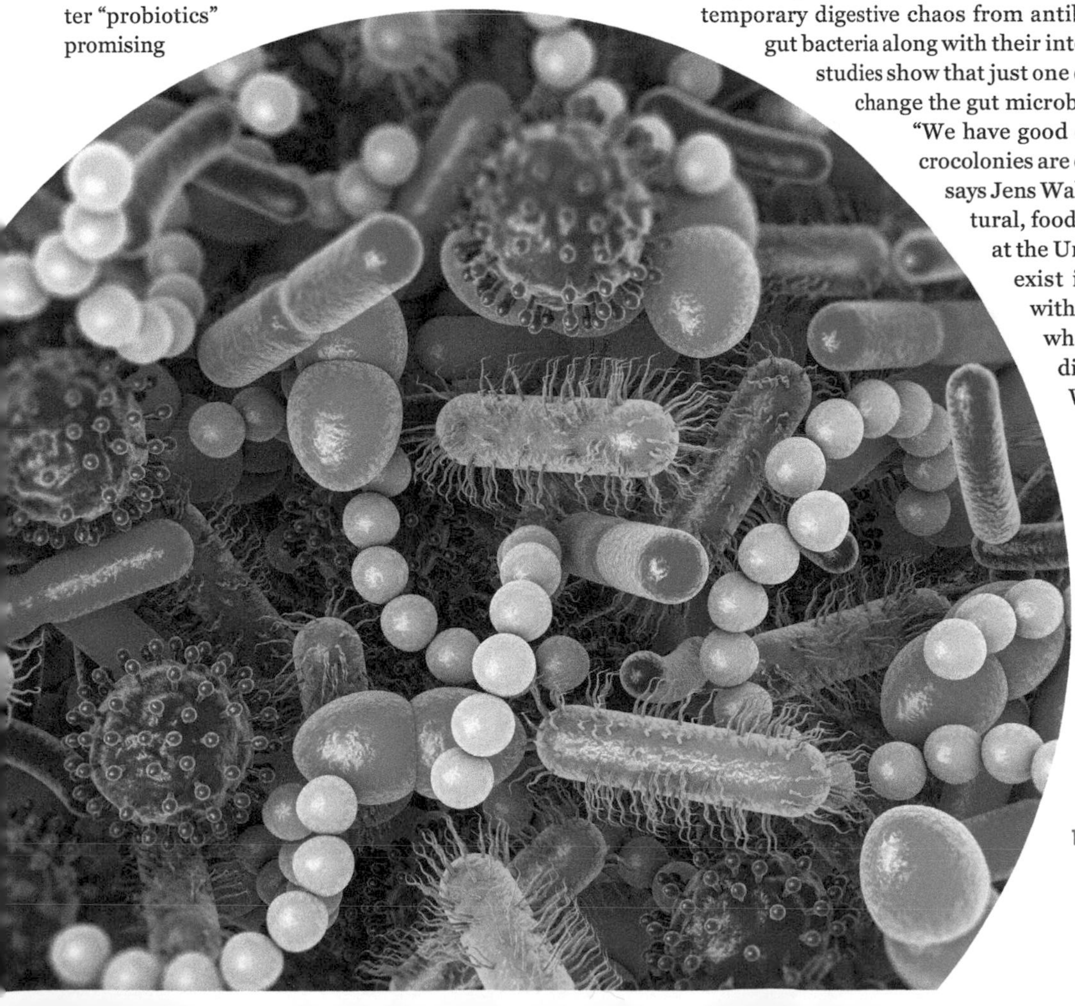

UP CLOSE AND PERSONAL:
A RENDERING OF
THE HUMAN MICROBIOME

ClinicalTrials.gov, where researchers must register medical studies, lists almost 1,500 microbiome-related research projects in various stages, and the National Institutes of Health's Human Microbiome Project has a library of over 32,000 microbiome samples available for study.

While the body has distinct microbiomes at different sites – for example, in the mouth and nose and on the skin – the one that's most often in the limelight is the gut microbiome, which aids digestion and secretes chemicals that travel through the bloodstream to all parts of the body.

"There are studies that link the microbiome with everything from autism to Alzheimer's," says Thomas Schmidt, head of the Michigan Microbiome Project at the University of Michigan–Ann Arbor, created to study how to engineer the gut microbiome to improve human health. "However, some of those relationships will be causal and others will just be coincidental, and we are in the stage of figuring it out." Gut bacteria aren't just active in the gut, he points out: The chemicals they create affect every aspect of our physical and mental health, and we've evolved to need those chemicals.

Schmidt studies one in particular called butyrate, made by bacteria in the large intestine. Butyrate is a preferred energy source for cells that line the intestine. The body can't make its own butyrate and counts on gut bacteria to do that job using fermentable fiber, which can't be broken down by the human digestive system. When cells don't get enough butyrate, they can malfunction and cause inflammation in the surrounding tissue, which may affect the body's other systems, too. That's why Schmidt encourages people to eat more fermentable fiber. Foods high in it include most fruits and vegetables, beans, oats and barley.

Friend or foe? Society has long villainized bacteria. Some types are harmful, of course, and the discovery of penicillin and other antibiotics has largely freed us from the epidemics they cause. But in our zeal to wipe them out, with antibacterial drugs, soaps, hand sanitizers and household cleaners, we inadvertently damage the good ones.

Dosing with antibiotics is the most obvious way to eradicate good bacteria, an excellent reason why doctors decline to prescribe antibiotics unless they're sure patients have a bacterial infection that really requires them. But anything people eat, drink or absorb through the skin can also change the microbiome. For example, studies of the common herbicide glyphosate suggest that it may alter the microbiome of bees and the gut microbiome of baby rats.

Perhaps the most widespread potential symptom of microbiome upheaval is the obesity epidemic, which afflicts almost 40% of U.S. adults. While the relationship is still unclear, researchers have found differences in the microbiomes of people with and without obesity. Infectious disease specialist

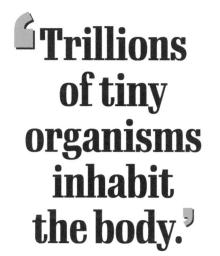

'Trillions of tiny organisms inhabit the body.'

Martin Blaser, who wrote "Missing Microbes: How the Overuse of Antibiotics Is Fueling Our Modern Plagues," believes many of today's major health ills, especially obesity, asthma and allergies, can be traced to microbiome disruptions caused in part by overreliance on antibiotics. He cites a Danish study suggesting that each course of antibiotics boosts the risk of developing inflammatory bowel disease during childhood by 14%.

The microbiome affects, and is affected by, medications in other ways, adds Blaser, director of the Center for Advanced Biotechnology and Medicine at Rutgers University: "If you give 100 people a drug, some will get better, some won't and some will get sick from it, and a big source of this variation has to do with the microbiome." Blaser expects that as we gain a more sophisticated understanding of this relationship, microbiome analysis will become part of choosing which drugs – and doses – are best matched to a patient's unique biology.

The only major microbiome development that's found a place in clinical practice is a fecal transplant to treat Clostridioides difficile, the stubbornly antibiotic-resistant and sometimes deadly bug known as "C.diff," which sickens almost half a million people each year, often during hospital stays when antibiotics weaken their native microbiomes.

A fecal transplant is just what it sounds like: Stool samples from a healthy volunteer are introduced into the infected person, either via the colon or swallowed in capsule form. The beneficial bacteria in the sample colonize the patient's intestines, displacing the harmful C. diff bacteria. Research suggests the treatment ousts the infection in up to 90% of patients after antibiotics have failed. "Fecal transplants have become the state of the art," Blaser says. "Thirty years ago if you told someone, 'We'll give you feces!' they would have laughed, but it's clearly correct."

Proceed with caution. The FDA still considers the treatment experimental and hasn't approved it for any use. But because fecal transplants have shown success against intractable C. diff. infections, the agency is not actively preventing them from being used in such cases, provided patients are aware of the risks and certain precautions are followed. The FDA updated those precautions in June to include additional testing of stool donations, following news that a patient had died after receiving a fecal transplant containing a drug-resistant strain of E.coli.

The promise of improving health with "natural"

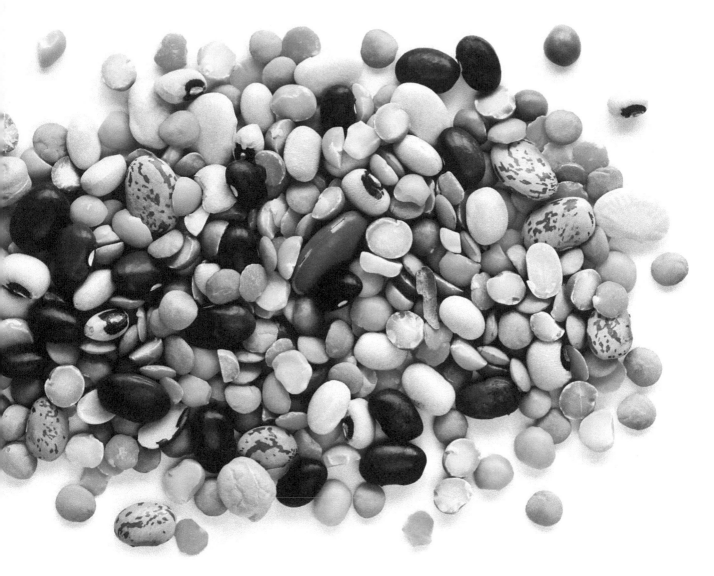

microbes has caused an explosion of "probiotic" products that often boast of containing multiple strains of beneficial live bacteria. Amazon alone stocks more than 3,000 probiotics.

But beware, says dietary supplement expert Pieter Cohen, assistant professor of medicine at Harvard Medical School and an internist at Cambridge Health Alliance. "Each live bacterium or fungus needs to be understood on its own," he says. "If there is research to suggest that a specific strain of a microorganism can be helpful in a specific clinical situation, then that specific strain should be the only live organism used to treat the condition."

No evidence. Cohen is concerned that probiotic makers aren't required to label their products transparently – with the strain of bacteria and the amount. Thus, consumers have no way to compare different probiotics or even be certain what's in them. "There is no evidence that all the different microorganisms sold as 'probiotics' in the U.S. are interchangeable, or even that they are beneficial."

Blaser agrees. "They are almost completely untested," he says. "The number of robust clinical trials is small.

▲ BEANS ARE ONE EXCELLENT SOURCE OF FERMENTABLE FIBER.

People are making money from these products, so why would they do a test that impedes their ability to make money?"

Recent studies suggest that OTC probiotics may affect the immune system unpredictably; one found that cancer patients taking probiotics didn't respond as well to immunotherapy as those who weren't.

Don't expect guidance from the FDA, at least for now. Close reading of probiotic labels reveals the products haven't been evaluated by the agency nor are they intended to "diagnose, treat, cure or prevent any disease." While the FDA is studying specific applications of specific organisms, it has not "approved any probiotic as a live biotherapeutic product," per a 2018 agency statement.

To nurture his gut microbiome, Schmidt focuses on upping his fermentable fiber and avoiding antibiotics generally. If he were facing hospitalization and the prospect of intravenous antibiotics, he says he'd store a fecal sample in the freezer to preserve his pre-hospital microbiome. "If I got a C.diff infection and needed a fecal transplant, I'd rather have my own bacteria, which work well in my body and are distinctive."

These moves may seem modest, given all the promise. But stay tuned, says Blaser: "The microbiome is a scientific and a medical frontier. I think a generation from now it will touch all areas of medicine." ●

by **Lisa Esposito**

WHAT IF, INSTEAD of languishing in front of a TV, people with dementia could step inside elaborately constructed sets designed to help them rekindle their pasts?

No, it's not a fantasy, nor a scene out of "Pleasantville." Across the country, some residential and adult day programs are diving deeply into the concept of reminiscence therapy – which uses photos, music, memorabilia and other tools – by creating immersive environments painstakingly designed to replicate moments from the distant past, when older people who now have dementia were teens or young adults in their prime.

The idea? To spark long-term memory that, perplexingly, is sometimes still tucked away in people with dementia.

In Chula Vista, California, a building has been transformed into a 9,000-square-foot indoor time capsule of a 1950s town. Launched in 2018, Glenner Town Square, an interactive senior day care center, currently has about 78 participants enrolled, many in their early 80s. Professional caregivers guide them through a series of storefronts: a diner with a jukebox where meals are served, an old-fashioned clinic with a registered nurse, a barber and beauty shop, a pet store, a movie theater playing classics, for example.

In the city hall, outfitted with vintage desks and manual typewriters, a former accountant taps into memories of her working years, performing never-forgotten tasks and reawakening a sense of purpose; staff engage with her as if she were the real town accountant. In the museum, curated by the San Diego Air & Space Museum, large model airplanes hang from the ceiling, sparking a flood of recollections for veterans with dementia, which, for one daughter, was particularly emotional, having never heard her father talk so freely about his military experience, says Scott Tarde, Glenner Town Square CEO. Other memory-jogging activities include: Tinkering with a 1959 T-Bird in the garage; browsing old-fashioned clothing and accessories at the '50s-style department store, reminiscing about styles of yesteryear. Cost: $95 a day.

GLENNER TOWN SQUARE IS A 9,000-SQUARE-FOOT TIME CAPSULE OF THE 1950S.

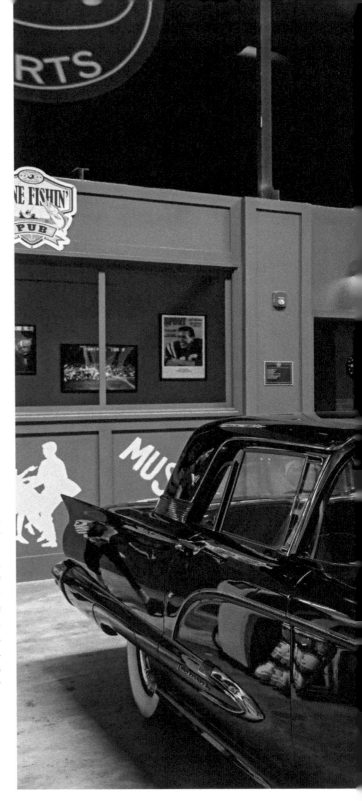

Bringing Memories

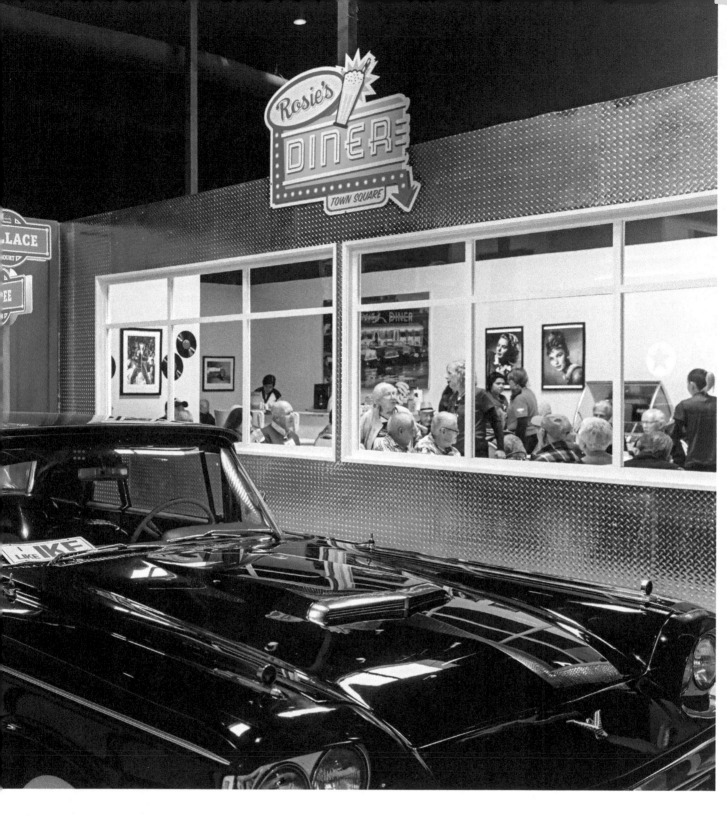

Back to Life

Reminiscence therapy offers people with dementia a link to the past

PHOTOGRAPHY BY **JENNIFER EMERLING** FOR USN&WR

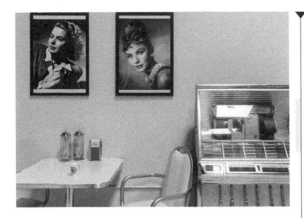

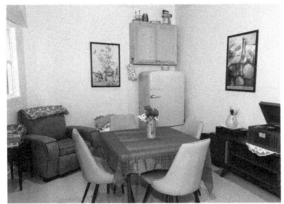

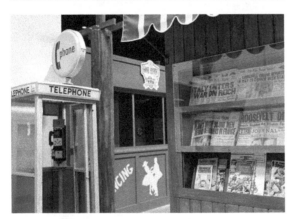

AN OLD-STYLE DINER COMPLETE WITH A JUKEBOX; A RECORD PLAYER; A PHONE BOOTH; AND GOLDEN ERA MOVIE POSTERS SET THE TONE IN THE IMMERSIVE INDOOR SENIOR CARE CENTER, WHERE PARTICIPANTS REKINDLE THE PAST.

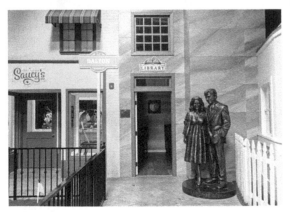

"It definitely made sense to me to create an environment that resonated strongly with people," Tarde says, "instead of just four walls and a television."

Outlook: intriguing. There is no cure for dementia, an umbrella term for the array of neurodegenerative conditions that can cause significant problems with memory, speech, thinking and behavior. Approximately 50 million people worldwide are living with it. Alzheimer's disease is far and away the most common form, and by 2060, U.S. rates of Alzheimer's and related dementias are projected to more than double. "Unfortunately, despite billions and billions in money spent by the federal government and by pharmaceutical companies, we still do not have what we call a disease-modifying agent for Alzheimer's disease – meaning something that really changes the course of the illness," says geriatric psychiatrist Daniel Bateman, a co-investigator at the Indiana Alzheimer Disease Center.

Bateman and other experts are intrigued by pioneering facilities that incorporate reminiscence therapy within specially designed environments – a bright spot in a pretty frustrating period in the dementia field. Quality-of-life initiatives have become increasingly vital as drugs to reverse disease or markedly ease symptoms aren't panning out. "It's cutting edge and it's exciting work," Bateman says. "One of the great pieces about the concept is that it really focuses on maintaining the dignity and the humanity of people with dementia, which can often be lost."

Immersive reminiscence therapy started in the 2000s with a unique Dutch village called Hogewey. The entire gated town is actually an imaginatively conceived long-term care facility. The inhabitants all have severe dementia, and are cared for by staffers who wear street clothes on-site, instead of uniforms. Group homes resemble housing of past decades and residents can move about the village's supermarket, barbershop, restaurant, courtyard and other amenities.

The notion that people with dementia could continue living seemingly independent lives, enjoying the outdoors and making their own choices in a familiar, stigma-free setting – instead of being largely restricted to a nursing home – captured worldwide media attention, and that of dementia-care innovators in the U.S. That this village sparked social engagement rather than the isolation so common among those with dementia stood out as a big advantage.

People suffering from dementia tend to withdraw from social engagements, conversations and everyday activities, explains Esther Oh, an associate professor in the division of geriatric medicine and gerontology at Johns Hopkins University School of Medicine. Reminiscence therapy, however, "really draws them out of [their] shell," says Oh, "because they're able to tap into their past and things they're very familiar with."

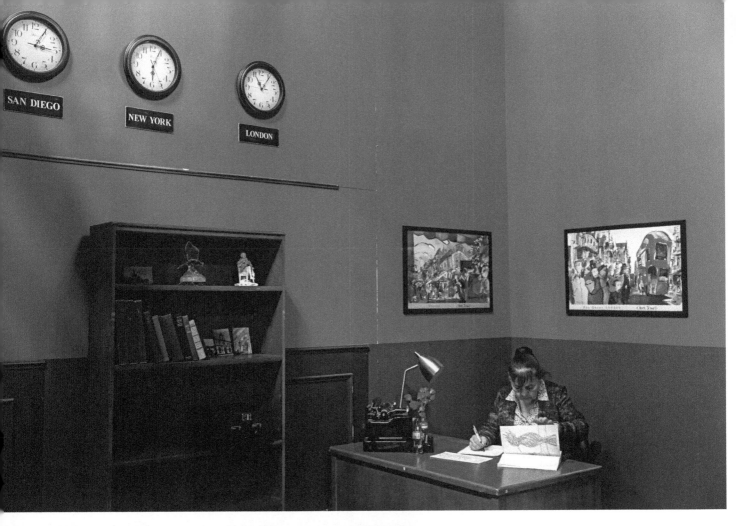

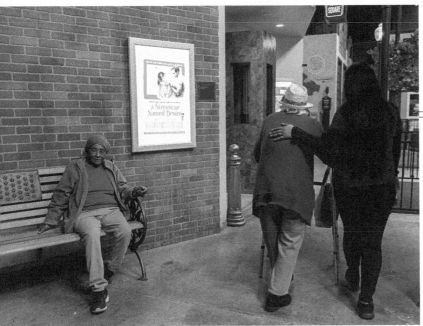

SUSIE HEAVILIN (TOP) "DOES THE NUMBERS"
TO CONNECT WITH HER FORMER IDENTITY AS AN
ACCOUNTANT. STAFF ENGAGE WITH HER AS IF SHE IS
THE REAL TOWN ACCOUNTANT.

CAREGIVERS ESCORT RESIDENTS ON DAILY ROUNDS OF
THE STOREFRONTS LINING THE SQUARE.

In March 2019, Margaret Nagy-Lagnese and her brother moved their 87-year-old mother, who has Alzheimer's, into Lantern of Chagrin Valley, one of a trio of long-term care facilities in Ohio designed to resemble the communities of residents' younger years. A few months in, they're satisfied with their decision.

Recalling familiar sights. When residents walk out their front doors to the porch, day is dawning with puffy, white clouds overhead. The grass is golf-course perfect. They enjoy a view complete with home sidings painted in familiar colors evoking sights of their youth. As the sun slowly sets, streetlights come on, easing residents into their nighttime routines.

But that sunlit sky? It's actually an LED-brightened and dimming ceiling. That luscious lawn? Textured green carpeting. Within the Main Street "storefronts," the focus isn't on retail but instead on structured activities for the long-term care

The approach may also counteract boredom. "One of the reasons why we have a lot of behavioral problems with dementia, quite frankly, is boredom," Oh adds. "There's nothing to do. They get very agitated. Occupying them with activities and things that really speak to their senses and their memory is a nonpharmacological method to alleviate some of the behavioral symptoms."

residents with dementia, who range from ages 64 to 99.

"It's amazing," Nagy-Lagnese says. "I laugh because my mom will say, 'It's really bright today – I need to go get my sunglasses to sit outside.'"

Certain amenities on indoor Main Street are especially effective at helping residents connect to their pasts – and to other people. For Nagy-Lagnese's mother, her small front porch allows her to invite fellow residents and visitors to stay and chat, awakening her lifelong bent for socializing. The nondenominational chapel enables the deeply religious Hungarian immigrant to maintain that piece of her identity.

Emerging evidence. Reminiscence therapy can take place anytime, anywhere, using objects from past eras to spark moments of crystal clarity. It's early to expect hard data on the effectiveness of immersive environments, but the core aspect of reminiscence therapy is backed by still-emerging evidence. "Reminiscence can be a good fit for people with dementia as it provides an opportunity to concentrate on those memories that are more intact, and focus on what that person can remember, rather than memory that is impaired," says Laura O'Philbin, a researcher with the Alzheimer Society of Ireland. She co-authored a 2018 Cochrane systematic review of studies on reminiscence therapy, which found that while its effects can vary, depending on how and where it's administered, "reminiscence can benefit people with dementia in the domains of quality of life, communication, mood and cognition," she says, even if the benefits are small.

Not all reminiscence therapy is created equal, and definitions and practices aren't universal, making it difficult to draw strong conclusions. "For example, some approaches involve individual therapy facilitated by a clinical psychologist, while others were a small group listening to music from the past once a week," O'Philbin says. "In my experience, people living with dementia typically really enjoy reminiscence and can feel a sense of pride when discussing their past. Different prompts stimulate animated discussion, and caregivers often learn something new about the person with dementia in the process."

However, not everyone may enjoy or be comfortable discussing the past. "For some, reminiscence may trigger memories that cause distress or upset. Although we found no evidence of this in our Cochrane review, it does occur," O'Philbin explains. Reminiscence facilitators must be prepared to manage negative responses sensitively, she says, and it can help to speak with a trusted relative or friend beforehand.

A simpler time. Immersive reminiscence environments rekindle the past in other ways, too. In Overland Park, Kansas, Mandy Shoemaker and her sister-in-law Michala Gibson, a nurse, always loved the idea of Hogewey, the Dutch dementia village. For local families, they envisioned a more familiar, farm-like environment. So Prairie Farmstead was born.

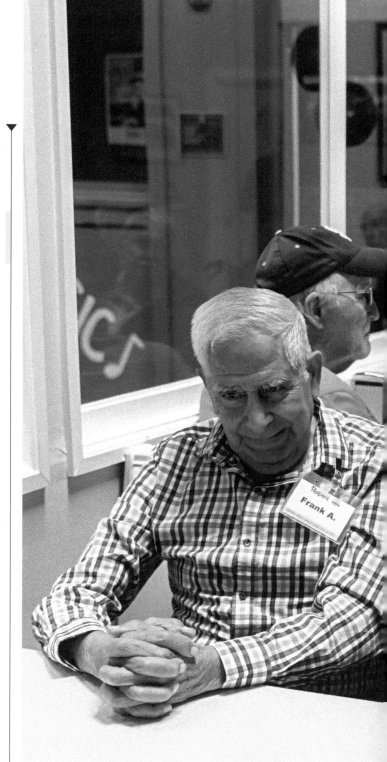

Two group homes sit on the farmstead. Eight residents with dementia live in each one and are overseen by professional caregivers.

"I would consider a lot of what we do reminiscence therapy," Shoemaker says, "because it evokes feelings from people's childhood." A barn with farm equipment, tractors, tools to sort, local farmers coming in to visit and greenery everywhere all feel familiar. Not to mention the animals.

Checking the chicken coop and finding newly laid eggs makes adults with dementia feel productive. The mini-pig, two full-grown goats and ducks waddling in a line make them smile. "We have a little baby goat right now, and he's literally five days old," Shoemaker says. "The kind of joy that residents experience because of

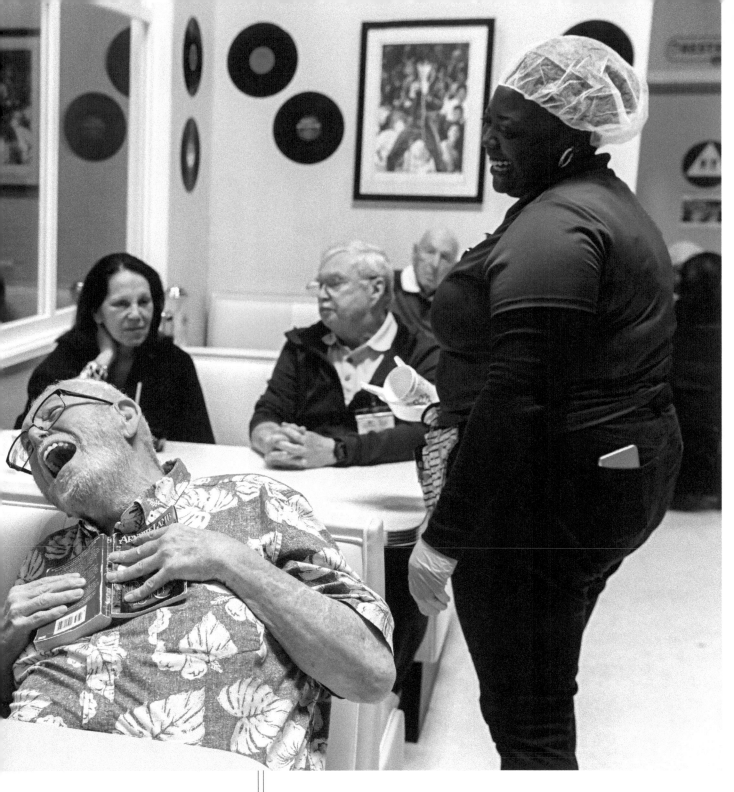

him is much more similar to the joy that you would feel as a child."

Martha Granstrom, born and raised in Kansas, was Prairie Farmstead's first resident. She lived at the Farmstead for about eight months, until her death in late 2018. She loved it, says Diane Conner, her daughter. Animals always mattered to Granstrom, notes Conner, describing a childhood filled with creatures nurtured by her mother. Decades later, it was Conner's turn to look out for her mom, who now had dementia. A bad experience with an institutional facility spurred Conner to find a better place. She recalls the ankle bracelet her mother had to wear, and a series of falls and other disturbing events. At that facility, the overriding emphasis was on keeping dementia patients quiet, calm and under control – and thus, easier to manage, she says. So Conner hired an outside caregiver to watch over her mom 24/7 when she couldn't be at the facility herself.

When she later found Prairie Farmstead, the difference was palpable. "They want you to be interacting," Connor says. "They want you to be outside. They want you to help cook. They want you to have daily chores. They want you to have a purposeful life." ●

It's Wise to Take

Making time for recovery is key to a successful exercise plan

by **Courtney Rubin**

RESEARCHERS HAVE spent years encouraging people to exercise regularly and vigorously. Now the big push is to get them to go at it gently – at least sometimes – and to take a break.

Why? It turns out that if you don't allow your muscles to recover between workouts, you could actually be decreasing your fitness – or worse. In people who exercise moderately to vigorously, experts say, not giving the muscles sufficient downtime can cause overtraining, physical and mental fatigue (hello, burnout), difficulty sleeping, decreased immunity, mood swings, and overuse injuries, such as stress fractures, muscle strains and joint pain. "We need to think of rest and recovery as an integral part of being fit and healthy, not just the time spent in the gym," says Michele Olson, a senior clinical professor of sport science at Alabama's Huntingdon College and a fellow of the American College of Sports Medicine.

Rebuilding required. Here's some physiology 101: Exercise is a catabolic event, meaning it causes breakdown in the body. The protein filaments within your muscle fibers, which help you produce force, are torn as your stores of fuels, including glucose, are depleted. Immediately after a workout, the body goes through an alarm stage – a matter of hours or an entire day, depending on how long and intense the exercise session – during which it is in a kind of shock, and immune function is suppressed.

Then comes the replenishment stage, when the body restores its fuels and mends muscle. Finally, during the compensation phase, rebuilding and progress happen, so you're able to run a bit faster or lift a bit more the next time.

But here's the hitch: If you keep working out without sufficient time to recover, you'll never make it to the compensation phase.

Gyms are racing to help you avoid this fate, building in a range of recovery activities from stretching and foam rolling (which for not-quite-understood reasons seems to

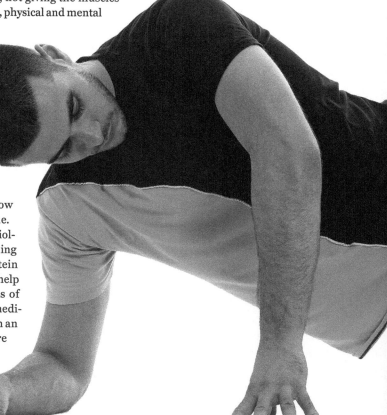

a Break

help loosen muscles and ease soreness) to very low-intensity exercise like an easy walk or cycle and educating members on the benefits of proper sleep. Equinox and other chains are now offering a whole category of recovery classes, with names like "Best Stretch Ever" and "MELT." Equinox also offers sleep coaching, while Crunch Fitness has introduced a Relax & Recover program that includes hydromassage in a water-powered bed that, for example, can work out kinks in your calves.

And Mile High Run Club, a New York-based chain of running gyms, features a "Recovery Room" stocked with compression sleeves, which zip up heel-to-hip and, when plugged in, use air to compress and knead legs. According to a 2016 review of studies published in the journal Sports Medicine, the garments help with recovery by increasing circulation and reducing muscle swelling. There are even entire gyms devoted to – wait for it – recovery, among them Stretch*d, LYMBR, Stretch U, and StretchLab, the last of which has some 50 locations in 17 states.

"Flexibility is really key to injury prevention," argues Amanda Freeman, CEO and co-founder of Stretch*d. But "when you're in a gym class, half the class is running out during the stretch portion, because they'd rather use the time to work out or to do something else."

Says David Reavy, a Chicago physical therapist: "Decreased range of motion means you'll be more apt to compensate with other muscles, which leads to increased chance of injury."

The trend toward going gentle, at least some of the time, is in part a reaction to the high-intensity exercise trend, which has people working out harder for spurts of time than they typically had before, Olson says. It's also a trickle down from professional sports, where smart recovery has become the last frontier – after better coaching, training, nutrition and gear – for athletes to legally enhance their performance.

"When you said 'recovery' 10 years ago, people would think it was from drugs or alcohol," says Gilad Jacobs, CEO of NormaTec, whose compression attachments are used by most of the country's pro sports teams. (LeBron James was one of the earliest adopters.) "Five years ago, it was post-operation." Now, he says, recovery means: "What can I do between my workouts actually to have gains?" The company's biggest area of growth: hobbyist athletes wanting to "become the best version of themselves," Jacobs explains.

"Active" recovery. There are a lot of expensive ways to recover – in part because people treat it as a luxury, like a manicure – but you don't need to spend any money at all to benefit. All you need to do is slow down. That doesn't mean you have to sit on the sofa for a day, though you can certainly do so if your muscles feel jellylike or are still sore. It does mean you should alternate hard workouts with easier ones, and sometimes very easy ones. Scientists call these easy workouts "active recovery," and they work by facilitating continued blood flow to the muscles, says Lance Dalleck, an associate professor of exercise and sport science at Western Colorado University. This promotes greater oxygen delivery and removal of metabolic byproducts that slow down recovery.

In the lab, scientists use precise exer-

FOAM ROLLING CAN HELP LOOSEN MUSCLES AND EASE SORENESS.

cise intensities to define active recovery – typically a percentage of "ventilatory threshold," the point at which breathing becomes hard and you feel like you can't take in as much air as you need. But at home or in the gym, Dalleck suggests using Rate of Perceived Exertion, or RPE, to guide your recovery. If 1 is just barely noticeable effort and 10 is gasping for breath, you want to be a 2, he says. This standard obviously will mean different things to different people, depending on how much and how hard they normally exercise.

It's tricky to be prescriptive about the specific amount of recovery you need – that's largely dependent on how hard you work out and what type of training you're doing, as well as how you feel. If you strength train, the American College of Sports Medicine recommends leaving 48 hours for recovery between workouts. If you do sweaty, breathless, high-intensity interval training, you'll need at least a day off before doing it again.

A proper stretch. The American College of Sports Medicine recommends static stretching – moving a limb to its full range of motion but not to the point of pain – at least two to three days per week. Each stretch should be held for about 30 seconds. Stretching should not be done cold – it should be done either after a few minutes of active warmup (meaning your breathing has quickened) or at the end of a workout. This is a change from old recommendations; it's been found that stretching before a warmup actually can reduce muscle strength and, in the case of running, speed. Sleep is, of course, essential to recovery; it's when muscles rebuild. Sleep is also when growth hormone is naturally released, which improves recovery.

You can also nudge your muscles to bounce back faster (and work more efficiently) by using recovery props, the most popular of which is the foam roller, which can be found in most gyms or bought online for as little as $5. Many physical therapists and gyms say that rollers iron out the fascia, the connective tissue that stretches over and through the muscles. But scientists don't think the foam roller is actually

> # One key target: the hip flexors, which get tight when you sit all day.

breaking down muscle adhesions – better known to you as sore points – and making the muscle more elastic. They think it's more likely that the rolling acts as a neural inhibition, making something happen at the spinal cord and brain level.

Mysterious mechanism. "We know foam rolling works, but it's probably on much more of a global system than a local one," says David Behm, a professor of human kinetics at Memorial University of Newfoundland in Canada, who has researched the subject. In a study, researchers rolled the opposite calf than the one with tender spots – and the pain went away. "We didn't even touch the calf with the pain," he says.

In previous studies, Behm and his fellow researchers found that after just two minutes of foam rolling the quadriceps, range of motion increased by 10 degrees (compared to less than 1 degree associated with doing nothing). In a separate study, they found that foam rolling performed twice on each muscle group for 60 seconds reduced muscle soreness for up to three days after exercise, increased the range of motion, and led to better performance in a vertical leap test.

Loosening up. You can foam-roll for five or 10 minutes before a workout – pro athletes foam roll every day – or you can do it on your off days as gentle recovery, Reavy says. He suggests focusing on the areas that are sore. If you're short on time, the one key area to target is your hip flexors, muscles that get tight when we sit all day. When they tighten up, they shut down your abdominals, your glutes, and your inner thighs, making you a prime candidate for back pain and also minimizing the effectiveness of your workout, because other muscles will have to compensate.

"One reason why people don't get results from their workouts is because the right muscles can't fire because they're too tight," Reavy says. "If you foam roll, you're going to feel better, and you're going to look better, because your workout will be more productive." ●

#1 Hospital
in Florida

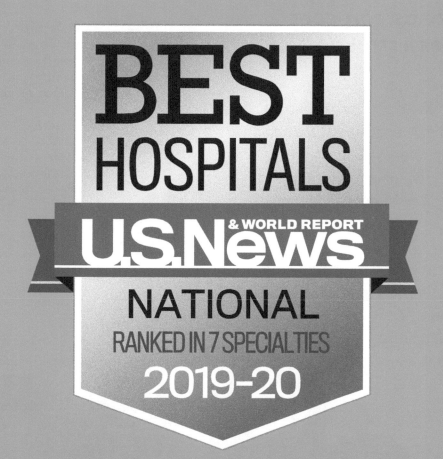

AdventHealth Orlando is honored to be the #1 hospital in the state of Florida with seven nationally ranked specialties and world-class physicians and caregivers comprising the most comprehensive care network in our region.

FeelHealthyFeelWhole.com

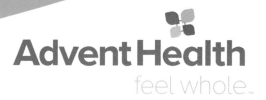

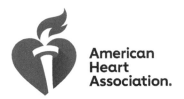

American
Heart
Association.

Commitment to Quality

Every 40 seconds, someone in America has a stroke or heart attack.

Make the time you have count by exploring your options for quality heart and stroke care for you and your loved ones. Every year, the American Heart Association® recognizes hospitals that demonstrate commitment to following treatment guidelines, and by doing so, it ensures that all Americans have access to the most current evidence-based care that saves lives and improves patient outcomes. Read more about the award categories and find a participating hospital near you.

 Heart disease and stroke are the No. 1 and No. 5 causes of death in the United States, respectively.

 Get With The Guidelines (GWTG) data registries represent 36% of all cardiovascular and stroke hospitalizations.

 More than 2,500 hospitals participate in the GWTG initiative, which ensures quality care for heart and stroke patients.

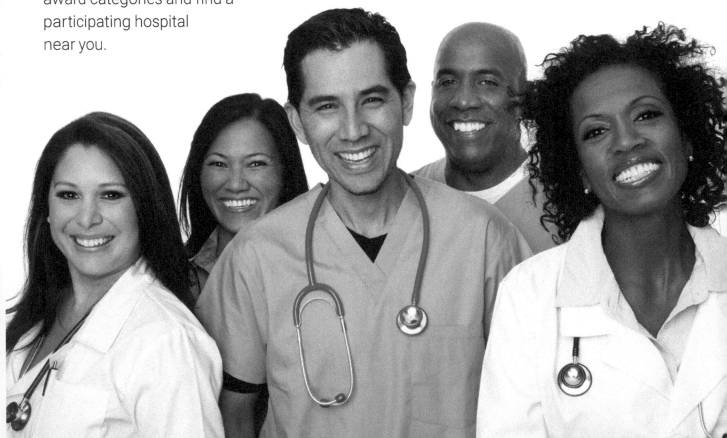

Key to the Awards

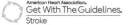 **American Heart Association. Get With The Guidelines.** Stroke

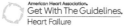 **American Heart Association. Get With The Guidelines.** Heart Failure

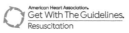 **American Heart Association. Get With The Guidelines.** Resuscitation

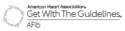 **American Heart Association. Get With The Guidelines.** AFib

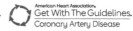 **American Heart Association. Get With The Guidelines.** Coronary Artery Disease

Gold Achievement
These hospitals are recognized for two or more consecutive calendar years of 85% or higher adherence on all achievement measures applicable to each program.

Silver Achievement
These hospitals are recognized for one calendar year of 85% or higher adherence on all achievement measures applicable to each program.

Gold Plus Achievement
These hospitals are recognized for two or more consecutive calendar years of 85% or higher adherence on all achievement measures applicable and 75% or higher adherence with additional select quality measures in heart failure, stroke and/or resuscitation.

Silver Plus Achievement
These hospitals are recognized for one calendar year of 85% or higher adherence on all achievement measures applicable and 75% or higher adherence with additional select quality measures in heart failure, stroke and/or resuscitation.

*These hospitals received Get With The Guidelines-Resuscitation awards from the American Heart Association for two or more patient populations.

 American Heart Association. Mission:Lifeline

 American Heart Association. Target: HF

American Heart Association. Target: Stroke

STEMI: Gold Receiving or Referring
These hospitals are recognized for two consecutive calendar years of 85% or higher composite adherence to all STEMI Receiving or Referring Center Performance Achievement indicators and 75% or higher compliance on each performance measure.

STEMI: Silver Receiving or Referring
These hospitals are recognized for one calendar year interval of 85% or higher composite adherence to all STEMI Receiving or Referring Center Performance Achievement indicators and 75% or higher compliance on each performance measure.

Target: Heart Failure and Target: Stroke Honor Roll
These hospitals are recognized for at least three consecutive months of 50% or higher adherence to all relevant measures in addition to current Bronze, Silver or Gold Get With The Guidelines - Heart Failure or Stroke recognition status.

STEMI: Gold Plus Receiving or Silver Plus Receiving
These hospitals are recognized for 75% or higher achievement of First Door-to-Device time of 120 minutes or less for transferred STEMI patient for two or more consecutive years (gold plus) or one consecutive calendar year (silver plus).

NSTEMI: Gold or Silver
These hospitals are recognized for achieving 65% adherence to Dual Antiplatelet prescription at discharge and 75% or higher compliance on each of the other four performance measures for two consecutive calendar years (gold) or one consecutive calendar year (silver).

Honor Roll - Elite Plus
These hospitals are recognized for at least a year of 75% or higher achievement of door-to-needle times within 60 minutes AND 50% achievement of door-to-needle times within 45 minutes in applicable stroke patients in addition to current Silver or Gold Get With The Guidelines - Stroke recognition status.

Honor Roll - Elite
These hospitals are recognized for at least a year of 75% or higher achievement of door-to-needle times within 60 minutes in applicable stroke patients in addition to current Silver or Gold Get With The Guidelines - Stroke recognition status.

American Heart Association.

Find Your Hospital Listed Alphabetically By State

For a searchable map of hospitals by region and across the U.S., visit heart.org/myhealthcare.

ALABAMA

Brookwood Baptist Medical Center, **Birmingham** .... (G+) (E)
Coosa Valley Medical Center, **Sylacauga** .... (G+) (HR)
Crestwood Medical Center, **Huntsville** .... (G) (G) (G)
Cullman Regional Medical Center, **Cullman** .... (G+)
Flowers Hospital, **Dothan** .... (G+)
Gadsden Regional Medical Center, **Gadsden** .... (G+) (HR)
Grandview Medical Center, **Birmingham** .... (G+) (HR) (G+) (E)
Huntsville Hospital, **Huntsville** .... (S) * (G+) (HR)
Marshall Medical Centers, **Guntersville** .... (G)
Medical Center Enterprise, **Enterprise** .... (S) (HR)
Mobile Infirmary, **Mobile** .... (G) (G) (G) (E)
North Alabama Medical Center, **Florence** .... (G+)
Princeton Baptist Medical Center, **Birmingham** .... (G+) (E)
South Baldwin Regional Medical Center, **Foley** .... (G+) (S+)
Southeast Alabama Medical Center, **Dothan** .... (G)
UAB Hospital, **Birmingham** .... (S+) (HR) (S) (G+) (E+)
USA Health University Hospital, **Mobile** .... (G+) (HR) (G+) (E+)
Walker Baptist Medical Center, **Jasper** .... (G)

ALASKA

Alaska Regional Hospital, **Anchorage** .... (G+) (HR)
Providence Alaska Medical Center, **Anchorage** .... (G+) (E+)

ARIZONA

Abrazo Arrowhead Campus, **Glendale** .... (G+) (E+)
Abrazo Central Campus, **Phoenix** .... (G+) (E+)
Abrazo Scottsdale Campus, **Phoenix** .... (S+) (HR)
Abrazo West Campus, **Goodyear** .... (G+) (E)
Banner Baywood Medical Center, **Mesa** .... (G+) (E+)
Banner Boswell Medical Center, **Sun City** .... (G+) (E+)
Banner Del E Webb Medical Center, **Sun City West** .... (G+) (E+)
Banner Desert Medical Center, **Mesa** .... (G+) (E+)
Banner Estrella Medical Center, **Phoenix** .... (G+) (E)
Banner Thunderbird Medical Center, **Glendale** .... (G+) (E+)
Banner University Medical Center Phoenix, **Phoenix** .... (G+) (E+)
Banner University Medical Center Tucson, **Tucson** .... (G+) (E)
Carondelet St. Mary's Hospital, **Tucson** .... (G+) (E+)
Dignity Health Chandler Regional Medical Center, **Chandler** .... (G+) (E+)
Dignity Health Mercy Gilbert Medical Center, **Gilbert** .... (G+) (E+)
Dignity Health St. Joseph's Hospital and Medical Center, **Phoenix** .... (G+) (HR) (G+) (E+)
HonorHealth Deer Valley Medical Center, **Phoenix** .... (G+) (E+)
HonorHealth John C. Lincoln Medical Center, **Phoenix** .... (G+) (E+)
HonorHealth Scottsdale Osborn Medical Center, **Scottsdale** .... (G+) (E+)
HonorHealth Scottsdale Shea Medical Center, **Scottsdale** .... (S+) (E+)
HonorHealth Scottsdale Thompson Peak Medical Center, **Scottsdale** .... (S+)
Mayo Clinic Hospital Arizona, **Phoenix** .... (G) (G+) (E+)
Mountain Vista Medical Center, **Mesa** .... (G+) (E)
Phoenix VA Healthcare System, **Phoenix** .... (G+)
The Carondelet Neurological Institute at St. Joseph's Hospital, **Tucson** .... (G+) (E+)
Tucson Medical Center, **Tucson** .... (S+) (G+) (E+)
Yuma Regional Medical Center, **Yuma** .... (G+) (E+)

ARKANSAS

Arkansas Heart Hospital, **Little Rock** .... (G)
Baptist Health - Fort Smith, **Fort Smith** .... (G+) (HR)
Baptist Health Medical Center, **Little Rock** .... (G+) (E+)
Baptist Health Medical Center - Arkadelphia, **Arkadelphia** .... (S) (HR)
Baptist Health Medical Center - Conway, **Conway** .... (G+) (HR)
CHI St. Vincent, **Little Rock** .... (G)
CHI St. Vincent Hot Springs, **Hot Springs** .... (G+) (HR)
Conway Regional Medical Center, **Conway** .... (S) (HR)
Forrest City Medical Center, **Forrest City** .... (G)
Johnson Regional Medical Center, **Clarksville** .... (S+)

Medical Center of South Arkansas, **El Dorado** .... (S) (HR)
Mercy Hospital Fort Smith, **Fort Smith** .... (S+)
Mercy Hospital Rogers, **Rogers** .... (G+)
Ouachita County Medical Center, **Camden** .... (S) (HR)
Saint Mary's Regional Medical Center, **Russellville** .... (S+) (E)
St. Bernards Five Rivers Medical Center, **Pocahontas** .... (G+) (HR) (G)
St. Bernards Medical Center, **Jonesboro** .... (G+) (S)
UAMS Medical Center, **Little Rock** .... (G+) (E+)
Washington Regional Medical Center, **Fayetteville** .... (G+) (E+)
White River Health System, **Batesville** .... (S)

CALIFORNIA

Adventist Health + Rideout, **Marysville** .... (G+) (E+)
Adventist Health Bakersfield, **Bakersfield** .... (G+) (E) (G)
Adventist Health Glendale, **Glendale** .... (G+) (E+)
Adventist Health Lodi Memorial, **Lodi** .... (S+) (E)
Adventist Health Simi Valley, **Simi Valley** .... (G+)
Adventist Health Ukiah Valley, **Ukiah** .... (G+) (HR)
Adventist Health White Memorial, **Los Angeles** .... (G+) (E+)
Alameda Hospital, **Alameda** .... (G+) (E+)
Alta Bates Summit Medical Center - Alta Bates Campus, **Berkeley** .... (S)
Alta Bates Summit Medical Center - Summit Campus, **Oakland** .... (S) (G+) (E+)
Alvarado Hospital Medical Center, **San Diego** .... (S+) (E)
Arrowhead Regional Medical Center, **Colton** .... (G+) (E+)
California Hospital Medical Center, **Los Angeles** .... (G+) (E+)
California Pacific Medical Center - Davies Campus, **San Francisco** .... (S)
California Pacific Medical Center - Mission Bernal Campus, **San Francisco** .... (S)
California Pacific Medical Center - Pacific Campus, **San Francisco** .... (S) (G+) (E)
Cedars-Sinai Marina del Rey Medical Center, **Marina del Rey** .... (S+)
Cedars-Sinai Medical Center, **Los Angeles** .... (G+) (E+)
Centinela Hospital Medical Center, **Inglewood** .... (G+) (HR) (S+) (E+)
CHA Hollywood Presbyterian Medical Center, **Los Angeles** .... (G+) (HR)
CHOC Children's Hospital, **Orange** .... (S+) *
Community Hospital of the Monterey Peninsula, **Monterey** .... (G+) (E+)
Community Memorial Hospital, **Ventura** .... (G+) (E+)
Community Regional Medical Center, **Fresno** .... (G+) (HR)
Corona Regional Medical Center, **Corona** .... (G+)
Desert Regional Medical Center, **Palm Springs** .... (G) (G+) (E+)
Desert Valley Hospital, **Victorville** .... (HR)
Dignity Health Arroyo Grande Community Hospital, **Arroyo Grande** .... (S+)
Dignity Health dba St. Mary Medical Center, **Long Beach** .... (G)
Dignity Health Dominican Hospital, **Santa Cruz** .... (HR) (G+) (E+)
Dignity Health French Hospital Medical Center, **San Luis Obispo** .... (S+)
Dignity Health Marian Regional Medical Center, **Santa Maria** .... (S+) (HR)
Dignity Health Memorial Hospital Bakersfield, **Bakersfield** .... (G+) (HR) (G+)
Dignity Health Mercy General Hospital, **Sacramento** .... (G+) (HR)
Dignity Health Mercy Hospital of Folsom, **Folsom** .... (G+) (E+)
Dignity Health Mercy Hospitals of Bakersfield, **Bakersfield** .... (G+) (HR)
Dignity Health Mercy Medical Center Merced, **Merced** .... (G+) (E)
Dignity Health Mercy Medical Center Redding, **Redding** .... (G+) (E)
Dignity Health Mercy San Juan Medical Center, **Carmichael** .... (G+) (E+)
Dignity Health Methodist Hospital of Sacramento, **Sacramento** .... (G+) (E+)
Dignity Health Northridge Hospital Medical Center, **Northridge** .... (G+) (E+)
Dignity Health Saint Francis Memorial Hospital, **San Francisco** .... (G+)
Dignity Health Sequoia Hospital, **Redwood City** .... (G+) (HR)
Dignity Health Sierra Nevada Memorial Hospital, **Grass Valley** .... (G+) (E)
Dignity Health St. Bernardine Medical Center, **San Bernardino** .... (G+) (HR)
Dignity Health St. John's Pleasant Valley Hospital, **Camarillo** .... (G+) (E)
Dignity Health St. John's Regional Medical Center, **Oxnard** .... (G+) (E+)
Dignity Health St. Joseph's Medical Center, **Stockton** .... (G+) (HR) (G)
Dignity Health St. Mary's Medical Center, **San Francisco** .... (G+) (E+)
Dignity Health Woodland Memorial Hospital, **Woodland** .... (G+) (E+)
Doctors Medical Center, **Modesto** .... (S) (G+) (G+) (E+) (G) (G)
Eden Medical Center, **Castro Valley** .... (G+) (E+)
El Camino Hospital, **Mountain View** .... (G+) (E+)

*These hospitals received Get With The Guidelines-Resuscitation awards from the American Heart Association for two or more patient populations.

Emanate Health: Foothill Presbyterian Hospital, **Glendora** .... (S+) (E)
Emanate Health: Inter-Community Hospital, **Covina** .... (HR)
Emanate Health: Queen of the Valley Hospital, **West Covina** ... (S) (HR) (G+) (S+)
Encino Hospital Medical Center, **Encino** .... (G+) (E+)
Enloe Medical Center, **Chico** .... (G+) (E+)
Fountain Valley Regional Hospital and Medical Center, **Fountain Valley** .... (G+) (G+) (E+)
Garfield Medical Center, **Monterey Park** .... (G+) (E+)
Good Samaritan Hospital, **Los Angeles** .... (G+) (E+)
Good Samaritan Hospital, **San Jose** .... (G+) (E+)
Hazel Hawkins Memorial Hospital, **Hollister** .... (E)
Henry Mayo Newhall Hospital, **Valencia** .... (E)
Hoag Hospital Irvine, **Irvine** .... (G+)
Hoag Memorial Hospital Presbyterian, **Newport Beach** .... (G+) (HR) (G+) (E+)
Huntington Hospital, **Pasadena** .... (G+) (E+)
JFK Memorial Hospital, **Indio** .... (G+)
John Muir Medical Center - Concord, **Concord** .... (G+) (G+) (E+)
John Muir Medical Center - Walnut Creek, **Walnut Creek** .... (G+) (E+)
Kaiser Foundation Hospital - Antioch, **Antioch** .... (S+) (G+) (E+)
Kaiser Foundation Hospital - Fremont , **Fremont** .... (G+) (E+)
Kaiser Foundation Hospital - Fresno, **Fresno** .... (S+) (G+) (E+)
Kaiser Foundation Hospital - Modesto, **Modesto** .... (G+) (E+)
Kaiser Foundation Hospital - Oakland, **Oakland** .... (G+) (E+)
Kaiser Foundation Hospital - Redwood City, **Redwood City** .... (G+) (E+)
Kaiser Foundation Hospital - Richmond, **Richmond** .... (G+) (E+)
Kaiser Foundation Hospital - Roseville, **Roseville** .... (G+) (G+) (E+)
Kaiser Foundation Hospital - Sacramento, **Sacramento** .... (S+) (G+) (E+)
Kaiser Foundation Hospital - San Diego Medical Center, **San Diego** .... (S+) (HR)
Kaiser Foundation Hospital - San Diego - Zion Medical Center, **San Diego** ..... (G+) (E+)
Kaiser Foundation Hospital - San Francisco, **San Francisco** .... (G+) (E+)
Kaiser Foundation Hospital - San Jose, **San Jose** .... (G+) (E+)
Kaiser Foundation Hospital - San Leandro, **San Leandro** .... (G+) (E+)
Kaiser Foundation Hospital - San Rafael, **San Rafael** .... (G+) (E+)
Kaiser Foundation Hospital - Santa Clara, **Santa Clara** .... (G+) (E+)
Kaiser Foundation Hospital - Santa Rosa, **Santa Rosa** .... (G+) (E+)
Kaiser Foundation Hospital - South Sacramento, **Sacramento** .... (G+) (E+)
Kaiser Foundation Hospital - South San Francisco, **South San Francisco** .. (G+) (G+) (E+)
Kaiser Foundation Hospital - Vacaville, **Vacaville** .... (S+) (G+) (E+)
Kaiser Foundation Hospital - Vallejo, **Vallejo** .... (G+) (G+) (E+)
Kaiser Foundation Hospital - Walnut Creek, **Walnut Creek** .... (G+) (E+)
Kaiser Foundation Hospital - West Los Angeles, **Los Angeles** .... (G+) (E+)
Kaiser Foundation Hospital Orange County, **Anaheim and Irvine** .... (G+) (E+)
Kaiser Foundation Hospital Woodland Hills, **Woodland Hills** .... (G+) (E+)
Kaiser Permanente - Downey Medical Center, **Downey** .... (G+) (E+)
Kaiser Permanente Baldwin Park Medical Center, **Baldwin Park** .... (G+) (E+)
Kaiser Permanente Fontana Medical Center, **Fontana** .... (G+) (E+)
Kaiser Permanente Los Angeles Medical Center, **Los Angeles** .... (G+) (E+)
Kaiser Permanente Moreno Valley Medical Center, **Moreno Valley** .... (G+) (E+)
Kaiser Permanente Ontario Medical Center, **Ontario** .... (G+) (E+)
Kaiser Permanente Panorama City Medical Center, **Panorama City** .... (G+) (E)
Kaiser Permanente Riverside Medical Center, **Riverside** .... (S+) (G+) (E+)
Kaiser Permanente South Bay Medical Center, **Harbor City** .... (G+) (E+)
Kaweah Delta Health Care District, **Visalia** .... (G+) (E)
Keck Hospital of USC, **Los Angeles** .... (G+)
Kern Medical, **Bakersfield** .... (G+)
La Palma Intercommunity Hospital, **La Palma** .... (S+) (HR)
Lakewood Regional Medical Center, **Lakewood** .... (S+) (HR)
Loma Linda University Children's Hospital, **Loma Linda** .... (G+) *
Loma Linda University Medical Center, **Loma Linda** .... (G+) (S+) (E+)
Loma Linda University Medical Center - Murrieta, **Murrieta** .... (G+) (E)
Long Beach Medical Center, **Long Beach** .... (G+) (HR) (G+) (E+)
Los Alamitos Medical Center, **Los Alamitos** .... (G+) (HR) (G+) (E+)
Los Robles Regional Medical Center, **Thousand Oaks** .... (G+) (E+)
Lucile Packard Children's Hospital Stanford, **Palo Alto** .... (G+) *
Marin General Hospital, **Greenbrae** .... (G+) (E+)
Memorial Care Saddleback Medical Center, **Laguna Hills** .... (G+) (E)
Memorial Hospital Los Banos, **Los Banos** .... (G+)
Memorial Medical Center, **Modesto** .... (S) (G+) (E+)
Methodist Hospital of Southern California, **Arcadia** .... (G+) (E+)
Mills-Peninsula Medical Center, **Burlingame** .... (S) (G+) (HR)
Mission Hospital Regional Medical Center, **Mission Viejo** .... (G+) (E+)
Montclair Hospital Medical Center, **Montclair** .... (S+) (HR)

NorthBay Healthcare Group, **Fairfield** .... (G+) (E)
Novato Community Hospital, **Novato** .... (S) (HR)
O'Connor Hospital, **San Jose** .... (G+) (HR)
Orange County Global Medical Center, **Santa Ana** .... (E+)
Oroville Hospital, **Oroville** .... (G+)
Palmdale Regional Medical Center, **Palmdale** .... (G+)
Paradise Valley Hospital, **National City** .... (S+) (S+) (E)
PIH Health Hospital - Whittier, **Whittier** .... (G+) (E+)
Placentia-Linda Hospital, **Placentia** .... (G+)
Pomona Valley Hospital Medical Center, **Pomona** .... (G+) (G+) (E+)
Providence Holy Cross Medical Center, **Mission Hills** .... (G+) (E)
Providence Little Company of Mary Medical Center San Pedro, **San Pedro** .... (G+)
Providence Little Company of Mary Medical Center Torrance, **Torrance** ...... (G+) (E+)
Providence Saint John's Health Center, **Santa Monica** .... (G+)
Providence St. Joseph Medical Center, **Burbank** .... (G+) (E+)
Providence Tarzana Medical Center, **Tarzana** .... (G+) (HR)
Redlands Community Hospital, **Redlands** .... (G+) (E)
Regional Medical Center of San Jose, **San Jose** .... (G+) (E+)
Riverside Community Hospital, **Riverside** .... (G+) (HR)
Riverside University Health System - Medical Center, **Moreno Valley** ... (S) (S+) (G+) (E+)
Ronald Reagan UCLA Medical Center, **Los Angeles** .... (G+) (HR) (G+) (E+)
Salinas Valley Memorial Healthcare System, **Salinas** .... (G+) (HR) (G+) (E) (S+)
San Antonio Regional Hospital, **Upland** .... (G+) (HR)
San Dimas Community Hospital, **San Dimas** .... (S) (HR)
San Joaquin General Hospital, **French Camp** .... (G+) (E+)
San Ramon Regional Medical Center, **San Ramon** .... (G+) (E+)
Santa Barbara Cottage Hospital, **Santa Barbara** .... (G+) (E+)
Santa Monica UCLA Medical Center and Orthopaedic Hospital, **Santa Monica** . (G+)
Scripps Green Hospital, **La Jolla** .... (G+)
Scripps Memorial Hospital Encinitas, **Encinitas** .... (G+) (E)
Scripps Memorial Hospital La Jolla, **La Jolla** .... (G+) (E+)
Scripps Mercy Hospital, **San Diego and Chula Vista** .... (G+) (HR)
Seton Medical Center, **Daly City** .... (G+) (HR)
Sharp Chula Vista Medical Center, **Chula Vista** .... (G+) (E+)
Sharp Grossmont Hospital, **La Mesa** .... (G+) (E+)
Sharp Memorial Hospital, **San Diego** .... (G+) (E+)
Shasta Regional Medical Center, **Redding** .... (S+) (HR)
Sherman Oaks Hospital, **Sherman Oaks** .... (S+) (HR) (G+) (HR)
SJH - Queen of the Valley Medical Center, **Napa** .... (G+) (HR)
Southwest Healthcare Systems: Inland Valley Medical Center & Rancho
    Springs Medical Center, **Wildomar and Murrieta** .... (G+) (E+)
St. Francis Medical Center, **Lynwood** .... (G+) (E)
St. Jude Medical Center, **Fullerton** .... (G+) (E+)
St. Louise Regional Hospital, **Gilroy** .... (G+) (E+)
Stanford Health Care, **Stanford** .... (S) (G+) (HR) (S+) (E+)
Sutter Amador Hospital, **Jackson** .... (S)
Sutter Auburn Faith Hospital, **Auburn** .... (S)
Sutter Coast Hospital, **Crescent City** .... (S)
Sutter Davis Hospital, **Davis** .... (S)
Sutter Delta Medical Center, **Antioch** .... (S)
Sutter Lakeside Hospital, **Lakeport** .... (S)
Sutter Medical Center Sacramento, **Sacramento** .... (S) (G+) (E)
Sutter Roseville Medical Center, **Roseville** .... (S)
Sutter Santa Rosa Regional Hospital, **Santa Rosa** .... (S) (G+) (E+)
Sutter Solano Medical Center, **Vallejo** .... (S)
Sutter Tracy Community Hospital, **Tracy** .... (S) (E+)
Temecula Valley Hospital, **Temecula** .... (G+) (E+)
Torrance Memorial Medical Center, **Torrance** .... (G+) (HR) (G) (G+) (HR) (G+) (S)
Tri-City Medical Center, **Oceanside** .... (G+) (S) (G+) (E+) (G) (G)
Twin Cities Community Hospital, **Templeton** .... (G+) (HR)
UC San Diego Health - Jacobs Medical Center, **La Jolla** .... (G+) (E+)
UC San Diego Health - UC San Diego Medical Center, **San Diego** .... (G+) (E+)
University of California Irvine Medical Center, **Orange** .... (G+) (HR) (G+) (E+)
University of California San Francisco (UCSF), **San Francisco** .... (G+) (E+)
University of California, Davis Medical Center, **Sacramento** .... (G+) (E)
USC Verdugo Hills Hospital, **Glendale** .... (G+) (HR)
VA Loma Linda Hospital, **Loma Linda** .... (S+)
Ventura County Medical Center/Santa Paula Hospital, **Ventura** .... (G+)
Washington Hospital Healthcare System, **Fremont** .... (G+) (HR)
Watsonville Community Hospital, **Watsonville** .... (G)

American Heart Association.

COLORADO

Boulder Community Health Foothills Hospital, **Boulder** .... G+ E+
Centura Health - Avista Adventist Hospital, **Louisville** .... G+
Centura Health - Castle Rock Adventist Hospital, **Castle Rock** .... G+ E+
Centura Health - Littleton Adventist Hospital, **Littleton** .... G+ E+
Centura Health - Longmont United Hospital, **Longmont** .... S+ E+
Centura Health - Parker Adventist Hospital, **Parker** .... G+
Centura Health - Penrose Hospital, **Colorado Springs** .... G G+ E+
Centura Health - Porter Adventist Hospital, **Denver** .... G+ E+
Centura Health - St. Anthony Hospital, **Lakewood** .... G+ HR E+ G+
Centura Health - St. Anthony North Hospital, **Westminster** .... G+ HR G+ HR
Denver Health Medical Center, **Denver** .... G
North Colorado Medical Center, **Greeley** .... S+ E
North Suburban Medical Center, **Thornton** .... G+ E+
Parkview Medical Center, **Pueblo** .... S+ HR G+ E+
Rose Medical Center, **Denver** .... G+ E+
SCL Health - Good Samaritan Medical Center, **Lafayette** .... G+ E
SCL Health - Lutheran Medical Center, **Wheat Ridge** .... G+ E+
SCL Health - Platte Valley Medical Center, **Brighton** .... G+ HR
SCL Health - Saint Joseph Hospital, **Denver** .... G+
SCL Health - St. Mary's Medical Center, **Grand Junction** .... G+ E+
Sky Ridge Medical Center, **Lone Tree** .... G+ E+
Swedish Medical Center, **Englewood** .... G+ HR
The Medical Center of Aurora, **Aurora** .... G+ E+
UCHealth – Medical Center of the Rockies, **Loveland** .... G HR E S+ S
UCHealth – Memorial Hospital , **Colorado Springs** .... G+ S+ G+ E+
UCHealth – Poudre Valley Hospital, **Fort Collins** .... G+ HR G+ E+
University of Colorado Hospital Authority, **Aurora** .... G G+ HR G+ E+

CONNECTICUT

Bridgeport Hospital, **Bridgeport** .... G HR
Connecticut Children's Medical Center, **Hartford** .... S
Danbury Hospital, Part of Western Connecticut Health Network,
   Danbury .... G+ HR G+
Eastern Connecticut Health Network, Manchester and Rockville, **Manchester** . G+
Greenwich Hospital, **Greenwich** .... G+ E+
Griffin Hospital, **Derby** .... S+
Hartford Hospital, **Hartford** .... G+ E+ G
Lawrence + Memorial Hospital, **New London** .... G+ E+
MidState Medical Center, **Meriden** .... G+ HR
Norwalk Hospital, **Norwalk** .... G+ HR S
Saint Francis Hospital and Medical Center, **Hartford** .... G+ HR G+
St. Vincent's Medical Center, **Bridgeport** .... G+ HR G+ HR
Stamford Hospital, **Stamford** .... G+ E G S
The Hospital of Central Connecticut, **New Britain** .... G+ E+ G+
The William W. Backus Hospital, **Norwich** .... S+ HR
UCONN Health / John Dempsey Hospital, **Farmington** .... G+ E+ E+
Waterbury Hospital, **Waterbury** .... G+ E+ G
Yale - New Haven Hospital, **New Haven** .... G+ E

DELAWARE

Bayhealth Medical Center - Kent General Hospital, **Dover** .... G+ G+ HR G
Bayhealth Medical Center Milford Memorial, **Milford** .... S G+ HR S
Beebe Healthcare, **Lewes** .... G+ S+ G+ HR S
Christiana Care Health Services, Inc., **Newark** .... G+ G+ E+ G S
Nanticoke Memorial Hospital, **Seaford** .... G+ G+ HR S
Saint Francis Hospital, **Wilmington** .... G+ HR

DISTRICT OF COLUMBIA

Howard University Hospital .... G+
MedStar Georgetown University Hospital .... G+ E+
MedStar Washington Hospital Center .... G+ E
Sibley Memorial Hospital .... G+ E+
The George Washington University Hospital .... G+ E+

FLORIDA

AdventHealth Altamonte Springs, **Altamonte Springs** .... G+ E+
AdventHealth Apopka, **Apopka** .... G+ HR

AdventHealth Celebration, **Celebration** .... G+ E+
AdventHealth Daytona Beach, **Daytona Beach** .... G+ E+
AdventHealth DeLand, **DeLand** .... G+ E+
AdventHealth East Orlando, **Orlando** .... G+ HR
AdventHealth Fish Memorial, **Orange City** .... G+ E+
AdventHealth Kissimmee, **Kissimmee** .... G+ E+
AdventHealth New Smyrna Beach, **New Smyrna Beach** .... G+ E+
AdventHealth North Pinellas, **Tarpon Springs** .... G+ HR
AdventHealth Ocala, **Ocala** .... G+
AdventHealth Orlando, **Orlando** .... G+ E+
AdventHealth Palm Coast, **Palm Coast** .... G+ E+
AdventHealth Tampa, **Tampa** .... G+ E+
AdventHealth Waterman, **Tavares** .... S+ E+
AdventHealth Wesley Chapel, **Wesley Chapel** .... G
AdventHealth Winter Park, **Winter Park** .... G+
AdventHealth Zephyrhills, **Zephyrhills** .... G+ E G+
Aventura Hospital and Medical Center, **Aventura** .... G+ E+
Baptist Hospital of Miami, **Miami** .... G+ E+
Baptist Medical Center - Jacksonville (Baptist Health), **Jacksonville** .... G+ E+
Baptist Medical Center - South (Baptist Health), **Jacksonville** .... G+
Bay Medical Center-Sacred Heart Health System, **Panama City** .... G+ E+ G S
Bayfront Health Port Charlotte Hospital, **Port Charlotte** .... S+ HR
Bayfront Health St. Petersburg, **St. Petersburg** .... G+ E+
Boca Raton Regional Hospital, **Boca Raton** .... G+ E+
Brandon Regional Hospital, **Brandon** .... G+ E+
Broward Health Coral Springs, **Coral Springs** .... G+ E+
Broward Health Medical Center, **Fort Lauderdale** .... G+ E+
Broward Health North, **Pompano Beach** .... G+ E+
Cape Canaveral Hospital, **Cocoa Beach** .... G+
Cape Coral Hospital, **Cape Coral** .... G+ E+
Capital Regional Medical Center, **Tallahassee** .... G+ E+
Central Florida Regional Hospital, **Sanford** .... S+ E+
Cleveland Clinic Florida, **Weston** .... G+ E+
Delray Medical Center, **Delray Beach** .... G+ E+
Doctors Hospital of Sarasota, **Sarasota** .... G+ E+ G+
Dr. P. Phillips Hospital, **Orlando** .... G+ E
Englewood Community Hospital, **Englewood** .... G+ HR G+ E+
Flagler Hospital, Inc., **Saint Augustine** .... G+ HR
FLORIDA MEDICAL CENTER a campus of North Shore, **Fort Lauderdale** .... G+ E+
Fort Walton Beach Medical Center, **Fort Walton Beach** .... G+ E+
Good Samaritan Medical Center, **West Palm Beach** .... G+ E
Gulf Breeze Hospital, **Gulf Breeze** .... S+ HR
Gulf Coast Medical Center, **Fort Myers** .... G+ E+
Halifax Health, **Daytona Beach** .... G+ E+
Health Park Medical Center, **Fort Myers** .... G+ E
Hialeah Hospital, **Hialeah** .... G+ G+
Holmes Regional Medical Center , **Melbourne** .... G+ HR
Holy Cross Hospital, **Fort Lauderdale** .... G+ HR G+ E+
Indian River Medical Center, **Vero Beach** .... G+ HR G+ E+
Jackson Memorial Hospital, **Miami** .... G+ E+
Jackson North Medical Center, **North Miami Beach** .... G+ E+
Jackson South Medical Center, **Miami** .... S+ E+
James A. Haley Veterans' Hospital, **Tampa** .... G+
JFK Medical Center, **Atlantis** .... G+ E+
Jupiter Medical Center, **Jupiter** .... G+
Kendall Regional Medical Center, **Miami** .... S+ E+
Lakeland Regional Health, **Lakeland** .... G+ E+
Lakewood Ranch Medical Center, **Bradenton** .... G+ E G
Largo Medical Center, **Largo** .... G G+ HR G+ E+ G+
Lee Memorial Hospital, **Fort Myers** .... G+ E+
Manatee Memorial Hospital, **Bradenton** .... G+ E+ G
Mease Countryside Hospital, **Safety Harbor** .... G+ HR G+
Mease Dunedin Hospital, **Dunedin** .... G+
Memorial Hospital, **Jacksonville** .... G+ HR G+ E+
Memorial Hospital Miramar, **Miramar** .... S+
Memorial Hospital Pembroke, **Pembroke Pines** .... G+
Memorial Hospital West, **Pembroke Pines** .... G+ E+
Memorial Regional Hospital, **Hollywood** .... G+ E+
Mercy Hospital, **Miami** .... G+ E
Morton Plant Hospital, **Clearwater** .... G+ E+

*These hospitals received Get With The Guidelines-Resuscitation awards from the American Heart Association for two or more patient populations.

Hospital	Badges
Morton Plant North Bay Hospital, **New Port Richey**	G+ HR
Mount Sinai Medical Center, **Miami Beach**	G+ HR G+ E+
NCH Healthcare System, **Naples**	G+ E+
Nicklaus Children's Hospital, **Miami**	G+ *
North Florida Regional Medical Center, **Gainesville**	G+ E+
North Shore Medical Center, **Miami**	G+ E+
Northside Hospital and Tampa Bay Heart Institute, **St. Petersburg**	HR G+ E+ G+
Northwest Medical Center, **Margate**	S+ E
Ocala Health, **Ocala**	G+ E+
Orange Park Medical Center, **Orange Park**	G G+ G+ G+ E+ G+
Orlando Health South Seminole Hospital, **Longwood**	S
Orlando Regional Medical Center, **Orlando**	G+ E+
Osceola Regional Medical Center, **Kissimmee**	S+ G+ E+
Palm Beach Gardens Medical Center, **Palm Beach Gardens**	G E+
Palmetto General Hospital, **Hialeah**	G+ E+
Palms of Pasadena Hospital, **South Pasadena**	G+ E+
Physicians Regional Healthcare System, **Naples**	G+ E+
Regional Medical Center Bayonet Point, **Hudson**	S+ E+
Rockledge Regional Medical Center, **Rockledge**	G+ E
Sacred Heart Health System, **Pensacola**	G+ G+ E
Sarasota Memorial Health Care System, **Sarasota**	G+ HR G+ E+
South Florida Baptist Hospital, **Plant City**	G+ HR
South Lake Hospital, **Clermont**	S HR
South Miami Hospital, **South Miami**	S+ E+
St. Anthony's Hospital, **St. Petersburg**	G+ E+ G
St. Joseph's Hospital, **Tampa**	G+ E+ G
St. Joseph's Hospital- North, **Lutz**	G
St. Mary's Medical Center, **West Palm Beach**	G+ E+
St. Vincent's Medical Center-Clay County, **Middleburg**	S+
St. Vincent's Medical Center-Riverside, **Jacksonville**	G+ HR
St. Vincent's Medical Center Southside, **Jacksonville**	G+ HR
Tallahassee Memorial HealthCare, **Tallahassee**	G+ E
Tampa General Hospital, **Tampa**	G+ E+
UF Health Shands Hospital, **Gainesville**	G+ E+
University of Miami Hospital, **Miami**	G+ E+
Venice Regional Bayfront Health, **Venice**	G+ E+
Viera Hospital, **Viera**	
Wellington Regional Medical Center, **Wellington**	G+ E+
West Boca Medical Center, **Boca Raton**	G+ HR G+ HR
West Florida Hospital, **Pensacola**	G+ E
West Kendall Baptist Hospital, **Miami**	G+
Westside Regional Medical Center, **Plantation**	G+ E+
Winter Haven Hospital, **Winter Haven**	G+ E+

GEORGIA

Hospital	Badges
Appling Healthcare System, **Baxley**	S+
AU Medical Center, **Augusta**	S+ HR G+ E+
Candler Hospital, **Savannah**	G+ E+
Cartersville Medical Center, **Cartersville**	G+ E+
Coliseum Medical Centers, **Macon**	S+
Doctors Hospital Augusta, **Augusta**	G+ E
Eastside Medical Center, **Snellville**	E+ E+
Emory Johns Creek Hospital, **Duluth**	G G
Emory Saint Joseph's Hospital, **Atlanta**	G+ E+ G G
Emory University Hospital, **Atlanta**	G+ E+ G G
Emory University Hospital Midtown, **Atlanta**	G+ HR G G
Fairview Park Hospital, **Dublin**	G+
Floyd Medical Center, **Rome**	G HR G+ E+
Grady Health System, **Atlanta**	G+ HR G+ E+
Gwinnett Medical Center, **Lawrenceville**	G+ E+ G+ G
Habersham Medical Center, **Demorest**	S S+
Hamilton Medical Center, **Dalton**	G+ E+
Meadows Regional Medical Center, **Vidalia**	S
Medical Center Navicent Health, **Macon**	G+ E+
Memorial University Medical Center, **Savannah**	G+ HR G+ E+
Midtown Medical Center, **Columbus**	G+ E+
Northeast Georgia Medical Center, **Gainesville**	G+ E+
Northside Hospital Atlanta, **Atlanta**	G+ G+ E+ G G
Northside Hospital Cherokee, **Canton**	G+ E+
Northside Hospital Forsyth, **Cumming**	G+ HR G+ E+ G G
Phoebe Putney Memorial Hospital, **Albany**	S+ G+ E

Hospital	Badges
Piedmont Athens Regional Medical Center, **Athens**	G+ E+
Piedmont Fayette Hospital, **Fayetteville**	S+ G+ E+
Piedmont Henry Hospital, **Stockbridge**	G+ E+
Piedmont Hospital, **Atlanta**	G+ E+
Piedmont Newnan Hospital, **Newnan**	G+ E+
Polk Medical Center, **Cedartown**	G+ E+
Redmond Regional Medical Center, **Rome**	G+ HR G+ E+
South Georgia Medical Center, **Valdosta**	G S G+ E+
Southern Regional Medical Center, **Riverdale**	G+ HR G
St. Francis Hospital, Inc., **Columbus**	G+ HR
St. Joseph's Hospital, **Savannah**	G+ E
St. Mary's Health Care System, **Athens**	G+ HR
Tanner Medical Center/Carrollton, **Carrollton**	G+ HR
University Hospital, **Augusta**	G G+ E+
Wellstar Cobb Hospital, **Austell**	G+ E+
Wellstar Douglas Hospital, **Douglasville**	G+ S+ E E S S
WellStar Kennestone Regional Hospital, **Marietta**	S+ S+ E+ E+ S
WellStar North Fulton Hospital, **Roswell**	G+ E+ S
WellStar Paulding Hospital, **Dallas**	S S
WellStar Spalding Regional Hospital, **Griffin**	G+ E+

HAWAII

Hospital	Badges
Adventist Health Castle, **Kailua**	G+ HR
Kaiser Foundation Hospital - Moanalua Medical Center, **Honolulu**	G+ G+ E
Kuakini Medical Center, **Honolulu**	G
Maui Memorial Medical Center, **Wailuku**	G+ HR G+ E
Pali Momi Medical Center, **Aiea**	G+ E
Straub Medical Center, **Honolulu**	G+ HR
The Queen's Medical Center Punchbowl, **Honolulu**	G G+ E+
The Queen's Medical Center West Oahu, **Ewa Beach**	G+ E+
Wahiawa General Hospital, **Wahiawa**	G+
Wilcox Medical Center, **Lihue**	G+ E+

IDAHO

Hospital	Badges
Eastern Idaho Regional Medical Center, **Idaho Falls**	G+ E+ G S
Kootenai Health, **Coeur d'Alene**	S S+ E+
St. Joseph Regional Medical Center, **Lewiston**	S

ILLINOIS

Hospital	Badges
Advocate BroMenn Medical Center, **Normal**	G+ HR S
Advocate Christ Medical Center, **Oak Lawn**	G+ E G
Advocate Condell Medical Center, **Libertyville**	G+ E
Advocate Good Samaritan Hospital, **Downers Grove**	G+ E G+
Advocate Good Shepherd Hospital, **Barrington**	G+ E
Advocate Illinois Masonic Medical Center, **Chicago**	G+ E
Advocate Lutheran General Hospital, **Park Ridge**	G+ E
Advocate Sherman Hospital, **Elgin**	G+ HR G+ E+ S
Advocate South Suburban Hospital, **Hazel Crest**	G+ E+
Advocate Trinity Hospital, **Chicago**	G+ HR
Alton Memorial Hospital, **Alton**	S+ E
AMITA Alexian Brothers Medical Center, **Elk Grove Village**	G+ E
AMITA Health Adventist Medical Center, Bolingbrook, **Bolingbrook**	S+ HR
AMITA Health Adventist Medical Center, La Grange, **La Grange**	G+ HR
AMITA Health St. Alexius Medical Center Hoffman Estates, **Hoffman Estates**	G+ E
Carle Foundation Hospital, **Urbana**	G G E
Community First Medical Center, **Chicago**	S+
Cook County Health, **Chicago**	S
Decatur Memorial Hospital, **Decatur**	G+ HR
Edward Hospital, **Naperville**	G+ E+
Herrin Hospital, **Herrin**	G+ HR G+
Holy Cross Hospital, **Chicago**	G+ E+
HSHS St. Elizabeth's Hospital, **O'Fallon**	G+ E S+ S
HSHS St. John's Hospital, **Springfield**	G+ HR G+ E+
Javon Bea Hospital- Rockton Ave, **Rockford**	G+ E+
Little Company of Mary Hospital and Health Care Centers, **Evergreen Park**	G+ E G
Loyola University Medical Center, **Maywood**	G+ HR S
MacNeal Hospital, **Berwyn**	G+ HR

American Heart Association.

(ILLINOIS CONTINUED)

Memorial Hospital of Carbondale, **Carbondale** .... G G+ HR G+ HR G+ S
Memorial Medical Center, **Springfield** .... G+ E+
Mercy Hospital & Medical Center, **Chicago** .... G+
MetroSouth Medical Center, **Blue Island** .... G+
Mount Sinai Hospital, **Chicago** .... G+
Northwest Community Hospital, **Arlington Heights** .... S G+ E
Northwestern Medicine Central DuPage Hospital, **Winfield** .... G+ HR S+ G+ E
Northwestern Medicine Delnor Hospital, **Geneva** .... HR G+ E
Northwestern Medicine Huntley, **Huntley** .... G+ E+
Northwestern Medicine Lake Forest Hospital, **Lake Forest** .... G+
Northwestern Medicine McHenry, **McHenry** .... G+ E+
Northwestern Memorial Hospital, **Chicago** .... S+ G+ E+ S
Norwegian American Hospital, **Chicago** .... S+ E+
OSF HealthCare Saint Anthony's Health Center, **Alton** .... G+ E+
OSF Saint Anthony Medical Center, **Rockford** .... G+ E+
OSF Saint Francis Medical Center, **Peoria** .... G+ E+
OSF St. Joseph Medical Center, **Bloomington** .... G+ E+
Palos Community Hospital, **Palos Heights** .... G
Presence Resurrection Medical Center, **Chicago** .... G+ E+ G
Presence Saint Francis Hospital, **Evanston** .... G+ HR
Presence Saint Joseph Hospital Chicago, **Chicago** .... G+
Presence Saint Joseph Hospital Elgin, **Elgin** .... G
Riverside Medical Center, **Kankakee** .... G+ HR
Rush Copley Medical Center, **Aurora** .... G+ HR
Rush Oak Park Hospital, **Oak Park** .... G+ E+
Rush University Medical Center, **Chicago** .... G+ E+ S
Silver Cross Hospital, **New Lenox** .... G+ E S
SSM Health Good Samaritan, **Mount Vernon** .... G+
Swedish American a Division of UW Health, **Rockford** .... G E
Swedish Covenant Hospital, **Chicago** .... G+
UChicago Medicine, **Chicago** .... S * G+ E+
UI Health Hospital & Clinics, **Chicago** .... G+ HR G+ E+
UnityPoint Health-Methodist, **Peoria** .... G+ HR
UnityPoint Health-Proctor, **Peoria** .... G+ G+
Vista Medical Center East, **Waukegan** .... S+ HR
West Suburban Medical Center, **Oak Park** .... G+

INDIANA

Baptist Health Floyd, **New Albany** .... G+ E+
Bluffton Regional Medical Center, **Bluffton** .... S+
Community Hospital, Community Healthcare System, **Munster** .... G+ HR
Community Hospital - North, **Indianapolis** .... G+ E+
Community Hospital East, **Indianapolis** .... G+ E+
Community Hospital of Anderson, **Anderson** .... G+ E
Community South, **Indianapolis** .... G+ E+
Deaconess, **Evansville** .... G+ E
Deaconess Gateway Hospital, **Newburgh** .... S+ HR
Elkhart General Hospital, **Elkhart** .... G+ E
Eskenazi Health, **Indianapolis** .... G+ E+
Franciscan Health Indianapolis, **Indianapolis** .... G+ HR G+ E+
Franciscan Health Lafayette East, **Lafayette** .... G+
Franciscan Health Michigan City, **Michigan City** ....
Good Samaritan, **Vincennes** .... S+
Indiana University Health Arnett, **Lafayette** .... S+ HR
Indiana University Health Ball Memorial Hospital, **Muncie** .... S G+ E
Indiana University Health Methodist Hospital, **Indianapolis** .... G+ G+ E+
IU Health Bloomington Hospital, **Bloomington** .... G+ HR
IU Health West Hospital, **Avon** .... G+ E+
Lutheran Hospital, **Fort Wayne** .... S G+ HR
Memorial Hospital, **South Bend** .... G+ HR
Memorial Hospital and Health Care Center, **Jasper** .... G+ E
Methodist Hospitals, Inc., **Gary** .... G+ E
Parkview Health, **Fort Wayne** .... G+
Porter Regional Hospital, **Valparaiso** .... G+
St. Mary Medical Center, **Hobart** .... G+ HR
St. Vincent Anderson Regional Hospital, **Anderson** .... G+ E
St. Vincent Evansville, **Evansville** .... G+
Union Hospital, **Terre Haute** .... G+ E

IOWA

Allen Hospital, **Waterloo** .... G+ G
CHI Health Mercy Hospital Council Bluffs, **Council Bluffs** .... S+ G
Genesis Medical Center, **Davenport** .... G+ E G G
Great River Medical Center, **West Burlington** .... S S+
Mary Greeley Medical Center, **Ames** .... S G+
Mercy Iowa City an affiliate of MercyOne, **Iowa City** .... G+ HR
Mercy Medical Center-Cedar Rapids, **Cedar Rapids** .... S+ E
MercyOne, **Sioux City** .... G+ HR G+ E G G
MercyOne Des Moines Medical Center, **Des Moines** .... G+ HR
MercyOne Dubuque Medical Center, **Dubuque** .... G+ HR
MercyOne North Iowa Medical Center, **Mason City** .... G+ HR G
Methodist Jennie Edmundson, **Council Bluffs** .... G G
Montgomery County Memorial Hospital, **Red Oak** .... S+
Myrtue Medical Center, **Harlan** .... S
Trinity Bettendorf, **Bettendorf** .... S+
UnityPoint Health -St. Luke's, **Sioux City** .... S+ HR G+ G
UnityPoint Health Trinity Regional Medical Center, **Fort Dodge** .... S+ E+ G S
University of Iowa Hospitals and Clinics, **Iowa City** .... G+ E+

KANSAS

AdventHealth Shawnee Mission, **Shawnee Mission** .... G+ HR S G+ E+ G+ S
Ascension Via Christi Hospital Pittsburg, Inc., **Pittsburg** .... G+ E+
Ascension Via Christi St. Francis, **Wichita** .... G+ E+
Centura Health - St. Catherine Hospital, **Garden City** .... G+ E
HaysMed. part of The University of Kansas Health, **Hays** .... G+ E
Hutchinson Regional Medical Center, **Hutchinson** .... G+
Lawrence Memorial Hospital, **Lawrence** .... G+ E+
Menorah Medical Center, **Overland Park** .... G+ E+
Olathe Medical Center, **Olathe** .... G+ E
Providence Medical Center, **Kansas City** .... G+ E+
Saint Luke's South Hospital, **Overland Park** .... G+ E+
Salina Regional Health Center, **Salina** .... G+ E+
Stormont-Vail HealthCare, **Topeka** .... G+ E+ G G
The University of Kansas Health System, **Kansas City** .... G+ HR G G
The University of Kansas Health System St. Francis Campus, **Topeka** .... G+ HR
Wesley Medical Center, **Wichita** .... G+ E+

KENTUCKY

Baptist Health LaGrange, **LaGrange** .... G+
Baptist Health Lexington, **Lexington** .... G+ HR G+ E+ S+
Baptist Health Louisville, **Louisville** .... G+ E+
Baptist Health Paducah, **Paducah** .... S+ S+ E+
Frankfort Regional Medical Center, **Frankfort** .... S+ E+
Hardin Memorial Health, **Elizabethtown** .... S+ E+
Highlands Regional Medical Center, **Prestonsburg** .... S+ HR
Jackson Purchase Medical Center, **Mayfield** .... S
Jewish Hospital, **Louisville** .... G+ E+ G+
King's Daughters Medical Center, **Ashland** .... G+ HR
Lake Cumberland Regional Hospital, **Somerset** .... G+ E
Norton Audubon Hospital, **Louisville** .... G
Norton Brownsboro Hospital, **Louisville** .... G+ E+ G
Norton Hospital, **Louisville** .... G+
Paul B. Hall Regional Medical Center, **Paintsville** .... G+
Pikeville Medical Center, Inc., **Pikeville** .... G+ HR
Saint Joseph Hospital, **Lexington** .... G+ E+
St. Elizabeth Edgewood, **Edgewood** .... G G+ HR G+ E+
St. Elizabeth Florence, **Florence** .... G G+ HR
St. Elizabeth Ft. Thomas, **Fort Thomas** .... G G+ HR G+ HR
Sts. Mary and Elizabeth Hospital, **Louisville** .... G+ E+
The Medical Center at Bowling Green, **Bowling Green** .... S+ HR G+ E+
University of Kentucky Hospital, **Lexington** .... G+ G+ E+
University of Louisville Hospital, **Louisville** .... G+ E+

LOUISIANA

Children's Hospital, **New Orleans** .... S
Christus Schumpert Medical Center, **Shreveport** .... S
East Jefferson General Hospital, **Metairie** .... G+ HR G+ E

American Heart Association.

Lakeview Regional Medical Center, a campus of Tulane Medical Center, Covington .... G+ HR
Ochsner LSU Health Shreveport, Shreveport .... G+ HR
Ochsner Medical Center - Kenner, Kenner .... G+ E+
Ochsner Medical Center - New Orleans, New Orleans .... G+ E
Our Lady of Lourdes Regional Medical Center, Lafayette .... G+ E
Our Lady of the Lake Regional Medical Center, Baton Rouge .... S+ G+ E+
Rapides Regional Medical Center, Alexandria ..... G + S + ★ G+ E+
Slidell Memorial Hospital, Slidell .... G+ E
St. Charles Parish Hospital, Luling .... S+
St. Francis Medical Center, Monroe .... G+ HR
St. Tammany Parish Hospital, Covington .... G+ HR
Terrebonne General Medical Center, Houma .... S+ E+ S+
Touro Infirmary, New Orleans .... G+ E
Tulane University Hospital and Clinic, New Orleans .... G+ E
University Medical Center New Orleans (UMCNO), New Orleans .. G+ E
West Jefferson Medical Center, Marrero .... G+ E
Willis-Knighton Pierremont Health Center, Shreveport .... S+ HR

MAINE

Central Maine Medical Center, Lewiston .... G+ HR
Eastern Maine Medical Center, Bangor .... G+ E+
Maine Medical Center, Portland .... G
MaineGeneral Medical Center, Augusta .... G
Mercy Hospital, EMHS member, Portland .... G+ HR S
Pen Bay Medical Center, Rockport .... S
York Hospital, York .... G+

MARYLAND

Adventist HealthCare Shady Grove Medical Center, Rockville .... G+ E+
Anne Arundel Medical Center, Annapolis .... G+ E G+
Atlantic General Hospital, Berlin .... S+ E
CalvertHealth Medical Center, Prince Frederick .... G+ HR
Carroll Hospital Center, Westminster .... G+ HR
Doctor's Community Hospital, Lanham .... G+ E
Frederick Memorial Hospital, Frederick .... G+ E
Greater Baltimore Medical Center, Baltimore .... G+ E
Holy Cross Germantown Hospital, Germantown .... G+ E+
Holy Cross Hospital, Silver Spring .... G+ E+
Howard County General Hospital, Columbia .... G+ E
Johns Hopkins Bayview Medical Center, Baltimore .... G+ E+
MedStar Franklin Square Medical Center, Baltimore ... G+ E+ G
MedStar Good Samaritan Hospital, Baltimore .... G+
MedStar Harbor Hospital, Baltimore .... S+
MedStar Montgomery Medical Center, Olney .... G+ E+
MedStar Southern Maryland Hospital Center, Clinton .... G+ E+
MedStar St. Mary's Hospital, Leonardtown .... S+ E
MedStar Union Memorial Hospital, Baltimore .... G+ E G+ G
Mercy Medical Center, Baltimore .... S+
Meritus Medical Center, Hagerstown .... S+ HR G+
Northwest Hospital, Randallstown .... G+ E
Peninsula Regional Medical Center, Salisbury .... G+ HR
Saint Agnes Hospital, Baltimore .... G+ E+
Sinai Hospital of Baltimore, Baltimore .... G+ E+ G
Suburban Hospital Johns Hopkins Medicine, Bethesda .... G+ HR S S
The Johns Hopkins Hospital, Baltimore .... G+ ★ G+ E+
Union Hospital of Cecil County, Elkton .... G+ E
University of Maryland Baltimore Washington Medical Center, Glen Burnie .... G+ E+ G
University of Maryland Charles Regional Medical Center, La Plata .... G+ E
University of Maryland Harford Memorial Hospital, Havre De Grace ...... G+ HR
University of Maryland Medical Center, Baltimore .... G+ E+
University of Maryland Prince George's Hospital Center, Cheverly .... G+ E+
University of Maryland Shore Medical Center at Easton, Easton .... G E S+
University of Maryland St. Joseph Medical Center, Towson .... G+ E+ G+ G
University of Maryland Upper Chesapeake Medical Center, Bel Air .... G+ E+
Washington Adventist Hospital, Takoma Park .... G+ E G
Western Maryland Health System, Cumberland ...... G+ E G G

MASSACHUSETTS

Addison Gilbert Hospital, Gloucester .... G+
Baystate Medical Center, Springfield .... G+ E+ S+
Baystate Noble Hospital, Westfield ....
Baystate Wing Hospital, Palmer .... S+ E
Berkshire Medical Center, Pittsfield .... G G+ HR G G+ E S
Beth Israel Deaconess Hospital - Needham, Needham .... G+ HR
Beth Israel Deaconess Hospital-Plymouth, Plymouth .... G+ E+
Beth Israel Deaconess Medical Center, Boston .... G+ HR G G+ E+
Beverly Hospital, Beverly .... G+ HR
Boston Children's Hospital, Boston .... G+ S+ ★
Boston Medical Center, Boston .... G+ E+
Brigham and Women's Faulkner Hospital, Boston .... G G+
Brigham and Women's Hospital, Boston .... G+ HR G+ E+
Cape Cod Hospital, Hyannis .... S+ HR
Cooley Dickinson Hospital, Northampton .... G+
Emerson Hospital, Concord .... G+
Fairview Hospital, Great Barrington .... S
Falmouth Hospital, member Cape Cod Healthcare, Falmouth ..... G
Good Samaritan Medical Center, Brockton .... G
Holy Family Hospital, Methuen .... S+ HR
Holyoke Medical Center, Holyoke .... G+ E+
Lahey Hospital & Medical Center, Burlington, Burlington .... G+ E
Massachusetts General Hospital, Boston .... S G+ E+
Mercy Medical Center, Springfield .... G+
MetroWest Medical Center - Framingham Union Hospital, Framingham .... G+ G+ HR G+ S
Milford Regional Medical Center, Milford .... G+
Mount Auburn Hospital, Cambridge .... G+ HR
Newton-Wellesley Hospital, Newton .... G G+ HR G+ E
North Shore Medical Center - Salem Hospital, Salem .... G+ HR
North Shore Medical Center - Union Hospital, Lynn .... G+
Norwood Hospital, A Steward Family Hospital, Norwood .... G+ HR
Saint Anne's Hospital, Fall River .... G+ HR
Saint Vincent Hospital, Worcester .... G+ HR
Signature Healthcare Brockton Hospital, Brockton .... G+ HR
South Shore Hospital, South Weymouth .... G
Southcoast Health Charlton Memorial Hospital, Fall River ..... G+ E
Southcoast Health St. Luke's Hospital, New Bedford .... G+ E
Southcoast Health Tobey Hospital, Wareham .... S+ HR
Steward St. Elizabeth's Medical Center, Brighton .... G+ HR G+ E
Sturdy Memorial Hospital, Attleboro .... G+ E+ G
Tufts Medical Center, Boston .... G+ E+
UMass Memorial - Marlborough Hospital, Worcester .... G G+ E+
UMass Memorial Medical Center, Worcester .... G G+ E+

MICHIGAN

Ascension St. John Hospital and Medical Center, Detroit .... G+ E
Beaumont Hospital, Grosse Pointe, Grosse Pointe .... G+ HR
Beaumont Hospital, Troy, Troy .... G+ HR
Borgess Medical Center, Kalamazoo .... G+ HR
Bronson Methodist Hospital, Kalamazoo .... G+ E+
Covenant HealthCare, Saginaw .... S+
DMC Harper University Hospital, Detroit .... S+
Garden City Hospital, Garden City .... S+ HR
Genesys Regional Medical Center, Grand Blanc .... G+ E
Henry Ford Allegiance Health, Jackson .... S+ E
Henry Ford Hospital and Health Network, Detroit .... G+ E+
Henry Ford Macomb Hospital, Clinton Township .... S+ E+
Henry Ford West Bloomfield Hospital, West Bloomfield .... G+ HR
Holland Hospital, Holland .... S+ E
Hurley Medical Center, Flint .... G+ E+
Lakeland Healthcare, Saint Joseph .... G+ E
Lapeer Regional Medical Center, Lapeer .... S+
McLaren - Flint, Flint .... G+ E
McLaren Bay Region, Bay City .... G+ E
McLaren Macomb, Mount Clemens .... G+ E
McLaren Northern Michigan, Petoskey .... G+ E+
McLaren Port Huron Hospital, Port Huron .... S+ E

(MICHIGAN CONTINUED)

Hospital	Awards
Mercy Health Saint Mary's, **Grand Rapids**	(G+) (E+)
Metro Health – University of Michigan Health, **Wyoming**	(G+) (E+)
Munson Medical Center, **Traverse City**	(G+) (E+)
ProMedica Bixby Hospital, **Adrian**	(S+)
ProMedica Monroe Regional Hospital, **Monroe**	(G+) (HR)
Sparrow Hospital, **Lansing**	(G+) (E+)
Spectrum Health Butterworth, **Grand Rapids**	(G+) (E+)
St. John Providence Hospital, **Southfield**	(S+) (E+)
St. John Providence Park Hospital, **Novi**	(S+) (E+)
St. Joseph Mercy Ann Arbor, **Ypsilanti**	(G+) (HR)
St. Joseph Mercy Oakland, **Pontiac**	(G+) (E+)
St. Mary Mercy Hospital, **Livonia**	(S+) (E)
St. Mary's of Michigan, **Saginaw**	(G+) (E)
University of Michigan Health System, **Ann Arbor**	(S) * (G+) (E+)

MINNESOTA

Hospital	Awards
CentraCare St. Cloud Hospital, **Saint Cloud**	(G+) (G+) * (S+) (G+) (G) (E+)
Essentia Health East. St. Mary's Medical Center, **Duluth**	(G+) (HR) (G+) (E+)
Hennepin County Medical Center, **Minneapolis**	(G) (G+) (E+)
Mayo Clinic Hospital, Saint Marys Campus, **Rochester**	(G+) (E+)
Mercy Hospital, **Coon Rapids**	(G+)
North Memorial Health Hospital, **Robbinsdale**	(G+) (E+)
Olmsted Medical Center, **Rochester**	(G+)
Park Nicollet Methodist Hospital, **Saint Louis Park**	(G+) (E+) (G+) (S)
Regions Hospital, **Saint Paul**	(G+) (E+) (S+) (S)
St. Luke's, **Duluth**	(G+) (G)

MISSISSIPPI

Hospital	Awards
Baptist Memorial Hospital - DeSoto, **Southaven**	(G+) (HR)
Baptist Memorial Hospital - North Mississippi, **Oxford**	(G+)
Forrest General Hospital, **Hattiesburg**	(G+) (HR) (G+) (S)
Gilmore Memorial Hospital, **Amory**	(G)
Greenwood Leflore Hospital, **Greenwood**	(S)
Magnolia Regional Health Center, **Corinth**	(S+)
Memorial Hospital at Gulfport, **Gulfport**	(G+) (E)
Merit Health Wesley, **Hattiesburg**	(G+) (HR) (G+)
Methodist Olive Branch Hospital, **Olive Branch**	(G+) (E+)
MS Baptist Medical Center, **Jackson**	(G+)
Ocean Springs Hospital, **Ocean Springs**	(G+) (E) (G)
OCH Regional Medical Center, **Starkville**	(G+) (E)
River Oaks Hospital, **Jackson**	(S)
Singing River Hospital, **Pascagoula**	(G+) (E) (G)
South Central Regional Medical Center, **Laurel**	(S+) (HR)
Southwest Mississippi Regional Medical Center, **McComb**	(S)
St. Dominic Memorial Hospital, **Jackson**	(G+) (E)
University of Mississippi Health Care, **Jackson**	(G+) (E+)

MISSOURI

Hospital	Awards
Barnes-Jewish Hospital, **St. Louis**	(S) (G+) (E+) (G) (S)
Belton Regional Medical Center, **Belton**	(G+) (E+)
Boone Hospital Center, **Columbia**	(G+) (E+) (G) (G)
Capital Region Medical Center, **Jefferson City**	(G+) (E)
Centerpoint Medical Center, **Independence**	(G+) (E+)
Christian Hospital, **St. Louis**	(S+) (HR)
Cox Medical Center Branson, **Branson**	(G+) (E)
Cox Medical Center South, **Springfield**	(S) (G+) (E+)
Cox Monett Hospital Inc, **Monett**	(G+)
Freeman Health System, **Joplin**	(S+) (S) (S)
Lake Regional Health System, **Osage Beach**	(G+) (E)
Lee's Summit Medical Center, **Lees Summit**	(S+) (E)
Liberty Hospital, **Liberty**	(G+) (HR)
Mercy Hospital Jefferson, **Crystal City**	(G+)
Mercy Hospital Joplin, **Joplin**	(S+)
Mercy Hospital South, **St. Louis**	(G+) (HR) (G+) (E+)
Mercy Hospital Springfield, **Springfield**	(G+) (E+)
Mercy Hospital St. Louis, **St. Louis**	(G+) (E+)
Mercy Hospital Washington, **Washington**	(S+) (E)
Missouri Baptist Medical Center, **St. Louis**	(S+) (E)

Hospital	Awards
Mosaic Life Care, **Saint Joseph**	(S) (G+) (E+)
Ozarks Medical Center, **West Plains**	(S+)
Phelps Health, **Rolla**	(S)
Research Medical Center, **Kansas City**	(G+) (HR) (G+) (E+) (S)
Saint Francis Medical Center, **Cape Girardeau**	(S+) (E)
Saint Luke's East Hospital, **Lees Summit**	(G+) (E+)
Saint Luke's Hospital of Kansas City, **Kansas City**	(HR) (G+) (E+)
Saint Luke's North Hospital, **Kansas City**	(G+) (E+)
Southeast Health, **Cape Girardeau**	(S+) (HR)
SSM Health DePaul Hospital, **Bridgeton**	(G+) (E+)
SSM Health Saint Louis University Hospital, **St. Louis**	(G+) (E+)
SSM Health St. Clare Hospital, **Fenton**	(G+) (E+)
SSM Health St. Joseph Hospital -St. Charles, **Saint Charles**	(G+) (E)
SSM Health St. Mary's Hospital, **St. Louis**	(G+) (E)
SSM St. Joseph Hospital Lake St. Louis, **Lake St Louis**	(G+) (E+)
St. Joseph Medical Center, **Kansas City**	(S+) (E)
St. Luke's Des Peres Hospital, **St. Louis**	(G+)
St. Luke's Hospital, **Chesterfield**	(G+) (E+)
St. Mary's Health Center, **Jefferson City**	(S+) (HR)
St. Mary's Medical Center, **Blue Springs**	(G+) (HR) (G+)
University of Missouri Health Care, **Columbia**	(G+) (HR)

MONTANA

Hospital	Awards
Benefis Health System, **Great Falls**	(G+) (HR) (G+)
Billings Clinic, **Billings**	(G+) (S)
Bozeman Health Deaconess Hospital, **Bozeman**	(S+) (E) (G+)
Kalispell Regional Healthcare, **Kalispell**	(G+) (HR) (G+) (HR) (G+) (G)
Providence St. Patrick Hospital, **Missoula**	(G+) (E) (G) (G)
St. Vincent Healthcare, **Billings**	(S)

NEBRASKA

Hospital	Awards
CHI Health Creighton University Medical Center Bergan Mercy, **Omaha**	(S+) (HR)
CHI Health Good Samaritan Hospital, **Kearney**	(G+) (HR)
CHI Health Immanuel Medical Center, **Omaha**	(S+) (E+)
CHI Health Lakeside Hospital, **Omaha**	(S+) (HR)
CHI Health St. Elizabeth, **Lincoln**	(G+) (E)
CHI Health St. Francis Medical Center, **Grand Island**	(S+) (E+)
Faith Regional Health Services, **Norfolk**	(G+) (HR)
Great Plains Health, **North Platte**	(G+) (E+) (G) (G)
Nebraska Medicine, **Omaha**	(G+) (E+)
Nebraska Medicine – Bellevue, **Bellevue**	(G+) (HR)
Nebraska Methodist Hospital, **Omaha**	(G+) (HR)
Regional West Medical Center, **Scottsbluff**	(G+) (E)

NEVADA

Hospital	Awards
Centennial Hills Hospital Medical Center, **Las Vegas**	(G+) (E) (G+)
Desert Springs Hospital Medical Center, **Las Vegas**	(G+) (HR) (S)
Dignity Health St. Rose Dominican Hospital - Rose de Lima Campus, **Henderson**	(G+)
Dignity Health St. Rose Dominican Hospital - San Martin Campus, **Las Vegas**	(G+)
Dignity Health St. Rose Dominican Hospital - Siena Campus, **Henderson**	(G+) (E) (G+)
Henderson Hospital, **Henderson**	(G) (S)
MountainView Hospital, **Las Vegas**	(G+) (E)
Northern Nevada Medical Center, **Sparks**	(G)
Renown Regional Medical Center, **Reno**	(G+) (HR) (G+) (E) (S)
Saint Mary's Regional Medical Center, **Reno**	(G+) (HR) (G+) (E)
Southern Hills Hospital & Medical Center, **Las Vegas**	(G+) (E+)
Spring Valley Hospital Medical Center, **Las Vegas**	(G+) (E+) (G)
Summerlin Hospital Medical Center, **Las Vegas**	(G+) (E+) (G)
Sunrise Hospital & Medical Center, **Las Vegas**	(G+) (E+)
University Medical Center of Southern Nevada, **Las Vegas**	(S) (G+) (HR)
Valley Hospital Medical Center, **Las Vegas**	(G+) (E) (G)

NEW HAMPSHIRE

Hospital	Awards
Catholic Medical Center, **Manchester**	(G+) (E+)
Concord Hospital, **Concord**	(G+) (E)
Dartmouth-Hitchcock Medical Center, **Lebanon**	(G) (G+) (G+) (E)

*These hospitals received Get With The Guidelines-Resuscitation awards from the American Heart Association for two or more patient populations.

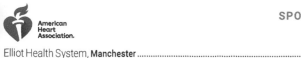

Elliot Health System, **Manchester** .... G+
Exeter Hospital, **Exeter** .... G
Parkland Medical Center, **Derry** ....
Portsmouth Regional Hospital, **Portsmouth** .... G+ E+
Southern New Hampshire Medical Center, **Nashua** ...... G+ HR
Wentworth-Douglass Hospital, **Dover** .... S G+

NEW JERSEY

Capital Health Regional Medical Center, **Trenton** .... G+ E
CarePoint Health - Bayonne Medical Center, **Bayonne** .... G+
CarePoint Health - Christ Hospital, **Jersey City** ...... G+ HR G+ E G+
CarePoint Health - Hoboken University Medical Center, **Hoboken** .... G+
CentraState Medical Center, **Freehold** .... G+ G+ E
Chilton Medical Center, **Pompton Plains** .... G+ E+
Cooper University Health Care, **Camden** .... G+ HR
Deborah Heart and Lung Center, **Browns Mills** .... G+ HR
Englewood Hospital and Medical Center, **Englewood** .... S
Hackensack Meridian Health Bayshore Medical Center, **Holmdel** .... G+ E
Hackensack Meridian Health Hackensack University Medical Center,
  Hackensack .... G+ E+
Hackensack Meridian Health Jersey Shore University Medical Center,
  Neptune .... G+ G+ E+
Hackensack Meridian Health JFK Medical Center, **Edison** ..... G+ E+
Hackensack Meridian Health Mountainside Medical Center, **Montclair** .... G+ HR
Hackensack Meridian Health Ocean Medical Center, **Brick** .... G+ E+
Hackensack Meridian Health Palisades Medical Center,
  North Bergen .... G+ HR G+ HR
Hackensack Meridian Health Raritan Bay Medical Center,
  Perth Amboy and Old Bridge .... G+ E
Hackensack Meridian Health Riverview Medical Center, **Red Bank** ..... G+ G+ E
Hackensack Meridian Health Southern Ocean Medical Center,
  Manahawkin .... G+ E+
HackensackUMC at Pascack Valley, **Westwood** .... S+ HR
Hackettstown Medical Center, **Hackettstown** .... G+ E+
Holy Name Medical Center, **Teaneck** .... G G+ E+
Hunterdon Healthcare, **Flemington** .... S S+ E+
Inspira Medical Center Elmer, **Elmer** ....
Inspira Medical Center Vineland, **Vineland** .... G+
Inspira Medical Center Woodbury, **Woodbury** .... G+
Jefferson Cherry Hill Hospital, **Cherry Hill** .... G+ E
Jefferson Stratford Hospital, **Stratford** .... G+ E
Jefferson Washington Township Hospital, **Turnersville** ..... G+ E+
Jersey City Medical Center RWJBarnabas Health, **Jersey City** ..... G+ E
Monmouth Medical Center, **Long Branch** .... G+ E+
Morristown Medical Center, **Morristown** .... G+ E+
Newark Beth Israel Medical Center, **Newark** .... G
Newton Medical Center, **Newton** .... G+ E+
Our Lady of Lourdes Medical Center, **Camden** .... G+ HR
Overlook Medical Center, **Summit** .... G+ E+
Penn Medicine Princeton Medical Center, **Plainsboro** ....
Robert Wood Johnson University Hospital, **New Brunswick** .... G+ E+
Robert Wood Johnson University Hospital Somerset, **Somerville** ... G+ HR
Saint Clare's Denville Hospital, **Denville** .... G+
Saint Clare's Hospital, **Denville and Dover** .... G+ HR
Saint Peter's University Hospital, **New Brunswick** ...... G+
St. Francis Medical Center, **Trenton** .... G+
St. Joseph's University Medical Center, **Paterson** ..... G+ E+ G+
St. Joseph's Wayne Medical Center, **Wayne** .... G+
St. Luke's Warren Hospital, **Phillipsburg** .... G+ E+
St. Mary's General Hospital, **Passaic** .... S+ HR
The Valley Hospital, **Ridgewood** .... G G+ E+
Trinitas Regional Medical Center, **Elizabeth** .... G
University Hospital, **Newark** .... G+ HR G+ E S
Virtua Memorial Hospital of Burlington County, **Mt. Holly** ..... S+

NEW MEXICO

Lovelace Medical Center, **Albuquerque** .... G+ HR G+ E+
MountainView Regional Medical Center, **Las Cruces** .... S+
Presbyterian Healthcare Services, **Albuquerque** ...... G+ E+ G+ G
University of New Mexico Hospitals, **Albuquerque** ...... G+ HR G+ E+ G

NEW YORK

Albany Med, **Albany** .... G+ HR G+ HR S
Albany Memorial Hospital, **Albany** .... G+
Arnot Ogden Medical Center, **Elmira** .... G+ E+
Auburn Community Hospital, **Auburn** .... G+ HR
Bassett Medical Center, **Cooperstown** .... G G+
BronxCare Health System, **Bronx** ...... G G+ HR G+ E+ G G
Brookdale University Hospital Medical Center, **Brooklyn** .... G+ E+
Catholic Health - Kenmore Mercy Hospital, **Buffalo** .... G+
Catholic Health - Mercy Hospital of Buffalo, **Buffalo** ..... G+ E S
Catholic Health - Mount St. Mary's Hospital, **Lewiston** ...... G+ HR
Catholic Health - Sisters of Charity Hospital, Sisters of Charity St. Joseph
  Campus, **Buffalo** .... G+
Catskill Regional Medical Center, **Harris** .... G+ E
Cayuga Medical Center, **Ithaca** .... S+ E
Cohen Children's Medical Center, **New Hyde Park** ...... G+ S+
Columbia Memorial Hospital, **Hudson** .... G+
Crouse Hospital, **Syracuse** .... G+ HR G+ E+ G
Ellenville Regional Hospital, **Ellenville** .... S
Ellis Medicine, **Schenectady** .... S+ G+ E+
Erie County Medical Center, **Buffalo** ....
F.F. Thompson Hospital, **Canandaigua** .... G+ HR
Faxton St. Luke's Healthcare, an affiliation of Mohawk Valley Health System,
  Utica .... G+ E
Gates Vascular Institute / Buffalo General Medical Center, **Buffalo** ..... G+ E+ S
Geneva General Hospital, **Geneva** .... G+
Glen Cove Hospital, **Glen Cove** .... G+ E
Good Samaritan Hospital, a Member of WMC Health Network, **Suffern** .... G+ E+
Good Samaritan Hospital Medical Center, **West Islip** ..... G+ HR
Guthrie Corning Hospital, **Corning** .... G+
HealthAlliance: Broadway Campus a Member of the WMC Health Network,
  Kingston .... HR
Highland Hospital, **Rochester** ...... G+ HR G+ HR
Huntington Hospital, **Huntington** .... G E S
Jamaica Hospital Medical Center, **Richmond Hill** ...... G+ G+ E+
John T. Mather Memorial Hospital, **Port Jefferson** ...... G+ E
Kingsbrook Jewish Medical Center, **Brooklyn** .... G+ HR
Lenox Hill Hospital, **New York** .... G+ E+ S
LIJ Medical Center at Forest Hills, **Forest Hills** .... G+ E
LIJ Valley Stream, **Valley Stream** .... G+ E
Long Island Community Hospital, **Patchogue** .... G+ E+
Long Island Jewish Medical Center, **New Hyde Park** ..... G+ HR
Maimonides Medical Center, **Brooklyn** .... G+ HR
Mercy Medical Center, **Rockville Centre** .... G+ E
MidHudson Regional Hospital of WMC Health, **Poughkeepsie** .... G+
Millard Fillmore Suburban Hospital, **Williamsville** ...... G+ HR
Montefiore Mount Vernon Hospital, **Mount Vernon** ..... G+
Montefiore Nyack Hospital, **Nyack** .... G+
Montefiore St. Luke's Cornwall, **Newburgh** .... G+ S
Mount Sinai Beth Israel, **New York** ...... G+ HR G+ E+ G
Mount Sinai Brooklyn, **Brooklyn** .... G+ HR
Mount Sinai Queens, **Astoria** .... G+ HR
Mount Sinai St. Luke's, **New York** .... G+
Mount Sinai St. Luke's & Mount Sinai West, **New York** ..... G+ HR
Nassau University Medical Center, **East Meadow** ...... HR G+ E+
New York Community Hospital, **Brooklyn** .... G+ E
Newark–Wayne Community Hospital, **Newark** .... G+
NewYork-Presbyterian Brooklyn Methodist Hospital, **Brooklyn** .... G+ E+
NewYork-Presbyterian Queens, **Flushing** .... G+ E G
NewYork-Presbyterian/Columbia University Medical Center, **New York** ..... G+ E+
New York Presbyterian/Hudson Valley Hospital, **Cortlandt Manor** ..... G+ E
NewYork-Presbyterian/Lawrence Hospital, **Bronxville** ..... G+ HR S
NewYork-Presbyterian/Lower Manhattan Hospital, **New York** ...... G+ E+
NewYork-Presbyterian/The Allen Hospital, **New York** ...... G+ E+
NewYork-Presbyterian/Weill Cornell Medical Center, **New York** .... G+ E+
Niagara Falls Memorial Medical Center, **Niagara Falls** ......
North Shore University Hospital, **Manhasset** .... G+ E+
Northern Dutchess Hospital, **Rhinebeck** .... G+
Northern Westchester Hospital, **Mount Kisco** ...... G+ E+
NYC Health + Hospitals/Bellevue, **New York** ..... G+ HR G G+ E+ G G

(NEW YORK CONTINUED)

NYC Health + Hospitals/Coney Island, **Brooklyn** .... G+ E
NYC Health + Hospitals/Elmhurst, **Elmhurst** .... S G+ E+
NYC Health + Hospitals/Harlem, **New York** .... G+ HR
NYC Health + Hospitals/Jacobi, **Bronx** .... S+ S G+ E+
NYC Health + Hospitals/Kings County, **Brooklyn** .... HR G G+ E+
NYC Health + Hospitals/Lincoln, **Bronx** .... G+ G+ E+
NYC Health + Hospitals/Metropolitan, **New York** .... G+
NYC Health + Hospitals/North Central Bronx, **Bronx** .... HR
NYC Health + Hospitals/Woodhull, **Brooklyn** .... G+
NYU Langone Hospital - Brooklyn, **Brooklyn** .... S G+ E+ S+
NYU Langone Tisch Hospital, **New York** .... G+ G+ E+ G
NYU Winthrop Hospital, **Mineola** .... G+ E+
Orange Regional Medical Center, **Middletown** .... G+
Our Lady of Lourdes Memorial Hospital, **Binghamton** .... G+ HR
Peconic Bay Medical Center, **Riverhead** .... G+ E+
Phelps Hospital, Northwell Health, **Sleepy Hollow** .... G+ E+
Plainview Hospital, **Plainview** .... G+ E
Putnam Hospital Center, **Carmel** .... G+
Richmond University Medical Center, **Staten Island** .... G+ E+ S
Rochester General Hospital, **Rochester** .... G+ E+
Rome Memorial Hospital, **Rome** .... G
Saint Joseph's Medical Center, **Yonkers** .... G+
Samaritan Hospital, **Troy** .... G+ E S
Saratoga Hospital, **Saratoga Springs** .... G
SBH Health System, **Bronx** .... G+ HR
South Nassau Communities Hospital, **Oceanside** .... G+ HR G+ E+
Southampton Hospital, **Southampton** .... G+ E+
Southside Hospital, **Bay Shore** .... G+ E+ G
St. Catherine of Siena Medical Center, **Smithtown** .... G+ E+
St. Charles Hospital, **Port Jefferson** .... G+
St. Francis Hospital, The Heart Center, **Roslyn** .... G+ HR G+ E+
St. John's Episcopal Hospital, **Far Rockaway** .... S+ G+
St. John's Riverside Hospital, **Yonkers** .... G+ E+
St. Joseph Hospital, **Bethpage** .... G+ E+
St. Peter's Hospital, **Albany** .... G+ E+
Staten Island University Hospital, **Staten Island** .... G+ E+
Stony Brook University Hospital, **Stony Brook** .... G+ G * S G+ E
Syosset Hospital, **Syosset** .... G+ HR
The Brooklyn Hospital Center, **Brooklyn** .... G+ HR G+ E+
The Mount Sinai Hospital, **New York** .... G+ HR G+ E+ G
UHS Wilson Medical Center, **Johnson City** .... G+ G+ HR
Unity Hospital, **Rochester** .... G+ E+
University Hospital of Brooklyn - SUNY Downstate Medical Center, **Brooklyn** .... G+
Upstate University Hospital, **Syracuse** .... G+ E+
UR Medicine / Noyes Health, **Dansville** .... S+ E
UR Medicine Strong Memorial Hospital, **Rochester** .... G+ HR G+ E+ G+
Vassar Brothers Medical Center, **Poughkeepsie** .... G+ HR S+
Westchester Medical Center, **Valhalla** .... G+ HR
White Plains Hospital, **White Plains** .... G+ HR
Wyckoff Heights Medical Center, **Brooklyn** .... G+ E

NORTH CAROLINA

Angel Medical Center, **Franklin** .... G+ E
Annie Penn Hospital, **Reidsville** .... S+ HR
Atrium Health Cleveland, **Shelby** .... G+ E
Atrium Health Lincoln, **Lincolnton** .... S+ E
Atrium Health Mercy , **Charlotte** .... G+
Atrium Health Pineville, **Charlotte** .... G+ E G+ G
Atrium Health Union, **Monroe** .... G+
Atrium Health University City, **Charlotte** .... G+ E+
Cape Fear Valley Medical Center, **Fayetteville** .... G G+ G G+ E+ G+ S
Carolinas HealthCare System Blue Ridge-Morganton, **Morganton** .... G+ HR
Carolinas HealthCare System NorthEast, **Concord** .... G+ E G+ G
Carolinas HealthCare System Stanly, **Albemarle** .... G+ HR
Carolinas Medical Center, **Charlotte** .... G+ E+ G+ G
CaroMont Regional Medical Center, **Gastonia** .... G+ E
Carteret Health Care Medical Center, **Morehead City** .... S G+ HR G+ G+ HR
Columbus Regional Healthcare, **Whiteville** .... E
Cone Health, **Greensboro** .... G+ G+ E+ G+ S
Duke Raleigh Hospital, **Raleigh** .... G+ E+

Duke Regional Hospital, **Durham** .... G+ E+
Duke University Hospital, **Durham** .... G+ HR E+
Durham VA HealthCare System, **Durham** .... G+ E+
FirstHealth Moore Regional Hospital - Richmond , **Rockingham** .... S+ E+
FirstHealth of the Carolinas Moore Regional Hospital, **Pinehurst** .... G+ E+
Frye Regional Medical Center, **Hickory** .... G+ HR G+ E G+ G
Granville Health System, **Oxford** .... G+ S+
Hugh Chatham Memorial Hospital, **Elkin** .... G+ E+
Iredell Memorial Hospital, **Statesville** .... G+
Mission Hospital McDowell, **Marion** .... G+ E+
Mission Hospitals, Inc., **Asheville** .... G+ E+
Nash UNC Health Care, **Rocky Mount** .... G+ HR G G
New Hanover Regional Medical Center, **Wilmington** .... G+ E+
Novant Health Forsyth Medical Center, **Winston-Salem** .... G+ HR G+ E+ G+
Novant Health Huntersville Medical Center, **Huntersville** .... G+ HR G+ E G
Novant Health Matthews Medical Center, **Matthews** .... G+ HR G+ E+
Novant Health Presbyterian Medical Center, **Charlotte** .... HR G+ E+ G+ G
Novant Health Rowan Medical Center, **Salisbury** .... HR G+ HR G+
Novant Health Thomasville Medical Center, **Thomasville** .... S+ E+
Onslow Memorial Hospital, **Jacksonville** .... G+ HR
Pardee UNC Health Care, **Hendersonville** .... G+
Transylvania Regional Hospital, **Brevard** .... S+ E
UNC Hospitals, **Chapel Hill** .... G+ G+ G
UNC Lenoir Health Care, **Kinston** .... S G+ E
UNC REX Healthcare, **Raleigh** .... G+ E+ G+ S
Vidant Beaufort Hospital, **Washington** .... S+ HR
Vidant Chowan Hospital, **Edenton** .... S+
Vidant Duplin Hospital, **Kenansville** .... S+
Vidant Edgecombe Hospital, **Tarboro** .... S+
Vidant Medical Center, **Greenville** .... G+ HR G S G+ HR G G
Vidant Roanoke-Chowan Hospital, **Ahoskie** .... S+
Wake Forest Baptist Health High Point Medical Center, **High Point** .... S+ G+ E
Wake Forest Baptist Health Lexington Medical Center, **Lexington** .... S+ E
Wake Forest Baptist Medical Center, **Winston-Salem** .... G+ E+
WakeMed Cary Hospital, **Cary** .... HR G+ E+
WakeMed Health & Hospitals - Raleigh Campus, **Raleigh** .... HR G+ E+
Wayne UNC Health Care, **Goldsboro** .... G+ HR

NORTH DAKOTA

Altru Health System, **Grand Forks** .... G+ E
CHI St. Alexius Health Bismarck, **Bismarck** .... G+ E S G
Essentia Health, **Fargo** .... S+ E+
Sanford Bismarck Medical Center, **Bismarck** .... G+ HR
Sanford Medical Center Fargo, **Fargo** .... G+ E+
Trinity Health, **Minot** .... G+ E+
West River Health Services, **Hettinger** .... S+

OHIO

Adena Health System, **Chillicothe** .... G+ HR
Ashtabula County Medical Center, **Ashtabula** .... G+
Atrium Medical Center, **Franklin** .... G+
Aultman Alliance Community Hospital, **Alliance** .... G
Aultman Hospital, **Canton** .... G+ HR G+
Blanchard Valley Health System, **Findlay** .... G+ E+
Cleveland Clinic, **Cleveland** .... G+ G+ * S+ G+ E+
Cleveland Clinic Akron General, **Akron** .... G+ E
Cleveland Clinic Fairview Hospital, **Cleveland** .... G+ E+
Cleveland Clinic Hillcrest Hospital, **Mayfield Heights** .... G+ E+
Cleveland Clinic Marymount Hospital, **Garfield Heights** .... G+ HR
Cleveland Clinic Medina Hospital, **Medina** .... G+ E
Cleveland Clinic South Pointe Hospital, **Warrensville Heights** .... S+ E
Cleveland Clinic Union Hospital, **Dover** .... G+ E
Fairfield Medical Center, **Lancaster** .... G+ E
Firelands Regional Medical Center, **Sandusky** .... S
Fisher Titus Medical Center, **Norwalk** .... G+ HR
Genesis Healthcare System, **Zanesville** .... G+ G+ E
Kettering Medical Center, **Dayton** .... G+ E+
Licking Memorial Hospital, **Newark** .... G G
Louis Stokes Cleveland VA Medical Center, **Cleveland** .... G+ HR
Marietta Memorial Hospital, **Marietta** .... S+ HR

*These hospitals received Get With The Guidelines-Resuscitation awards from
the American Heart Association for two or more patient populations.

American Heart Association.

Hospital	Badges
Mercy Health - Anderson Hospital, **Cincinnati**	(G+)(S+)(HR)
Mercy Health - Fairfield Hospital , **Fairfield**	(G+)(HR)(E)
Mercy Health - St. Elizabeth Youngstown Hospital, **Youngstown**	(G+)(HR)(G+)(E+)
Mercy Health Clermont Hospital, **Batavia**	(G+)
Mercy Medical Center, **Canton**	(G+)(HR)(G+)(E)(G)
Miami Valley Hospital, **Dayton**	(G+)(E+)
Mount Carmel Health System, **Columbus**	(G+)(E)
Mount Carmel St. Ann's, **Westerville**	(G+)(E)
OhioHealth Marion General Hospital, **Marion**	(G+)(E)
OhioHealth Riverside Methodist Hospital, **Columbus**	(G+)(E+)
ProMedica Flower Hospital, **Sylvania**	(G+)(E+)
ProMedica Toledo Hospital, **Toledo**	(G+)(E+)
Southwest General Health Center, **Middleburg Heights**	(G)(G+)(E+)(G+)(G)
Summa Akron City Hospital, **Akron**	(G+)(E+)
Sycamore Medical Center, **Miamisburg**	(G+)(E)
The Jewish Hospital Mercy Health, **Cincinnati**	(S+)(G+)(HR)
The MetroHealth System, **Cleveland**	(G)(G+)(HR)(G+)(E+)
The Ohio State University Wexner Medical Center, **Columbus**	
The University of Toledo Medical Center, **Toledo**	(G+)(HR)(G+)(E)
UH Regional Hospitals, Bedford Medical Center and Richmond Medical Center, **Richmond Heights**	
University Hospitals Ahuja Medical Center, **Beachwood**	(S+)(HR)
University Hospitals Cleveland Medical Center, **Cleveland**	(G+)(E+)
University Hospitals Elyria Medical Center, **Elyria**	(G+)(E)
University Hospitals Geauga Medical Center, **Chardon**	(G+)(E)
University Hospitals Parma Medical Center, **Parma**	(G+)(E)
University Hospitals Portage Medical Center , **Ravenna**	(S+)(E)
University Hospitals St. John Medical Center, **Cleveland**	(G+)(E+)
University of Cincinnati Medical Center, **Cincinnati**	(G+)(HR)(G+)(E+)(G+)
Upper Valley Medical Center, **Troy**	(S+)(E+)
West Chester Hospital, **West Chester**	(S+)(G+)(HR)(G)
West Hospital, **Cincinnati**	(G+)(HR)(E)
Western Reserve Hospital, LLC, **Cuyahoga Falls**	

OKLAHOMA

Hospital	Badges
Hillcrest Hospital South, **Tulsa**	(S+)(E+)
Hillcrest Medical Center, **Tulsa**	(S+)(HR)(G+)(E+)
INTEGRIS Baptist Medical Center, **Oklahoma City**	(G+)(E)
INTEGRIS Southwest Medical Center, **Oklahoma City**	(G+)(E)
Jane Phillips Medical Center, **Bartlesville**	(G)(S)
McAlester Regional Health Center, **McAlester**	(G+)(E)
Mercy Hospital Oklahoma City Comprehensive Stroke Center, **Oklahoma City**	(G+)(E+)
Norman Regional Health System, **Norman**	(G+)(E+)(G+)(G)
Saint Francis Hospital, **Tulsa**	(G+)(E+)
St. Anthony Hospital, **Oklahoma City**	(G+)(HR)
St. John Medical Center, **Tulsa**	(G+)(E+)
St. Mary's Regional Medical Center, **Enid**	(S+)(E)
Stillwater Medical Center, **Stillwater**	(G+)(E)

OREGON

Hospital	Badges
Adventist Health Tillamook, **Tillamook**	(S+)
Asante Rogue Regional Medical Center, **Medford**	(G+)(S)
Good Samaritan Regional Medical Center, **Corvallis**	(G+)(E)
Kaiser Foundation Hospital Sunnyside, **Clackamas**	(G+)(E)
Kaiser Foundation Hospital Westside, **Hillsboro**	(G+)
Legacy Emanuel Medical Center, **Portland**	(G+)(E+)
Legacy Meridian Park Medical Center, **Tualatin**	(G+)(HR)
Legacy Mount Hood Medical Center, **Gresham**	(G+)(E+)
Oregon Health & Science University, **Portland**	(G+)(HR)
PeaceHealth Sacred Heart Medical Center RiverBend, **Springfield**	(G+)(E+)
Providence Hood River Memorial Hospital, **Hood River**	(G+)(HR)
Providence Medford Medical Center, **Medford**	(G+)(E)(G)
Providence Newberg Medical Center, **Newberg**	(G+)(E)
Providence Portland Medical Center, **Portland**	(G+)(E+)(G+)
Providence Seaside Hospital, **Seaside**	(G+)
Providence St. Vincent Medical Center, **Portland**	(G+)(E+)(G)(S)
Providence Willamette Falls Medical Center, **Oregon City**	(G+)(E+)
Samaritan Albany General Hospital, **Albany**	(G+)(HR)
Samaritan North Lincoln Hospital, **Lincoln City**	(S+)
Samaritan Pacific Communities Hospital, **Newport**	(G+)
Sky Lakes Medical Center, **Klamath Falls**	(G+)(HR)
St. Anthony Hospital, **Pendleton**	(S+)(E)
St. Charles Medical Center- Bend, **Bend**	(G+)
Tuality Healthcare, **Hillsboro**	(G+)

PENNSYLVANIA

Hospital	Badges
Abington Hospital-Jefferson Health, **Abington**	(G+)(G+)(E+)(G+)
Allegheny General Hospital, **Pittsburgh**	(G+)(HR)(G+)(E+)
Allegheny Valley Hospital, **Natrona Heights**	(G+)(HR)(S+)
Aria Health, **Philadelphia**	(G+)(E+)(G+)
Brandywine Hospital Tower Health, **Coatesville**	(S+)(HR)
Bryn Mawr Hospital, **Bryn Mawr**	(G+)(HR)(G)
Butler Memorial Hospital, **Butler**	(G+)
Carlisle Regional Medical Center, **Carlisle**	(G+)
Chambersburg Hospital, **Chambersburg**	(G+)(HR)(G+)(HR)
Chester County Hospital, **West Chester**	(S+)(HR)(G+)(G)
Chestnut Hill Hospital, **Philadelphia**	(G+)(E+)
Conemaugh Memorial Medical Center, **Johnstown**	(G)(G+)(E+)
Crozer-Chester Medical Center, **Upland**	(G+)(E+)
Delaware County Memorial Hospital, **Drexel Hill**	(G+)
Doylestown Hospital, **Doylestown**	(G+)(HR)(G)(G+)(E+)(G+)(S)
Einstein Medical Center Montgomery, **East Norriton**	(G+)(E+)
Einstein Medical Center - Philadelphia, **Philadelphia**	(G+)(E+)
Evangelical Community Hospital, **Lewisburg**	(G+)
Excela Health Latrobe, **Latrobe**	(G+)(HR)
Excela Health Westmoreland, **Greensburg**	(G+)(HR)
Forbes Hospital, **Monroeville**	(G+)(HR)(G+)(E)
Geisinger Community Medical Center, **Scranton**	(G+)(E+)(G+)
Geisinger Holy Spirit, **Camp Hill**	(G)(G+)(G+)
Geisinger Medical Center, **Danville**	(G+)(E+)(G+)
Geisinger Wyoming Valley, **Wilkes Barre**	(G+)(HR)(G+)
Grand View Health, **Sellersville**	(S)(G)(HR)(G+)(HR)
Hahnemann University Hospital, **Philadelphia**	(G+)(HR)(S)
Heritage Valley Beaver, **Beaver**	(G+)(E)
Heritage Valley Sewickley, **Sewickley**	(G+)
Holy Redeemer Hospital, **Meadowbrook**	(G)
Indiana Regional Medical Center, **Indiana**	(S)
Jeanes Hospital - Temple University Health System, **Philadelphia**	(G+)
Jefferson Hospital, **Clairton**	(G+)(G+)
Lankenau Medical Center, **Wynnewood**	(G+)(HR)(G+)
Lansdale Hospital, **Lansdale**	(G+)(HR)
Lehigh Valley Health Network Cedar Crest, **Allentown**	(G+)(E+)
Lehigh Valley Health Network Muhlenberg, **Bethlehem**	(G+)(E+)
Lehigh Valley Hospital- Hazleton, **Hazleton**	(G+)(HR)(G+)(HR)
Lehigh Valley Hospital - Schuylkill, **Pottsville**	(G+)(HR)
Lehigh Valley Pocono, **East Stroudsburg**	(G)(HR)
Lower Bucks Hospital, **Bristol**	(G+)
Memorial Hospital, York, PA, **York**	(S+)(E)
Mercy Fitzgerald Hospital, **Darby**	(G)(G+)(E)
Mercy Philadelphia Hospital, **Philadelphia**	(G+)
Monongahela Valley Hospital, **Monongahela**	(G)(G+)(HR)(G+)(HR)(G)
Moses Taylor Hospital, **Scranton**	(S+)(E)
Mount Nittany Medical Center, **State College**	(G+)(HR)
Nazareth Hospital, **Philadelphia**	(G+)(HR)(E)
Paoli Hospital, **Paoli**	(G+)(G)
Penn Highlands DuBois, **DuBois**	(G+)(G)
Penn Medicine Lancaster General Hospital, **Lancaster**	(G+)(E+)
Penn Presbyterian Medical Center, **Philadelphia**	(G+)
Penn State Hershey Medical Center, **Hershey**	(G+)(HR)(S)(G+)(E+)
Pennsylvania Hospital, **Philadelphia**	(S)(G+)(E+)
Phoenixville Hospital, **Phoenixville**	(G+)(HR)
Pinnacle Health System - West Shore Hospital, **Mechanicsburg**	(G+)
Pottstown Hospital, **Pottstown**	(G+)
Reading Hospital, **West Reading**	(G+)(HR)(G+)(E+)(G)
Regional Hospital of Scranton, **Scranton**	(G)(E)(S)
Riddle Hospital, **Media**	(G)(E)(G)
Robert Packer Hospital, **Sayre**	(G+)
Sacred Heart Hospital, **Allentown**	(G+)
Saint Vincent Health System, **Erie**	(S+)(HR)(G+)(HR)
Sharon Regional Hospital, **Sharon**	(G+)(HR)
St. Clair Hospital, **Pittsburgh**	(G+)(E+)

American Heart Association.

(PENNSYLVANIA CONTINUED)

St. Joseph Regional Health Network, **Reading** ...... G+ HR G+ E S
St. Luke's Hospital - Anderson Campus, **Easton** ...... G+ E
St. Luke's Hospital Quakertown Campus, **Quakertown** ...... G+ E+
St. Luke's Monroe Campus, **Stroudsburg** ...... S+ E+
St. Luke's University Hospital, **Bethlehem** ...... G+ E+
St. Mary Medical Center, **Langhorne** ...... G G+ E+ G
Suburban Community Hospital , **Norristown** ...... G+ G+ E
Temple University Hospital, **Philadelphia** ...... G+ E+
The Children's Hospital of Philadelphia, **Philadelphia** ...... G
The Good Samaritan Health System, **Lebanon** ...... G+ HR G+ E
The Hospital of the University of Pennsylvania, **Philadelphia** ...... G+ G+ E+ S+
Thomas Jefferson University Hospital, **Philadelphia** ...... G+ E+
Uniontown Hospital, **Uniontown** ...... G+ E
UPMC Altoona, **Altoona** ...... G+ E+
UPMC East, **Monroeville** ...... G+ E+
UPMC Hamot, **Erie** ...... G+ HR G+ E+
UPMC Horizon, **Greenville** ...... S+
UPMC Mercy Pittsburgh, **Pittsburgh** ...... G+ E+
UPMC Northwest, **Seneca** ...... G+ E
UPMC Passavant, **Pittsburgh** ...... G+ HR
UPMC Pinnacle Hanover, **Hanover** ...... G+ HR
UPMC Pinnacle Harrisburg, Community and West Shore Campuses, **Harrisburg** ...... G+ HR G+ HR S+
UPMC Presbyterian, **Pittsburgh** ...... G+ E+
UPMC Shadyside, **Pittsburgh** ...... G+ E+
UPMC Somerset , **Somerset** ...... S+
UPMC St. Margaret, **Pittsburgh** ...... G+
Washington Health System, **Washington** ...... G+ E
Wayne Memorial Hospital, **Honesdale** ...... S
Waynesboro Hospital, **Waynesboro** ...... S+ HR
WellSpan Ephrata Community Hospital and the Center for Heart Care, **Ephrata** ...... G+ HR G+ E
WellSpan Gettysburg Hospital, **Gettysburg** ...... G+ HR G+ E
WellSpan Health - York Hospital, **York** ...... G+ HR G+ G+ E
West Penn Allegheny Health System, **Pittsburgh** ...... G+ HR
Wilkes Barre General Hospital, **Wilkes Barre** ...... S+ E

PUERTO RICO

Hospital HIMA San Pablo Bayamon, **Bayamon** ...... G+ HR
Hospital HIMA - San Pablo - Caguas, **Caguas** ...... G+ HR G+ E+

RHODE ISLAND

Kent Hospital, **Warwick** ...... G+ HR
Landmark Medical Center, **Woonsocket** ...... G+
Newport Hospital, **Newport** ...... G+
Our Lady of Fatima Hospital, **North Providence** ...... G
Rhode Island Hospital, **Providence** ...... G+ E+
South County Hospital, **Wakefield** ...... G+
The Miriam Hospital, **Providence** ...... G+ E

SOUTH CAROLINA

Aiken Regional Medical Center, **Aiken** ...... G+ E
AnMed Health, **Anderson** ...... G G+ HR
Beaufort Memorial Hospital, **Beaufort** ...... G+ E G
Bon Secours St. Francis-Downtown, **Greenville** ...... G+ HR G+ E+
Bon Secours St. Francis Hospital, **Charleston** ...... G+ E+
Coastal Carolina Hospital, **Hardeeville** ...... G+ E+
Conway Medical Center, **Conway** ...... G+ E+
East Cooper Medical Center, **Mount Pleasant** ...... S+ HR
Grand Strand Medical Center, **Myrtle Beach** ...... G+ E+
Lexington Medical Center, **West Columbia** ...... G+ G+ E+ G S
McLeod Regional Medical Center, **Florence** ...... G+ E+
Mount Pleasant Hospital, **Mount Pleasant** ...... S+ HR
MUSC Health, **Charleston** ...... G+ E+
MUSC Health Florence Medical Center, **Florence** ...... S
MUSC Health Lancaster Medical Center, **Lancaster** ...... G+ E+
Piedmont Medical Center, **Rock Hill** ...... G+ HR G+ G+ E
Prisma Health Baptist Hospital, **Columbia** ...... S S+
Prisma Health Baptist Parkridge Hospital, **Columbia** ...... S+

Prisma Health Greenville Memorial Hospital, **Greenville** ...... G+ E+
Prisma Health Greer Memorial Hospital, **Greer** ...... G+ E
Prisma Health Richland Hospital, **Columbia** ...... G+ G * G+ E+ G+
Ralph H. Johnson VA Medical Center, **Charleston** ...... S+
Regional Medical Center of Orangeburg & Calhoun Counties, **Orangeburg** ...... G+ E
Roper Hospital, **Charleston** ...... G+ E+
Self Regional Healthcare, **Greenwood** ...... G+ HR
Spartanburg Medical Center - Mary Black Campus, **Spartanburg** ...... G+ HR
Summerville Medical Center, **Summerville** ...... G+ HR
Tidelands Georgetown Memorial Hospital, **Georgetown** ...... G+ E+
Tidelands Waccamaw Community Hospital, **Murrells Inlet** ...... G+ E+
Trident Medical Center, **Charleston** ...... G+ E+

SOUTH DAKOTA

Avera St. Luke's Hospital, **Aberdeen** ...... G+
Rapid City Regional Hospital, **Rapid City** ...... G+ E
Sanford USD Medical Center, **Sioux Falls** ...... G

TENNESSEE

Baptist Memorial Hospital Memphis, **Memphis** ...... S+ E+
Blount Memorial Hospital, **Maryville** ...... S+ E
Bristol Regional Medical Center, **Bristol** ...... S HR G G
CHI Memorial, **Chattanooga** ...... S+ E
Erlanger East Hospital, **Chattanooga** ...... S+
Erlanger Health System, **Chattanooga** ...... G+ E+
Fort Sanders Regional Medical Center, **Knoxville** ...... G+ E+ G+
Holston Valley Medical Center, **Kingsport** ...... G G
Jackson-Madison County General Hospital, **Jackson** ...... G+ E+
LeConte Medical Center, **Sevierville** ...... G+
Methodist Healthcare University Hospital, **Memphis** ...... G+ E+
Methodist LeBonheur Healthcare, **Memphis** ...... G+
Methodist Medical Center, **Oak Ridge** ...... G+ S
Morristown-Hamblen Healthcare System, **Morristown** ...... S+
Newport Medical Center, **Newport** ...... S+
North Knoxville Medical Center, **Powell** ...... G+ E+
Parkridge Medical Center, **Chattanooga** ...... S
Parkwest Medical Center, **Knoxville** ...... G+ S
Saint Francis Hospital - Memphis, **Memphis** ...... G+ E
Saint Thomas Midtown Hospital, **Nashville** ...... G+ E+
Saint Thomas Rutherford Hospital, **Murfreesboro** ...... G+ E
Saint Thomas West Hospital, **Nashville** ...... G+ E+
St. Francis Hospital - Bartlett, **Bartlett** ...... G+ E+
Sumner Regional Medical Center, **Gallatin** ...... G+ E
The University of Tennessee Medical Center, **Knoxville** ...... G+ G+ E+
TriStar Centennial Medical Center, **Brentwood** ...... G+ E+
TriStar Hendersonville Medical Center, **Hendersonville** ...... S+
TriStar Horizon Medical Center, **Dickson** ...... S+ HR
TriStar Skyline Medical Center, **Nashville** ...... S+ E+
TriStar Southern Hills Medical Center, **Nashville** ...... G+ HR
TriStar Summit Medical Center, **Hermitage** ...... G+ E+
Turkey Creek Medical Center, **Knoxville** ...... S+
Vanderbilt University Medical Center, **Nashville** ...... G+ E+

TEXAS

AdventHealth - Central Texas, **Killeen** ...... G HR G+
Baptist Health System, **San Antonio** ...... G+ HR
Baylor All Saints Medical Center, **Fort Worth** ...... G+ E
Baylor Jack and Jane Hamilton Heart and Vascular Hospital, **Dallas** ...... S+ S
Baylor Scott & White Lake Pointe, **Rowlett** ...... G+
Baylor Scott & White, Marble Falls, **Marble Falls** ...... S+ E+
Baylor Scott & White Medical Center - Centennial, **Frisco** ...... S+
Baylor Scott & White Medical Center - College Station, **College Station** ...... G+ E
Baylor Scott & White Medical Center - Grapevine, **Grapevine** ...... G+ E+
Baylor Scott & White Medical Center - Hillcrest, **Waco** ...... G+ HR
Baylor Scott & White Medical Center - Irving, **Irving** ...... G+ E
Baylor Scott & White Medical Center - McKinney, **McKinney** ...... G+
Baylor Scott & White Medical Center - Round Rock, **Round Rock** ...... G+ E+
Baylor Scott & White Medical Center - Temple, **Temple** ...... G+ E+
Baylor Scott & White Medical Center Lakeway, **Lakeway** ...... S+
Baylor Scott & White Medical Center of Plano, **Plano** ...... S+

*These hospitals received Get With The Guidelines-Resuscitation awards from the American Heart Association for two or more patient populations.

Baylor Scott & White The Heart Hospital - Plano, **Plano** ...... G+ HR
Baylor University Medical Center at Dallas, **Dallas** ...... G+ E+
Ben Taub Hospital, **Houston** ...... S G+ E+ G+ G
Brazosport Regional Health System, **Lake Jackson** ...... G+ HR
BSA Health System, **Amarillo** ...... G+ HR
Cedar Park Regional Medical Center, **Cedar Park** ...... G+ HR
Central Texas Medical Center, **San Marcos** ...... G+ HR
CHI St. Joseph Health Regional, **Bryan** ...... G+ G+ E+ S+ S
CHI St. Luke's Health – Baylor St. Luke's Medical Center, **Houston** ...... G+ E
CHI St. Luke's Health – The Woodlands Hospital, **The Woodlands** ...... G+ E+ S G
CHI St. Luke's Health Memorial Lufkin, **Lufkin** ...... G+ E
Children's Medical Center Dallas, **Dallas** ...... S+ *
CHRISTUS Good Shepherd Health System - Longview, **Longview** ...... G+ E+
CHRISTUS Good Shepherd Medical Center - Marshall, **Marshall** ...... G+ E+
CHRISTUS Santa Rosa Health, **San Antonio** ...... G+ HR
CHRISTUS Southeast Texas Health System - St. Elizabeth, **Beaumont** ...... G+ E+
CHRISTUS Spohn Hospital Corpus Christi - Shoreline, **Corpus Christi** ...... G+ E
CHRISTUS St. Michael Health System, **Texarkana** ...... G+ E+
CHRISTUS St. Michael Hospital-Atlanta, **Atlanta** ...... S+ E
Citizens Medical Center, **Victoria** ...... G+ E+ G
Connally Memorial Medical Center, **Floresville** ...... G
Corpus Christi Medical Center, **Corpus Christi** ...... G+ E
Covenant Medical Center, **Lubbock** ...... G+ E
Cuero Regional Hospital, **Cuero** ...... G+
Cypress Fairbanks Medical Center, **Houston** ...... G+ E+
Dallas Regional Medical Center, **Mesquite** ...... S+
Del Sol Medical Center, **El Paso** ...... G+ E
Dell Seton Medical Center at The University of Texas, **Austin** ...... G+ E+
DeTar Healthcare System, **Victoria** ...... G+ E+ S+ S
Doctors Hospital at Renaissance, **Edinburg** ...... G+ HR G+ E
Doctors Hospital of Laredo, **Laredo** ...... S+ HR
HCA Houston Healthcare - Clear Lake, **Webster** ...... G+ E+ G
HCA Houston Healthcare-Southeast, **Pasadena** ...... G+ S
HCA Houston Healthcare Conroe, **Conroe** ...... G+ E+ G+
HCA Houston Healthcare Kingwood, **Kingwood** ...... G+ E+
HCA Houston Healthcare North Cypress, **Cypress** ...... G+ E+ G+ G
HCA Houston Healthcare Northwest, **Houston** ...... G+ E+
HCA Houston Healthcare Tomball, **Tomball** ...... S+
HCA- West Houston Medical Center, **Houston** ...... G+ E+
Heart Hospital of Austin, **Austin** ...... S+
Hendrick Medical Center, **Abilene** ...... G+ E+ S S
Houston Methodist Baytown Hospital, **Baytown** ...... G+ G+ E
Houston Methodist Clear Lake Hospital, **Nassau Bay** ...... G+ E+
Houston Methodist Hospital, **Houston** ...... S+ G+ E+
Houston Methodist Sugar Land Hospital, **Sugar Land** ...... G+ E+
Houston Methodist The Woodlands Hospital, **The Woodlands** ...... G+ E
Houston Methodist West Hospital, **Houston** ...... G+ E+
Houston Methodist Willowbrook Hospital, **Houston** ...... G+ E+
Huntsville Memorial Hospital, **Huntsville** ...... G+ E+
JPS Health Network, **Fort Worth** ...... G+ E+
Knapp Medical Center, **Weslaco** ...... G+ HR
Las Palmas Medical Center, **El Paso** ...... G+
Medical Center Hospital, **Odessa** ...... S+ G+ HR
Medical City Dallas, **Dallas** ...... G G+ *
Methodist Charlton Medical Center, **Dallas** ...... G+ HR G+
Methodist Dallas Medical Center, **Dallas** ...... G+ E S
Methodist Hospital, **San Antonio** ...... G+ E+
Methodist Mansfield Medical Center, **Mansfield** ...... G+ E+ G+
Methodist Richardson Medical Center, **Richardson** ...... G+ HR G+
Methodist Stone Oak Hospital, **San Antonio** ...... G+ E+
Metropolitan Methodist Hospital, **San Antonio** ...... S+ G+ E+
Midland Memorial Hospital, **Midland** ...... S
Nacogdoches Medical Center, **Nacogdoches** ...... S+ S
Northeast Methodist Hospital, **San Antonio** ...... G+ E
OakBend Medical Center, **Richmond** ...... G+
Parkland Health & Hospital System, **Dallas** ...... G+ G+ E G
Providence Health Center, **Waco** ...... G+ HR
Resolute Health Hospital , **New Braunfels** ...... S+ E+
Rio Grande Regional Hospital, **McAllen** ...... G+ E+ S
Seton Medical Center Austin, **Austin** ...... G+ E
Seton Medical Center Hays, **Kyle** ...... G+ E

Seton Medical Center Williamson, **Round Rock** ...... G+ HR
Shannon Medical Center, **San Angelo** ...... G+ G+ G G
South Texas Health System, **Edinburg** ...... S+ E+
Southwest General Hospital, **San Antonio** ...... G+ E+
St. David's Georgetown Hospital, **Georgetown** ...... G
St. David's Medical Center, **Austin** ...... G+ E+ G
St. David's North Austin Medical Center, **Austin** ...... G+ HR G G
St. David's Round Rock Medical Center, **Round Rock** ...... G+ E G+
St. David's South Austin Medical Center, **Austin** ...... S+ HR G+ E G
St. Joseph Medical Center, **Houston** ...... G+ E+
Texas Health Arlington Memorial Hospital, **Arlington** ...... G+ HR G+ E
Texas Health Denton, **Denton** ...... S+ E+ G+
Texas Health Fort Worth, **Fort Worth** ...... G+ E+
Texas Health Heart and Vascular Hospital, **Arlington** ...... G+ HR
Texas Health Huguley Hospital Fort Worth South, **Burleson** ...... S
Texas Health Hurst Euless Bedford, **Bedford** ...... G S
Texas Health Presbyterian Hospital Dallas, **Dallas** ...... G+ HR S
Texas Health Presbyterian Hospital Plano, **Plano** ...... S+ HR G
Texoma Medical Center, **Denison** ...... G+ E+
The Hospitals of Providence East Campus, **El Paso** ...... G+ HR
The Hospitals of Providence Memorial Campus, **El Paso** ...... S+
The Hospitals of Providence Sierra Campus, **El Paso** ...... G+ HR
The Hospitals of Providence Transmountain Campus, **El Paso** ...... G+
The University of Texas Medical Branch - Galveston Campus, **Galveston** ...... G G+ E+
Titus Regional Medical Center, **MT Pleasant** ...... G+ E+
United Regional Healthcare System, **Wichita Falls** ...... G+ E
University Health System, **San Antonio** ...... G+ E+
University Medical Center of El Paso, **El Paso** ...... G+ E+
UT Health - Tyler, **Tyler** ...... G+ HR
UT Southwestern Medical Center, **Dallas** ...... G+ E+
Valley Baptist Medical Center-Brownsville, **Brownsville** ...... G+ E+
Valley Baptist Medical Center-Harlingen, **Harlingen** ...... G+ E+
Valley Regional Medical Center, **Brownsville** ...... G+ E+ S
Wadley Regional Medical Center, **Texarkana** ...... G+ E
Wise Health System, **Decatur** ...... S+ S

UTAH

American Fork Hospital, **American Fork** ...... S+ E+
Davis Hospital and Medical Center, **Layton** ...... G+ E
Dixie Regional Medical Center, **Saint George** ...... G+ E+
Intermountain Medical Center, **Murray** ...... G+ E+
Jordan Valley Medical Center/JVMC-West Valley Campus/Mountain Point Medical Center, a Campus of JVMC, **West Jordan** ...... G+ E
Lakeview Hospital, **Bountiful** ...... G+ E+
McKay-Dee Hospital, **Ogden** ...... G+ E+
Mountain View Hospital - Payson, **Payson** ...... G+
Ogden Regional Medical Center, **Ogden** ...... G+ E+
St. Mark's Hospital, **Salt Lake City** ...... G+ E+
Timpanogos Regional Hospital, **Orem** ...... G+
University of Utah Health, **Salt Lake City** ...... G+ HR G+ E+
Utah Valley Hospital, **Provo** ...... G+ E+

VERMONT

The University of Vermont Medical Center, **Burlington** ...... G+

VIRGINIA

Augusta Health, **Fishersville** ...... S G+ HR
Bon Secours DePaul Medical Center, **Norfolk** ...... G+ E+ G
Bon Secours Mary Immaculate Hospital, **Newport News** ......
Bon Secours Maryview Medical Center, **Portsmouth** ...... G+ E+ G+
Bon Secours Memorial Regional Medical Center, **Mechanicsville** ...... G+ HR G+
Bon Secours Rappahannock General Hospital, **Kilmarnock** ...... G+ HR
Bon Secours Richmond Community Hospital, **Richmond** ...... S+ HR
Bon Secours St. Francis Medical Center, **Midlothian** ...... G+ HR G+
Bon Secours St. Mary's Hospital, **Richmond** ...... G+ HR G+ HR G
Carilion Roanoke Memorial Hospital, **Roanoke** ...... G+ HR
Centra Lynchburg General Hospital, **Lynchburg** ...... G+ E+ E+
Centra Southside Community Hospital, **Farmville** ...... S+ E
Chesapeake Regional Medical Center, **Chesapeake** ...... G+ G
Fauquier Hospital, **Warrenton** ...... S+

American Heart Association.

(VIRGINIA CONTINUED)

Inova Alexandria Hospital, **Alexandria**............................ G+ E G+ S
Inova Fair Oaks Hospital, **Fairfax** .... G+ E
Inova Fairfax Hospital, **Falls Church** .... G+ E+ G+ S
Inova Loudoun Hospital, **Leesburg**........................... G+ E+ S+
Inova Mount Vernon Hospital, **Alexandria** .... G+ E+
John Randolph Medical Center, **Hopewell** .... G+ G+ HR
Mary Washington Hospital, **Fredericksburg**.............. G+ E
Novant Health UVA Health System Haymarket Medical Center, **Haymarket**....... G+
Novant Health UVA Health System Prince William Medical Center,
 Manassas... G+ HR G+ HR
Reston Hospital Center, **Reston** .... G+ E+
Riverside Regional Medical Center, **Newport News**.......... G+ E+
Sentara CarePlex Hospital, **Hampton** .... S+ E+
Sentara Leigh Hospital, **Norfolk**............................... G+ E+ G
Sentara Louise Obici Memorial Hospital, **Suffolk** .... G+ E+
Sentara Martha Jefferson Hospital, **Charlottesville**..... G+ E+
Sentara Norfolk General Hospital/Sentara Heart Hospital, **Norfolk**.......... G+ E+
Sentara Northern Virginia Medical Center, **Woodbridge** ..... G+ E+ S+
Sentara Princess Anne Hospital, **Virginia Beach** .... G+ E+
Sentara RMH Healthcare, **Harrisonburg** .... S+ E+ S+
Sentara Virginia Beach General Hospital, **Virginia Beach** .... G+ E+ S+
Sentara Williamsburg Regional Medical Center, **Williamsburg** .... S+ E+
Southside Regional Medical Center, **Petersburg**.............. S+
StoneSprings Hospital Center, **Dulles**....................... G+
The University of Virginia Health System, **Charlottesville**......... G+ HR G+ E+ G
Twin County Regional Healthcare, **Galax** .... G+ E+
VCU Community Memorial Hospital, **South Hill**........... G+ E+
Virginia Commonwealth University Medical Center, **Richmond** .... G+ E+
Virginia Hospital Center, **Arlington**......................... S+ E
Winchester Medical Center, **Winchester**.................... G

WASHINGTON

Confluence Health-Central Washington Hospital, **Wenatchee** .... G+ E+ G+
EvergreenHealth Medical Center, **Kirkland** .... G+ E+
EvergreenHealth Monroe, **Monroe** .... G+ HR
Harborview Medical Center, **Seattle** .... G+ E+ G
Harrison Medical Center, **Bremerton**........................ S+ HR G+ E+
Highline Medical Center, **Burien**............................... G+ E+
Jefferson Healthcare, **Port Townsend** .... S G+
Legacy Salmon Creek Medical Center, **Vancouver** ..... G+ HR
MultiCare Deaconess Hospital, **Spokane**................... G+ E+
MultiCare Good Samaritan Hospital, **Puyallup**............ G+ E
MultiCare Valley Hospital, **Spokane Valley**................ S+ G
Northwest Hospital & Medical Center, **Seattle**............ G+
Overlake Medical Center, **Bellevue**.......................... G+ E
PeaceHealth Southwest Medical Center, Stroke & Telestroke Program,
 Vancouver .... G+ E
PeaceHealth St. John Medical Center, **Longview** .... G+ HR
PeaceHealth St. Joseph Medical Center, **Bellingham** ... G+ E+
Providence Centralia Hospital, **Centralia**.................. G+
Providence Regional Medical Center Everett, **Everett** ..... G+ E+
Providence Sacred Heart Medical Center & Children's Hospital, **Spokane** ..... G+ E+
Providence St. Mary Medical Center, **Walla Walla** .... G+
Providence St. Peter Hospital, **Olympia** .... G+ S G+ E+
Saint Anthony Hospital, **Gig Harbor** .... G+ E+
Seattle Children's Hospital, **Seattle** .... S+ *
Seattle VA Medical Center, **Seattle** .... S+ HR
Skagit Valley Hospital, **Mount Vernon**...................... G+ E
St. Clare Hospital, **Lakewood** .... G+
St. Joseph Medical Center, **Tacoma**.......................... S+ HR G+ E+
Swedish Edmonds, **Edmonds** .... G+ E+
Swedish Medical Center - Cherry Hill Campus, **Seattle**........ G+ E+
Swedish Medical Center - First Hill Campus, **Seattle** .... S
Swedish Medical Center - Issaquah Campus , **Issaquah**........ G+

Trios Health, **Kennewick**.. G+ HR
University of Washington Medical Center, **Seattle** .... S+
UW Medicine | Valley Medical Center, **Renton** .... G+
UW Medicine | Valley Medical Center, **Renton** ....
Virginia Mason Medical Center, **Seattle**..................... G+ E+ G
Virginia Mason Memorial Hospital, **Yakima**................. G+ S G+ HR

WEST VIRGINIA

Cabell Huntington Hospital, **Huntington** .... G+ S+ G+ E+
CAMC General Hospital, **Charleston** .... S S E
Mon Health Medical Center, **Morgantown** .... G+
Ohio Valley Medical Center, Inc., **Wheeling**................ G+
Raleigh General Hospital, **Beckley** .... S
St. Mary's Medical Center, **Huntington**...................... G+ G G+ HR
United Hospital Center, **Bridgeport** .... G+ G+ G+ E
West Virginia University Hospital, Inc., **Morgantown** ...... G+ HR G+ E
Wheeling Hospital, **Wheeling** .... G+

WISCONSIN

Ascension All Saints Hospital, **Racine** .... G+ G+ E
Ascension Columbia St. Mary's Hospital Milwaukee, **Milwaukee** ..... G+
Ascension Columbia St. Mary's Hospital Ozaukee, **Mequon** .... G+ HR
Ascension NE Wisconsin- Mercy Campus, **Oshkosh**.......... G+
Ascension NE Wisconsin- St. Elizabeth Campus, **Appleton** .... G+ E
Ascension SE Wisconsin Hospital - Elmbrook Campus, **Brookfield** .... G+ HR
Ascension St. Joseph Hospital, **Milwaukee**................. G+ HR
Aspirus Wausau Hospital, **Wausau**............................ G+ E
Aurora BayCare Medical Center, **Green Bay** .... G G+ HR G+ E+
Aurora Lakeland Medical Center, **Elkhorn** .... G+ HR G+ E
Aurora Medical Center - Grafton, **Grafton**.................. G+ G+ HR
Aurora Medical Center - Kenosha, **Kenosha**............... G+ HR G+ E
Aurora Medical Center - Oshkosh, **Oshkosh**............... S+ G+ E+
Aurora Medical Center Manitowoc County, **Two Rivers** ..... G+ HR S+ E+
Aurora Medical Center Summit, **Summit** .... G+ G+ E
Aurora Medical Center Washington County, **Hartford** .... G+
Aurora Memorial Hospital Burlington, **Burlington** .... G+
Aurora Sheboygan Memorial Medical Center, **Sheboygan**...... G+ E+
Aurora Sinai Medical Center, **Milwaukee**.................... G+ HR G+ E+
Aurora St. Luke's Medical Center, **Milwaukee** .... G+ HR G+ E+
Aurora St. Luke's South Shore, **Cudahy** .... G+ HR G+ E+
Aurora West Allis Medical Center, **West Allis** .... G+ HR E+
Bellin Memorial Hospital, **Green Bay**......................... G+ E
Beloit Memorial Hospital, **Beloit** ....
F & MCW – Community Memorial Hospital, **Menomonee Falls**...... S
Froedtert Hospital, **Milwaukee**.................. G+ HR S+ ★ G+ E+
Gundersen Lutheran Medical Center, **La Crosse**.......... G+ E+
Marshfield Medical Center, **Marshfield** .... G+ E+
Mayo Clinic Health System in Eau Claire, **Eau Claire**...... G+
Mayo Clinic Health System LaCrosse, **La Crosse** .... G+ E
Mercy Hospital and Trauma Center, **Janesville**............ G+ E
Oconomowoc Memorial Hospital, **Oconomowoc** .... G+
SSM Health St. Clare Hospital, **Baraboo**.................... G+ HR
SSM Health St. Mary's Hospital - Madison, **Madison** ..... G+ E+
St. Agnes Hospital, **Fond Du Lac** .... G+ G+ HR
St. Mary's Janesville Hospital, **Janesville**.................. G+ HR
ThedaCare Regional Medical Center-Neenah, **Neenah** ..... G+ HR
United Hospital System - St. Catherine's Medical Center Campus,
 Pleasant Prairie... G+ HR
United Hospital System Inc, **Kenosha** .... S
UnityPoint Health -Meriter, **Madison** .... G G+ E
University of Wisconsin Hospital, **Madison** .... G+ E+ G S
Waukesha Memorial Hospital, **Waukesha**.................. G+ E

WYOMING

Cheyenne Regional Medical Center, **Cheyenne** .... G+ S G+ E
Wyoming Medical Center, **Casper** .... G+ E+

This content is available online at **https://custom.usnewsbrandfuse.com/american-heart-association**

---

*These hospitals received Get With The Guidelines-Resuscitation awards from the American Heart Association for two or more patient populations.

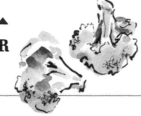

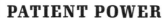
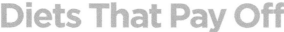

Diets That Pay Off

U.S. News puts 41 eating plans through their paces

AS STRUGGLING DIETERS have learned, losing weight is tough, and most diets don't deliver. This is why U.S. News produces its Best Diets rankings, based on the views of a panel of nationally recognized experts (Page 102) who considered the effectiveness of some of the best-known eating plans, whether the aim is to lose weight, improve heart health, or manage diabetes.

Our panelists reviewed the research, added their own fact-finding, and rated the diets from 1 to 5 (the top score) in a number of areas: short-term weight loss (the likelihood of losing significant weight during the first 12 months); long-term weight loss (the likelihood of maintaining significant weight loss for two years or more); diabetes prevention and management; heart health (effectiveness at preventing cardiovascular disease and reducing risk for heart patients); ease of compliance; nutritional completeness (how well a plan meets federal dietary guidelines); and safety (whether, for example, it omits key nutrients).

Which plan can help you achieve your goals? Check out the results in these pages. For more on the plans, visit usnews.com/bestdiets.

How the Plans Compare Overall

Forty-one diets were rated from 1 to 5 on multiple measures. Rank is based on a score compiled from panelists' average scores for each measure. The results:

Rank	Diet	Overall score	Short-term weight loss	Long-term weight loss	For diabetes	For heart health	Nutrition	Safety	Easy to follow
1	Mediterranean	4.2	2.9	3.1	3.8	4.4	4.8	4.9	3.8
2	DASH	4.1	3.0	3.3	3.5	4.3	4.8	4.8	3.3
3	Flexitarian	4.0	3.5	3.3	3.5	3.9	4.6	4.7	3.5
4	MIND	3.9	2.8	2.8	3.3	4.0	4.6	4.7	3.4
4	WW (Weight Watchers)	3.9	3.9	3.4	3.4	3.3	4.6	4.5	3.5
6	Mayo Clinic	3.8	3.2	3.1	3.5	3.5	4.5	4.4	3.0
6	Volumetrics	3.8	3.7	3.3	3.5	3.3	4.5	4.5	2.9
8	TLC	3.7	3.0	2.7	3.0	4.0	4.6	4.6	2.7
9	Nordic	3.6	2.8	3.2	3.0	3.3	4.6	4.5	2.4
9	Ornish	3.6	3.4	3.1	3.4	4.4	4.1	4.2	1.9
11	Fertility	3.5	2.5	2.3	3.1	3.1	4.2	4.2	3.3
11	Jenny Craig	3.5	3.8	3.0	3.4	3.1	3.8	3.9	3.1
11	Vegetarian	3.5	3.2	3.0	3.1	3.7	4.0	4.1	2.6
14	Asian	3.4	2.8	2.9	2.7	3.0	4.2	4.3	2.5
15	Anti-Inflammatory	3.3	2.6	2.4	3.0	3.5	3.8	4.0	2.6
15	Flat Belly	3.3	3.2	2.5	2.7	3.2	3.9	3.9	2.8
15	Nutritarian	3.3	3.2	2.7	3.3	3.5	3.7	3.9	1.9
15	Spark Solution	3.3	3.2	2.6	2.6	2.7	4.1	4.2	2.4
19	Engine 2	3.2	3.6	3.0	3.3	3.8	3.1	3.5	1.9
20	Eco-Atkins	3.1	3.5	2.6	2.9	3.3	3.4	3.4	2.1
20	South Beach	3.1	3.5	2.5	2.8	2.7	3.4	3.5	2.8
20	Vegan	3.1	3.6	3.2	3.4	4.0	2.8	3.3	1.5
23	Biggest Loser	3.0	3.8	2.3	2.9	2.9	3.5	3.4	2.3
23	Glycemic Index	3.0	2.7	2.2	2.8	2.5	3.7	3.8	2.0
23	Nutrisystem	3.0	3.7	2.5	3.0	2.6	3.1	3.5	2.5
23	Zone	3.0	3.2	2.5	2.7	2.8	3.5	3.6	2.2
27	Abs	2.9	2.8	2.0	2.5	2.5	3.4	3.6	2.7
27	Macrobiotic	2.9	2.9	2.7	3.0	3.3	2.9	3.3	1.7
27	SlimFast	2.9	3.8	2.5	2.8	2.5	2.9	3.1	2.7
30	HMR Program	2.8	4.1	2.3	2.8	2.6	2.9	3.0	2.4
31	Optavia	2.7	3.9	2.2	2.9	2.8	2.6	2.9	2.1
32	Alkaline	2.5	2.3	1.9	2.1	2.3	2.7	3.1	2.0
33	Fast	2.4	3.1	2.1	2.2	2.3	2.7	2.5	2.0
33	Paleo	2.4	3.0	2.3	2.6	2.0	2.3	2.8	1.9
33	Raw Food	2.4	3.6	2.9	2.9	2.9	2.1	2.2	1.1
33	Supercharged Hormone	2.4	2.9	2.0	2.2	2.1	2.7	2.8	2.0
37	Atkins	2.2	3.9	2.2	2.7	2.0	1.8	2.2	1.9
38	Keto	2.1	3.9	2.3	2.8	2.1	1.4	1.9	1.4
38	Whole30	2.1	3.0	1.8	2.0	1.8	2.0	2.6	1.5
40	Body Reset	2.0	2.8	1.4	1.6	1.7	2.1	2.7	1.7
41	Dukan	1.9	3.2	2.0	2.1	1.5	1.6	2.2	1.4

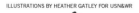

Best Weight Loss Diets

Diets are ranked by the average of the scores experts assigned them for producing short- and long-term results.

Rank	Diet	Avg. score
1	WW (Weight Watchers)	3.7
2	Volumetrics	3.5
3	Flexitarian	3.4
3	Jenny Craig	3.4
3	Vegan	3.4
6	Engine 2	3.3
6	Ornish	3.3
6	Raw Food	3.3
9	HMR Program	3.2
9	Mayo Clinic	3.2
9	SlimFast	3.2

Best Diets for the Heart

With these plans, you can take aim at cholesterol, blood pressure or triglycerides, as well as weight.

Rank	Diet	Avg. score
1	Mediterranean	4.4
1	Ornish	4.4
3	Dash	4.3
4	MIND	4.0
4	TLC	4.0
4	Vegan	4.0
7	Flexitarian	3.9
8	Engine 2	3.8
9	Vegetarian	3.7
10	Anti-Inflammatory	3.5
10	Mayo Clinic	3.5
10	Nutritarian	3.5

The Expert Panel

Twenty-five panelists reviewed detailed assessments of the U.S. News list of 41 diets and rated them on a number of key measures, described on Page 101.

Louis Aronne
Professor of metabolic research at Weill Cornell Medical College

Kathie Beals
Associate professor, clinical, division of nutrition, University of Utah

Amy Campbell
Nutrition and wellness consultant and writer

Lawrence Cheskin
Director, Johns Hopkins Weight Management Center

Michael Dansinger
Founding director of the Diabetes Reversal Program at Tufts Medical Center

Michael Davidson
Director of preventive cardiology, University of Chicago Medical Center

Meredith Dillon
Registered dietitian specializing in pediatric Type 1 and Type 2 diabetes at Children's National Medical Center

Teresa Fung
Professor of nutrition, Simmons College

Hollie Gelberg
Clinical/research dietitian at the Department of Veterans Affairs Greater Los Angeles Healthcare System

Andrea Giancoli
Nutrition communications consultant

Michael Greger
Physician, author and internationally recognized speaker on nutrition, food safety and public health issues

Stephan Guyenet
Neurobiologist and writer who specializes in the role of the brain in eating behavior and body fatness

David Katz
Director, Yale-Griffin Prevention Research Center

Penny Kris-Etherton
Distinguished professor of nutrition, Pennsylvania State University

JoAnn Manson
Professor of women's health, Harvard Medical School

Yasmin Mossavar-Rahmani
Associate professor of clinical epidemiology and population health, Albert Einstein College of Medicine

Elisabetta Politi
Nutrition director, Duke Diet and Fitness Center

Rebecca Reeves
Adjunct assistant professor, University of Texas School of Public Health

Eric Rimm
Professor of epidemiology and nutrition, and director of the Program in Cardiovascular Epidemiology at the Harvard T.H. Chan School of Public Health

Susan Roberts
Professor of nutrition, Tufts University and founder of the iDiet weight loss program

Lisa Sasson
Clinical associate professor of nutrition, food studies and public health, New York University

Laurence Sperling
Founder and director of the Heart Disease Prevention Center at Emory University

Anne Thorndike
Assistant professor of medicine at Harvard Medical School and an associate physician at Massachusetts General Hospital

Jill Weisenberger
Author, health and wellness coach, and internationally recognized expert in nutrition and diabetes

Adrienne Youdim
Associate clinical professor of medicine, UCLA David Geffen School of Medicine, Cedars Sinai Medical Center

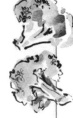

Best Diabetes Diets

These plans scored highest for both managing and preventing the condition.

Rank	Diet	Avg. score
1	Mediterranean	3.8
2	DASH	3.5
2	Flexitarian	3.5
2	Mayo Clinic	3.5
2	Volumetrics	3.5
6	Jenny Craig	3.4
6	Ornish	3.4
6	Vegan	3.4
6	WW (Weight Watchers)	3.4
10	Engine 2	3.3
10	Mind	3.3
10	Nutritarian	3.3

Best Plant-Based Diets

These diets emphasize minimally processed foods from plants and are good bets for weight loss.

Rank	Diet	Avg. score
1	Mediterranean	4.2
2	Flexitarian	4.0
3	Nordic	3.6
3	Ornish	3.6
5	Vegetarian	3.5
6	Asian	3.4
7	Anti-Inflammatory	3.3
7	Nutritarian	3.3
9	Engine 2	3.2
10	Eco-Atkins	3.1
10	Vegan	3.1

Best Commercial Diets

Nutritional value, ease of use and safety are counted, as well as weight loss effectiveness.

Rank	Diet	Avg. score
1	WW (Weight Watchers)	3.9
2	Jenny Craig	3.5
3	Nutritarian	3.3
4	South Beach	3.1
5	Biggest Loser	3.0
5	Nutrisystem	3.0
5	Zone	3.0
8	SlimFast	2.9
9	HMR Program	2.8
10	Optavia	2.7

Easiest-to-Follow Diets

The ranking is based on ease of use and a diet's ability to deliver weight loss and good nutrition.

Rank	Diet	Avg. score
1	Mediterranean	3.8
2	Flexitarian	3.5
2	WW (Weight Watchers)	3.5
4	MIND	3.4
5	DASH	3.3
5	Fertility	3.3
7	Jenny Craig	3.1
8	Mayo Clinic	3.0
9	Volumetrics	2.9
10	Flat Belly	2.8
10	South Beach	2.8

ILLUSTRATIONS BY HEATHER GATLEY FOR USN&WR

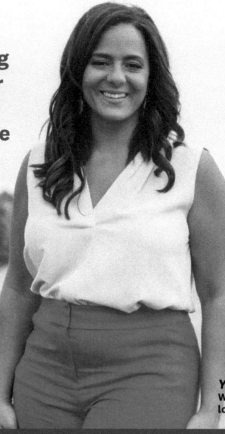
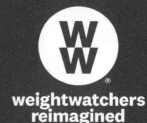

Eating Under the Microscope

13 weeks. 13 strangers. One big goal: to advance the science of weight loss

by **Katherine Hobson**

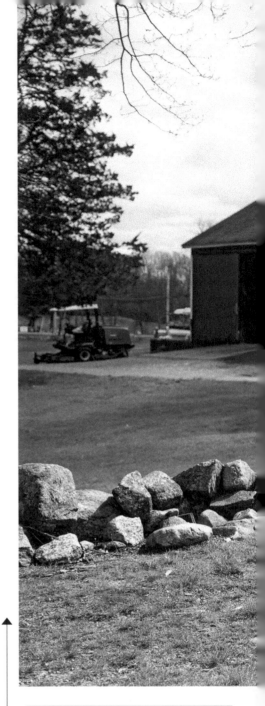

FOR MANY, THE JOURNEY from normal life to a stint living with strangers in a secluded conference center began with a Facebook ad. "JOIN OUR WEIGHT LOSS DIET STUDY!" it beckoned. "Lose 15% of your weight and stay for 3 months at a wooded lakefront retreat in Massachusetts."

"I thought it was fake," says Charisse Shields, a 33-year-old actress, recalling the promised perks: "free housing, gourmet meals and up to $10,000." But she discovered the study was, in fact, entirely legit and being led by prominent researchers at Boston Children's Hospital and Indiana University–Bloomington. By late April 2019, she and 12 fellow participants in the ambitious "FB4" study were preparing to leave the cocoon of the Warren Conference Center and Inn, where they'd spent the previous 13 weeks eating every morsel on their carefully calibrated plates in an attempt to answer a fundamental question in the science of weight loss: Which diet helps keep the pounds off?

"Many people can lose weight over the short term," says FB4 study director Cara Ebbeling, co-director of the Boston Children's obesity prevention center. What's tough is maintaining that loss over time. So before ever checking into the Inn, Shields and the others had to gradually lose at least 12% of their body weight, over about three months, by eating prepackaged, very-low-carb meals that the researchers provided. For Shields, this involved dodging abundant free food on a job site, where she became known as the lady who toted

The Three Diets

The FB4 study looks at whether the balance of nutrients affects metabolism and body fatness. All three study diets get about 20% of their calories from protein.

- **Very-low-carb**
  About 75% fat, 5% carbs.
  That means yes to nuts and bacon; no to dinner rolls and pasta.

- **High-carb with some added sugar but no refined grains**
  About 25% fat, 55% carbs, including veggies and whole grains; about 20% of total calories come from added sugars (such as jelly beans and gummy bears).

- **High-carb with no added sugar and some refined grains**
  About 25% fat, 55% carbs; about half of grains come from refined sources like crackers and rice cereal.

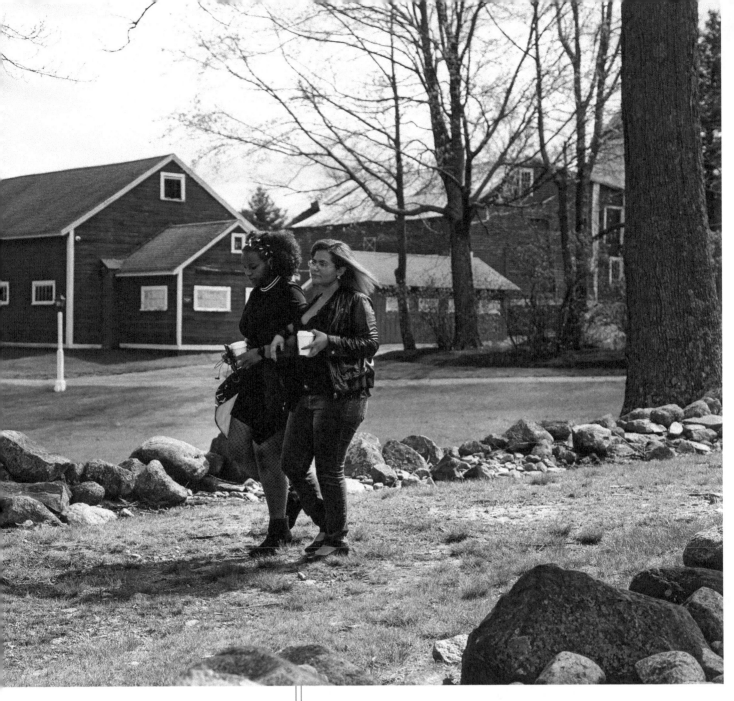

PARTICIPANTS STROLL THE STUDY GROUNDS IN ASHLAND, MASSACHUSETTS.

her study grub around in search of a microwave.

Restrictive diets are no picnic. Compounding matters: Once people lose weight, they burn fewer calories – a physiological slump that can undermine even valiant efforts. Thus the weight-maintenance focus of the roughly $13 million study, which is enrolling adults nationwide who are at least moderately overweight. Specifically, it's examining whether what people eat vs. simply how many calories impacts metabolism and body fat. Is there a sweet-spot ratio of carbs, protein and fat that can help prevent weight regain, when the body seems wired to self-sabotage?

When FB4 participants first arrive, they're assessed to estimate how many daily calories their newly slimmed bodies burn. Then they're randomly assigned to one of three diets (box, Page 104) with individualized calorie counts based on those measurements: very-low-carb; high-carb with some added sugar; and high-carb with no added sugar. The two high-carb variations are designed to tease out whether sugar is uniquely harmful to weight control, says pediatric endocrinologist David Ludwig, co-director of BCH's obesity prevention center and an FB4 principal investigator.

No crumbs left behind. Serving three meals a day that conform to the prescribed diets, with quantities painstakingly calculated to match each person's specific caloric burn rate, that taste good, and that provide variety enough to avert deadly boredom, wasn't what the resort's staff was used to. "We're a hospitality company," says Warren Conference Center and Inn General Manager Kim Sternick. But FB4 requires measuring ingredients down to at least the gram. Each meal is built around common elements, then tweaked to meet the diets' stringent requirements. Consider a taco-themed lunch: The very-low-carb group gets 80% lean ground beef with a romaine lettuce wrap, steamed cauliflower and walnuts; the high-carb, high-starch group gets a soft taco with 90% lean beef, tortilla chips, cauliflower with farro, and

FROM TOP: ELLEN WEBBER FOR USN&WR; GETTY IMAGES

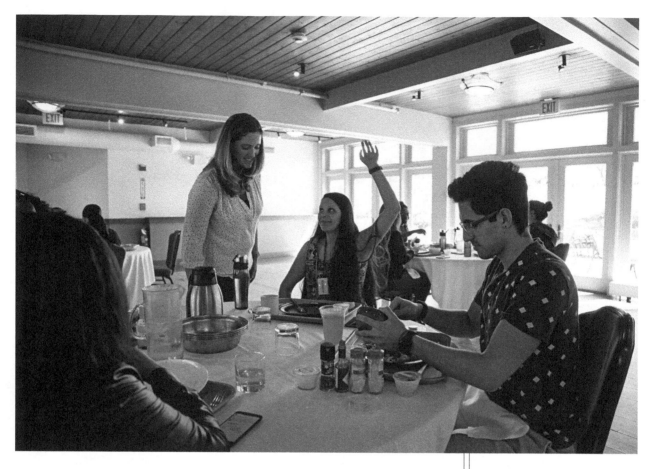

raisins, while the high-carb, high-sugar group gets all that – minus the chips – plus Kool-Aid and jelly beans.

About those jelly beans: They're actually assorted Jelly Bellys, and no, you can't pick out the flavors you hate, nor can you skip or swap any other component of your meals. Participants are monitored to ensure every crumb – every drop of sauce – is scraped off the plate with a spatula and consumed. People with food allergies are excluded from FB4, and unrepentant picky eaters need not apply. Study dietitians did cede to common food aversions, leaving grapefruit, cilantro and mushrooms off the menu. Sanctioned spices – e.g., curry, paprika, cinnamon and hot pepper sauce – are available. Coffee is allowed (sweetened only with stevia) but with a daily limit on caffeinated cups. Celebrating a birthday? Expect tea with the flavor of confetti cake. Because exercise also influences calorie burn, everyone must log at least 30 daily minutes (90 max) at a mild to moderate clip. Participants wear an activity

**CLEAN-PLATE CLUB:
A STUDY DIETITIAN INSPECTS
TO MAKE SURE EVERY SINGLE
MORSEL HAS BEEN EATEN.**

tracker, another tracker to gauge sleep, and a continuous glucose monitor to measure blood sugar response to meals. In their free time, they work remotely; take classes online; practice hobbies; read. Yoga, career coaching, workshops and other activities are offered. Since FB4 is longer than a typical residential controlled feeding study – lingo for testing diets under conditions that assure only the prescribed foods are eaten – organizers take care to make the experience enjoyable. (The $10,000 for finishing the study doesn't hurt.)

A weighty issue. If this all seems over the top, it's because the question of how to handle obesity and its attendant chronic diseases is urgent. The proportion of U.S. adults with obesity has climbed from about 13% in the 1960s to nearly 40%. But precisely why is subject to intense debate. Ludwig and others propose that a longstanding hypothesis known as the carbohydrate-insulin model may explain why simply restricting calories doesn't work for everyone. Here's the idea in a

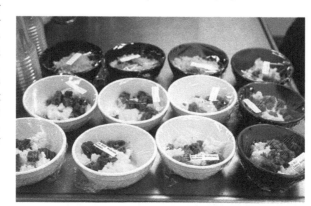

**ONE MEAL, THREE VARIATIONS,
AND ABSOLUTELY NO SWAPS OR
SKIPPED INGREDIENTS ALLOWED**

WHEN A LEGACY OF INNOVATION AND COMPASSION COMBINES WITH THE EVOLVING NEEDS OF THE COMMUNITY, THE RESULT IS SOMETHING SPECIAL.

El Camino Hospital is now El Camino Health, a comprehensive healthcare provider dedicated to the well-being of the people we serve. Our commitment to offering advanced, personalized care is tailored to reflect the specific needs of our communities. Among them: South Asian Heart Center, ASPIRE: After-School Program Interventions and Resiliency Education® and leadership in LGBTQ healthcare equality.

As we strive to deliver the most personal care possible, by offering more locations for more care options, we're working tirelessly to redefine what you should expect from your healthcare partner.

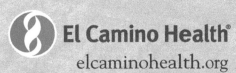

El Camino Health®

elcaminohealth.org

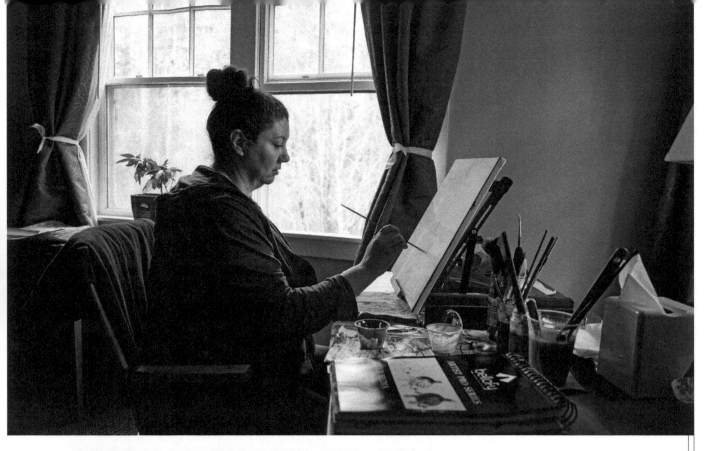

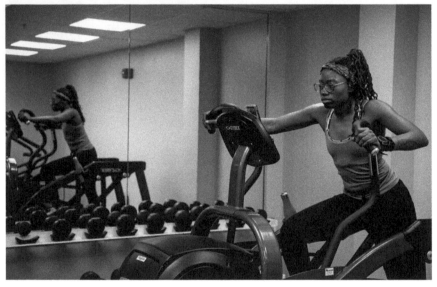

arriving in cohorts – will be crunched and the results eventually published.

The question of which diet works best is really two different questions, says Tanya Halliday, assistant professor of kinesiology at the University of Utah: "Are we interested in the biology and physiology, or do we mean what diet is best in the current environment that we live in?" FB4 addresses the physiology piece, but not under real-world conditions; then there are studies like DIETFITS, where participants got dietary advice and behavior-change tips over 22 group sessions but were on their own for food shopping, prep and eating. For that trial, researchers randomly assigned 609 adults classified as overweight or obese to either a low-fat or healthy low-carb diet for a year. Neither diet delivered a weight-loss advantage, nor did genetic patterns or insulin resistance, also considered, relate to success.

A real-world problem. This kind of experiment can show how diets do in the real world, where researchers can't really control whether participants follow diets to a T or accurately report what they're eating. Researchers trade off the rigor and tight supervision of controlled feeding studies for the broader applicability of real-world trials, says Christopher Gardner, director of nutrition studies at Stanford Prevention Research Center and lead author of DIETFITS, whose results were published in 2018.

nutshell: When carbs, particularly highly processed ones, hit the bloodstream, they cause a rush of insulin that socks away calories in fat cells, leaving too few for the rest of the body. As a result, a diet heavy on processed carbs makes people hungrier and prone to overeating. And resisting that hunger can slow down metabolism, Ludwig explains.

Last fall, Ludwig, Ebbeling and colleagues published results of the Framingham State Food Study, which examined this question under different research conditions; they found that a low-carb diet increased calorie burn among adults trying to maintain weight loss. Other researchers dispute the carbohydrate-insulin model (although they say processed carbs may drive obesity for other reasons). The debate is ongoing, and FB4 stands to contribute. The study is slated to end in 2021, after which data from a planned 125 participants – who will continue

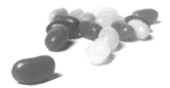

Both study types are necessary. "If we understand the mechanism, we can optimize it," says neuroscience and obesity researcher Stephan Guyenet. "At least in theory, we could design diets that are better than what we currently use." If a certain macronutrient balance emerges as superior, people might be more motivated to change their diets, and you'd have "the basis for more scientifically informed public health advice and policy," Ludwig says.

What's often lost in the diet wars is that individuals are individual – no one approach will likely work for all. "The diet educators were stunned" in DIETFITS to see how people thrived and failed on completely opposite diets, possibly owing to differences in satiety, Gardner says. That's why two people can eat a cheesy veggie omelet or steel-cut oatmeal with berries and have wholly different responses: immediate fullness or hunger pangs demanding seconds. And countless other factors influence the "ideal" diet – from taste preferences and cultural traditions to what's easy, affordable and available. A 2014 review published jointly by three major health organizations concluded that as long as people burn off more calories than they take in, weight loss can happen on virtually any diet. The best diet is one that revolves around whole foods and vegetables, while limiting refined grains and sugar. If everyone ate that way, Gardner bets we'd "solve 50%" of the obesity problem.

A CLINICAL RESEARCH SPECIALIST RUNS A BOD POD TEST TO MEASURE BODY COMPOSITION.

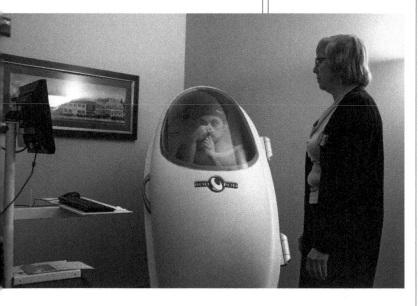

Regardless of the diet, experts generally agree: It would be great if research could serve up a better recipe for making new habits stick long term. And that's the challenge awaiting FB4 participants, who'll have to maintain their weight loss on their own steam, using new insights coupled with some phone-based nutritional counseling sessions. Charisse Shields now knows she can eat more than she thought, provided her meals are balanced and the food quality, high. Gillian Cotton-Graves, 19, vows to join a gym and eat more mindfully. Carla Zelinksi, 38, will focus on moderate carbs while getting consistent, but not extreme, exercise. Cosetta Medina, 34, no longer craves bread and will aim for nutrient-dense meals. Dan Alban, 23, plans moderation, plus more cauliflower. They say the three-month hiatus from their usual routines to reflect on their dietary habits and life overall has been a "gift." Notes Medina: "I'm so proud of all of us." ●

*For more details or to apply to be part of **FB4**, visit childrenshospital.org/fb4study*

Overprocessed and Overeaten

FROZEN MEALS. Sugary cereals. Soda. It's no secret: Highly processed foods are thought to fuel obesity, but there hasn't been direct evidence of a link to overeating and weight gain. Until now. A recent study finds that heavy consumption of these foods causes excess calorie intake and weight gain, while eating whole foods – those in their natural state – produces the opposite effect. Researchers at the National Institute of Diabetes and Digestive and Kidney Diseases recruited 20 adults to spend 28 days as inpatients. Half were assigned to a diet drawing over 80% of calories from ultra-processed foods (think: packaged meals, snacks and soft drinks) and half to a diet supplying over 88% of calories from whole foods, like fruits and veggies, meat, eggs and dairy. People could eat as much as they wanted but meals were matched for calories and for carbs, protein, fat, sugar and sodium. After two weeks, the groups switched diets.

The contrast was striking. On average, participants devoured about 500 more daily calories on the ultraprocessed diet and gained about 2 pounds, whereas they dropped 2 pounds on the unprocessed regimen.

Why? Something about whole-food meals may cause the gut to tell the brain: "Eat less," says lead author Kevin Hall, noting that hunger hormones were lower and appetite-taming hormones were higher on the unprocessed diet.

The ultraprocessed foods were also softer, easier to chew and swallow, and eaten more quickly, so it's possible that by the time the brain received fullness signals, participants had already overeaten. The takeaway may sound simple, but it's more complicated than trying to tax processed foods or telling everyone to eat foods in their natural state. Moreover, ultraprocessed foods are generally cheaper than whole foods and require less time and know-how to safely prepare. "A lot of thought needs to go into this," says Hall, who's planning further studies to test the link. *–K.H.*

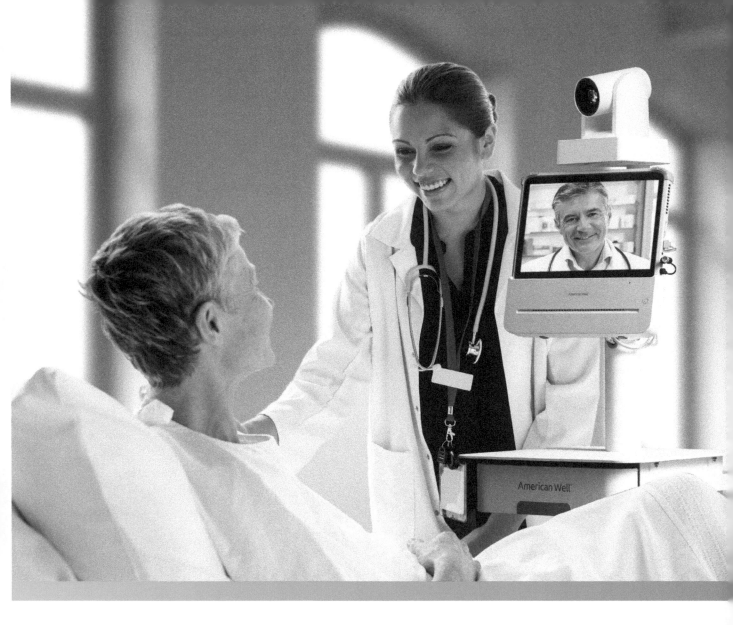

CHAPTER 3

BEST
HOSPITALS
U.S.News & WORLD REPORT
2019-20

Best Hospitals

Best Hospitals

HONOR ROLL

BEST
HOSPITALS
U.S.News & WORLD REPORT
HONOR ROLL
2019-20

The 21 medical centers below excel in treating patients with complex diagnoses and those with relatively routine needs.

Each is nationally ranked in eight or more of the 16 Best Hospitals specialties and is rated "high performing" in most or all of nine common procedures and conditions (full ratings at usnews.com/best-hospitals). Honor Roll standing is based on points. A hospital that was ranked No. 1 in all specialties and rated high performing in all procedures and conditions would have received 448 points. The 20 highest scorers (21 because of a tie) qualified for the Honor Roll.

1 Mayo Clinic
Rochester, Minn.
417 points

2 Massachusetts General Hospital
Boston, 369 points

3 Johns Hopkins Hospital
Baltimore
354 points

4 Cleveland Clinic
333 points

5 New York-Presbyterian Hospital-Columbia and Cornell
New York, 313 points

6 UCLA Medical Center
Los Angeles
309 points

7 UCSF Medical Center
San Francisco
306 points

8 Cedars-Sinai Medical Center
Los Angeles, 305 points

9 NYU Langone Hospitals
New York
252 points

10 Northwestern Memorial Hospital
Chicago, 232 points

11 U. of Michigan Hospitals-Michigan Medicine
Ann Arbor, 227 points

12 Stanford Health Care-Stanford Hospital
Palo Alto, Calif.,
226 points

13 Brigham and Women's Hospital
Boston, 215 points

14 Mount Sinai Hospital
New York
212 points

15 UPMC Presbyterian Shadyside
Pittsburgh, 202 points

16 Keck Hospital of USC
Los Angeles
200 points

17 University of Wisconsin Hospitals
Madison, 186 points

18* Hospitals of the University of Pennsylvania-Penn Presbyterian
Philadelphia, 185 points

18* Mayo Clinic-Phoenix
185 points

20* Houston Methodist Hospital
178 points

20* Yale New Haven Hospital
New Haven, Conn.
178 points

*Denotes a tie

A Guide to the Rankings

How we identified 165 outstanding hospitals in 16 specialties

by **Ben Harder**

THE MISSION of the Best Hospitals annual rankings, now in their 30th year, remains the same as always: to help guide patients who need an especially high level of care to the right place. These are patients whose surgery or condition is complex. Or whose advanced age, physical infirmity or existing medical condition puts them at heightened risk.

Such people account for a small fraction of hospital patients, but they add up to millions of individuals, and most hospitals may not be able to meet their needs. A hospital ranked by U.S. News in cardiology and heart surgery, say, is likely to have the experience and expertise to operate safely on a patient 85 or 90 years old with a leaky heart valve. Some community hospitals cannot supply the special techniques and precautions needed, and should instead send such a patient to a hospital that can. Many community hospitals do that. But not all.

The following pages offer hospital rankings in 16 specialties, from cancer to urology. Of 4,656 hospitals evaluated this year, only 165 performed well enough to be ranked in any specialty. In 12 of 16 specialties, analysis of objective data from the federal government and other sources generated the main factors determining whether a hospital was ranked. Some kinds of data, such as death rates, are intimately related to quality. Numbers of patients and the balance of nurses to patients are examples of data that are also important, although the quality connection may seem less evident. To capture medical experts' opinions, we also factored in results from annual surveys of specialist physicians who were asked to name hospitals they consider best in their specialty at handling difficult cases.

Hospitals in the other four specialties (ophthalmology, psychiatry, rehabilitation and rheumatology) were ranked solely on the basis of the annual physician surveys. That's because so few patients die in these specialties that mortality rates, which

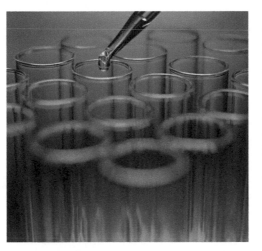

carry heavy weight in the 12 other specialties, mean little.

Based on input from experts and medical studies, we have revised the methodology over time to improve the rankings' usefulness to consumers. This year, we added two quality measures in the 12 data-driven specialties that matter to many people: patient experience ratings, and how successful each hospital is at discharging patients to their home (as opposed to a nursing home or other facility). We also removed certain factors, including post-operative bleeding and accidental lacerations, that many health care professionals consider to be unreliable. More detail on the methodology is available at usnews.com/best-hospitals.

To be considered for ranking in the 12 data-driven specialties, a hospital had to meet any of four criteria: It had to be a teaching hospital, or be affiliated with a medical school, or have at least 200 beds, or have at least 100 beds and offer at least four out of eight advanced medical technologies. This year 2,728 hospitals met that test.

The hospitals next had to meet a volume requirement in each specialty – a minimum number of Medicare inpatients from 2015 to 2017 who received certain procedures and treatment for specific conditions. The minimum number of patients for cardiology and heart surgery, for example, was 1,931, of which 800 had to be surgical. A hospital that fell short was still eligible if it was nominated in the specialty by at least 1% of the physicians responding to the expert opinion survey.

At the end of the process, 1,870 hospitals remained candidates for ranking in at least one specialty. Each received a U.S. News score of 0 to 100 based on four elements, described below. The 50 top performers in each of the 12 specialties were ranked. Scores and data for the rest are at usnews.com. The four elements and their weights in brief:

Patient outcomes (37.5%). Success at keeping patients alive and getting them home was judged by the proportion of Medicare inpatients with certain conditions in 2015, 2016

Canon — a bright future in healthcare.

Healthcare IT

Offering leading-edge
diagnostic support systems
and network solutions
utilizing ICT.

Diagnostic Imaging Systems

Meeting clinical needs with
high resolution imaging
from CT, MRI, X-ray and
Ultrasound systems.

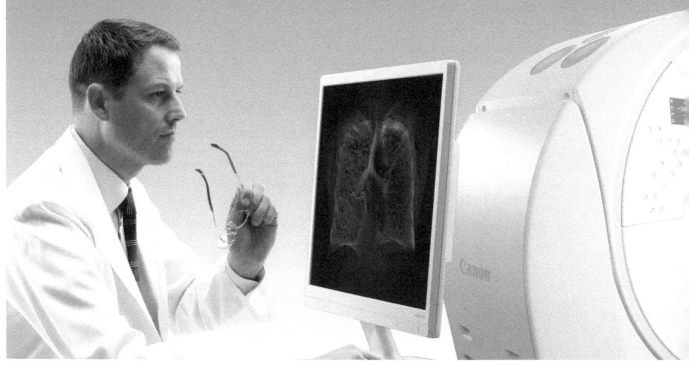

Images are for illustrative purposes only.

It has been more than one year since Canon welcomed Canon Medical into the Canon Group.

One thing hasn't changed. The patient is always at the heart of everything we do. Canon Medical's philosophy, "Made for Life," embodies our mission in healthcare to improve the lives of people wherever they are in the world.

Our cutting-edge solutions in medical imaging and in-vitro diagnostics are built around delivering the best possible care. Driven by a commitment to data science research and collaboration, we continue to develop intelligent IT platforms to transform the healthcare problems of today into the solutions of tomorrow.

Caring for life — now and into the future.

In-vitro Diagnostic Systems

Supporting examination workflows with high resolution and rapid analysis of blood and other specimens taken from patients.

Canon

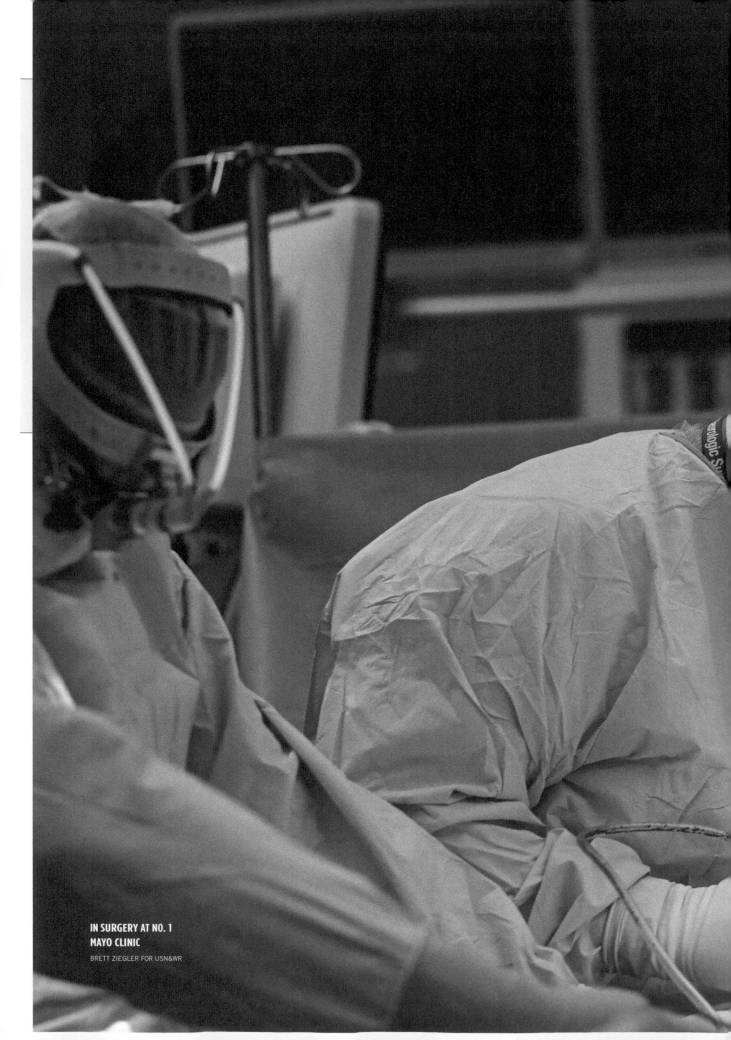

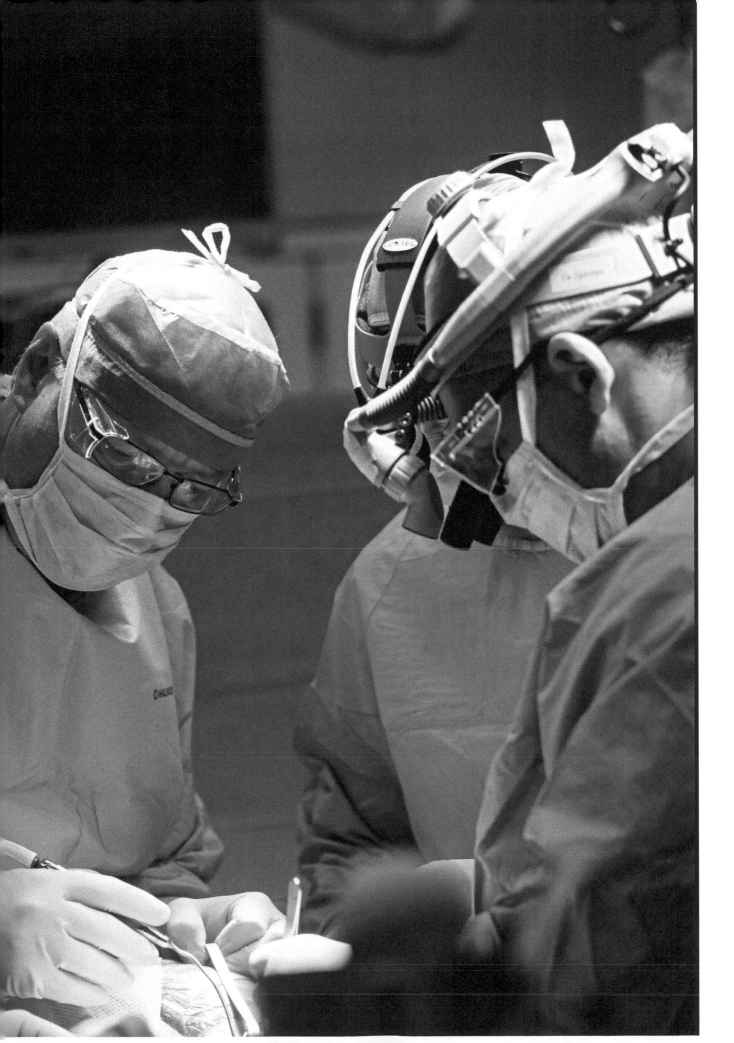

and 2017 who died within 30 days of admission or were discharged to another health care facility. Both rates were adjusted to account for the severity of patients' illnesses, the complexity of their care, and risk-elevating factors such as advanced age, obesity, high blood pressure and poverty (as reflected by whether they received Medicaid).

A widely used approach to so-called risk adjustment was employed to adjust each patient's risk in calculating odds of a good outcome. To avoid penalizing institutions that receive the sickest patients, we excluded from our analysis patients transferred into a hospital from another hospital. In the tables that follow, a score of 10 indicates the best chance of survival or discharge to home (and 1 the worst) relative to other hospitals.

Patient experience (5%). Most hospitals are required to assess patients' satisfaction with their experience using a survey known as the Hospital Consumer Assessment of Healthcare Providers and Systems, or HCAHPS. The score reflects how many patients had a positive overall experience during hospitalization.

Other care-related indicators (30%). The balance of patients per nurse and the hospital's number of patients – an indicator of its degree of experience in a specialty – are examples of these factors.

Expert opinion (27.5%). Specialists were asked to name up to five hos-

USNEWS.COM/BESTHOSPITALS

Visit usnews.com regularly while researching your health care choices, as U.S. News often adds content aimed at helping patients and families make decisions about their medical care. We also update the Best Hospitals, Best Children's Hospitals and Best Regional Hospitals data on the website when new data become available.

pitals that they consider best in their area of expertise for patients with the most difficult medical problems. In the 2019 survey alone, responses were tallied from some 24,000 physicians.

The figures shown under "% of specialists recommending hospital" in the tables are the average percentages of specialists in 2017, 2018 and 2019 who recommended a hospital.

In the four survey-based specialties, a hospital had to be cited by at least 5% of responding physicians in the latest three years of U.S. News surveys to be ranked. That created lists of 11 hospitals in psychiatry, 12 in ophthalmology, 12 in rehabilitation and 14 in rheumatology.

If you've consulted past editions of Best Hospitals, you may notice that a hospital you're considering has risen or fallen in the rankings. A decline shouldn't automatically be interpreted as a decline in performance; rather, it may be because U.S. News revised the methodology, as was the case this year.

No hospital, no matter how excellent, is best for every patient. You'll want to add your own fact-gathering to ours and consult with your doctor or other health professional. ●

A Glossary of Terms

Discharge to home score: reflects proportion of patients who, at discharge, went home rather than to a nursing home or other facility.

FACT accreditation level: hospital meets Foundation for the Accreditation of Cellular Therapy standards as of March 1, 2019, for harvesting and transplanting stem cells from a patient's own bone marrow and tissue (level 1) and from a donor (level 2) to treat cancer.

NAEC epilepsy center: designated by the National Association of Epilepsy Centers as of March 1, 2019, as a regional or national referral facility (level 4) for staffing, technology and training in epilepsy care.

NCI cancer center: designated by the National Cancer Institute as of March 1, 2019, as a clinical or comprehensive cancer hospital.

NIA Alzheimer's center: designated by the National Institute on Aging as of March 5, 2019, as an Alzheimer's Disease Center, indicating high quality of research and clinical care.

Number of patients: estimated number of Medicare inpatients in 2015, 2016 and 2017 who received certain high-level care as defined by U.S. News. Based on an adjustment to the number of such patients with traditional Medicare insurance. In geriatrics, only patients ages 75 and older are included.

A Nurse Magnet hospital: recognized by the American Nurses Credentialing Center as of February 1, 2019, for nursing excellence.

Nurse staffing score: relative balance of nonsupervisory registered nurses (inpatient and outpatient) to average daily number of all pa-

tients. Inpatient staffing receives greater weight. Agency and temporary nurses are not counted.

Patient experience: percentage of patients who responded positively to a survey about the overall quality of their stay.

Patient services score: number of services offered out of the number considered important to quality (such as genetic testing in cancer and an Alzheimer's center in geriatrics).

% of specialists recommending hospital: percentage of physicians responding to U.S. News surveys in 2017, 2018 and 2019 who named the hospital as among the best in their specialty for especially challenging cases and procedures, setting aside location and cost.

Rank: based on U.S. News score except in ophthalmology, psychiatry, rehabilitation and rheumatology, where specialist recommendations determine rank.

Survival score: reflects patient survival rate in the specialty within 30 days of admission.

Technology score: reflects availability of technologies considered important to a high quality of care, such as PET/CT scanner in pulmonology and diagnostic radio-isotope services in urology.

Transparency score: indicates whether hospital publicly reports heart outcomes through the American College of Cardiology and the Society of Thoracic Surgeons.

Trauma center: indicates Level 1 or 2 trauma center certification. Such a center can care properly for the most severe injuries.

U.S. News score: summary of quality of hospital inpatient care. In most specialties, survival is worth 30%, discharge to home 7.5%, operational quality data such as nurse staffing and patient volume 30%, specialists' recommendations 27.5%, and patient experience 5%.

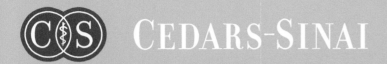
CEDARS-SINAI

HONORED TO BE AMONG THE TOP 10 HOSPITALS IN THE NATION.

Cedars-Sinai is proud to be ranked in the top 10 of
U.S. News & World Report's Best Hospitals
Honor Roll, and to be among the very best in multiple
specialties. Thank you for trusting us to deliver
the expert care you and your family deserve, when
you need it most.

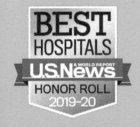

RANKED #8 OVERALL IN THE NATION

RANKED #2 IN THE NATION FOR GASTROENTEROLOGY & GI SURGERY

RANKED #3 IN THE NATION FOR CARDIOLOGY & HEART SURGERY

RANKED #3 IN THE NATION FOR ORTHOPEDICS

RANKED #4 IN THE NATION FOR PULMONOLOGY

RANKED #8 IN THE NATION FOR GYNECOLOGY

RANKED #10 IN THE NATION FOR NEPHROLOGY

ALSO RANKED AMONG THE NATION'S BEST IN:

CANCER

DIABETES & ENDOCRINOLOGY

EAR, NOSE & THROAT

GERIATRICS

NEUROLOGY & NEUROSURGERY

UROLOGY

1-800-CEDARS-1   cedars-sinai.org

Cancer

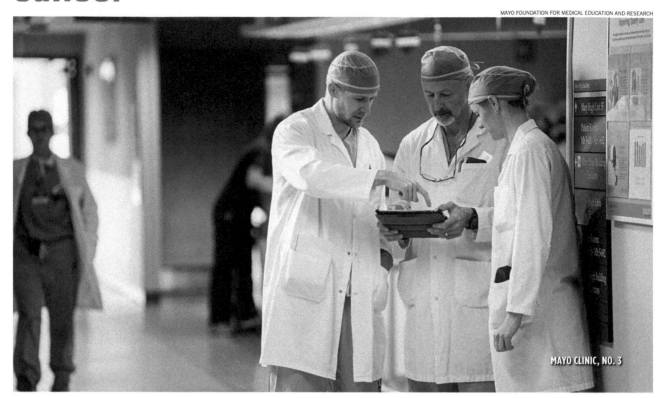

MAYO FOUNDATION FOR MEDICAL EDUCATION AND RESEARCH

MAYO CLINIC, NO. 3

Rank	Hospital	U.S. News score	Survival score (10=best)	Discharge to home score (10=best)	Patient experience (% positive responses)	Number of patients	Nurse staffing score (higher is better)	NCI cancer center	FACT accreditation level (2=best)	Patient services score (8=best)	% of specialists recommending hospital
1	University of Texas MD Anderson Cancer Center, Houston	100.0	10	10	95%	13,804	1.8	Yes	2	8	48.4%
2	Memorial Sloan-Kettering Cancer Center, New York	94.7	10	10	93%	8,383	2.1	Yes	2	8	45.7%
3	Mayo Clinic, Rochester, Minn.	84.6	10	10	94%	5,457	2.8	Yes	2	8	20.4%
4	Johns Hopkins Hospital, Baltimore	81.8	10	10	92%	2,489	2.2	Yes	2	8	17.6%
5	Dana-Farber/Brigham and Women's Cancer Center, Boston	72.5	10	10	96%	4,087	2.2	Yes	2	8	26.0%
6	Cleveland Clinic	71.5	10	9	93%	3,248	2.5	Yes	2	8	7.4%
7	UPMC Presbyterian Shadyside, Pittsburgh	71.4	10	10	89%	5,019	2.1	Yes	2	8	3.8%
8	H. Lee Moffitt Cancer Center and Research Institute, Tampa	71.2	10	10	94%	4,247	1.3	Yes	2	7	7.4%
8	Massachusetts General Hospital, Boston	71.2	10	10	93%	4,135	2.4	Yes	2	8	10.6%
10	Northwestern Memorial Hospital, Chicago	70.4	10	10	92%	2,292	1.9	Yes	2	8	2.3%
11	City of Hope Helford Clinical Research Hosp., Duarte, Calif.	68.8	10	10	95%	3,098	2.5	Yes	2	7	4.3%
12	Cedars-Sinai Medical Center, Los Angeles	67.1	10	10	92%	3,347	2.5	No	2	8	1.3%
12	UCSF Medical Center, San Francisco	67.1	10	10	93%	3,098	2.7	Yes	2	8	4.8%
14	Roswell Park Comprehensive Cancer Center, Buffalo	67.0	10	10	94%	1,746	1.9	Yes	2	8	2.2%
15	Seattle Cancer Care Alliance/U. of Washington Medical Ctr.	66.2	10	10	92%	2,172	2.1	Yes	2	8	6.4%
16	University of Maryland Medical Center, Baltimore	65.2	10	10	88%	1,113	2.8	Yes	2	8	0.6%
17	Siteman Cancer Center, St. Louis	64.0	10	10	90%	4,291	2.2	Yes	2	8	3.7%
18	Hosps. of the U. of Pennsylvania-Penn Presby., Philadelphia	63.7	10	7	91%	3,965	2.5	Yes	2	8	5.9%
19	NYU Langone Hospitals, New York, N.Y.	63.1	10	10	89%	2,248	2.3	Yes	2	8	2.3%
20	Ohio State University James Cancer Hospital, Columbus	62.7	10	8	95%	4,222	2.1	Yes	2	7	5.1%
21	UCLA Medical Center, Los Angeles	62.5	10	10	92%	2,759	3.1	Yes	2	8	5.3%
21	USC Norris Cancer Hosp.-Keck Med. Ctr. of USC, Los Angeles	62.5	10	10	94%	1,875	2.9	Yes	2	8	0.9%
23	Jefferson Health-Thomas Jefferson U. Hospitals, Philadelphia	62.1	10	10	89%	2,461	2.0	Yes	2	8	1.6%
24	Beth Israel Deaconess Medical Center, Boston	61.7	10	8	89%	1,894	1.6	Yes	2	8	2.7%

(CONTINUED ON PAGE 124)

Terms are explained on Page 118.

More @ usnews.com/besthospitals

City of Hope is ranked the
leading cancer hospital in California
by U.S. News & World Report and,
most important, by Gus Perez, cancer survivor.

© 2019 City of Hope

We are honored to have the highest U.S. News ranking in the state, yet it's our patient's health and well-being that provides us with the only validation we need.

Remission, our only rest point.

A full cure, the only goal.

Our patients are at the forefront of everything we do and every decision we make.

That's why we're committed to delivering the best clinical care possible from relentless research and innovative treatments to unparalleled compassion for every City of Hope patient.

At City of Hope, we'll continue to put cancer patients and their families first.

That won't stop until we stop cancer.

Discover more at CityofHope.org

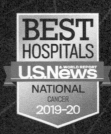

BEST HOSPITALS
U.S.News WORLD REPORT
NATIONAL
CANCER
2019-20

City of Hope®

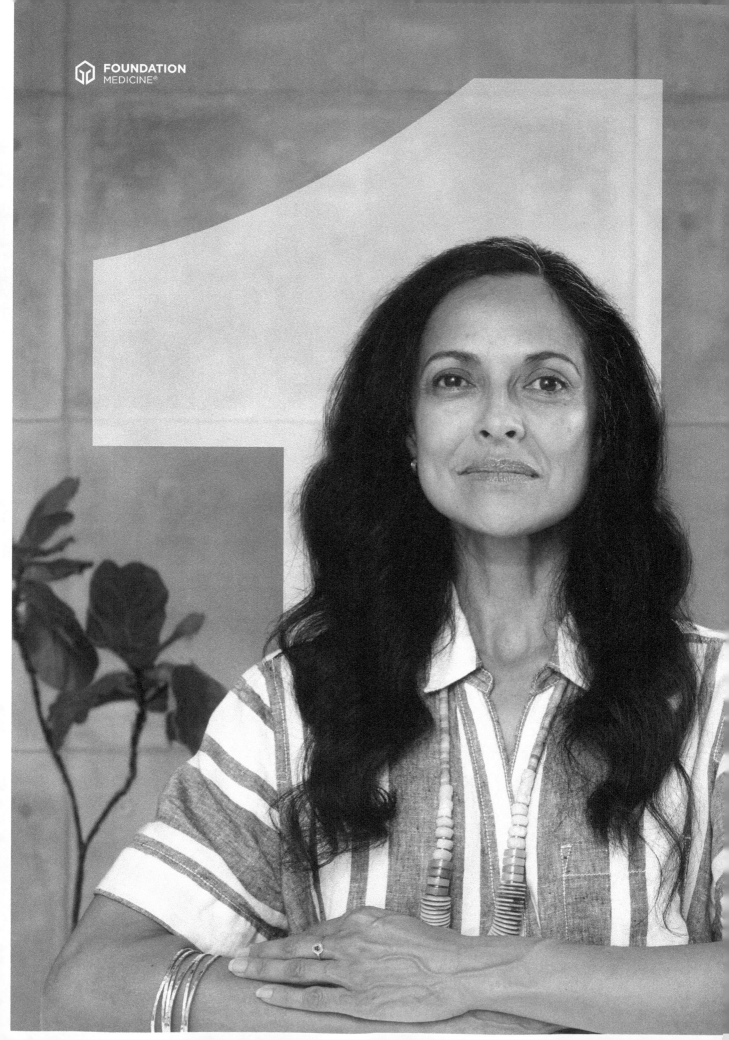

I'm the one facing **cancer.** And now it's **personal.**

Every cancer is unique. Your treatment plan should be too.

1 in 3 people in the United States will be diagnosed with cancer in their lifetime.[1] Yesterday, that was someone else. Today, that's me. So now it's personal. And because my cancer is advanced, I know to start with the FoundationOne®CDx test.

The first FDA-approved test of its kind, FoundationOne CDx uses comprehensive genomic profiling (CGP) to help my doctor understand what makes my cancer unique. So we can create a treatment plan that's as personalized as possible.

If you or a loved one ever face advanced cancer, ask your doctor to start with step one.

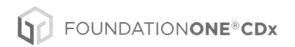 FOUNDATION**ONE**®CDx

Learn more at
StartWithStepOne.com/test

1.888.870.1811 | Rx only

FoundationOne CDx is a test intended to help doctors identify which cancer patients may benefit from certain treatments or clinical trial options. Use of the test does not guarantee that you will be matched to a treatment or clinical trial, or that all relevant alterations will be detected. Some patients may require a biopsy, which could pose a risk. See our website for the full labeling, including indications for use and safety information.

Cancer (CONTINUED)

Rank	Hospital	U.S. News score	Survival score (10=best)	Discharge to home score (10=best)	Patient experience (% positive responses)	Number of patients	Nurse staffing score (higher is better)	NCI cancer center	FACT accreditation level (2=best)	Patient services score (8=best)	% of specialists recommending hospital
25	Stanford Health Care-Stanford Hospital, Palo Alto, Calif.	61.6	10	10	90%	3,348	2.9	Yes	2	8	5.4%
26	University of Virginia Medical Center, Charlottesville	61.0	10	10	90%	1,239	2.0	Yes	2	8	0.6%
27	University of North Carolina Hospitals, Chapel Hill	60.8	10	10	92%	2,028	1.6	Yes	2	8	2.1%
28	UC Davis Medical Center, Sacramento, Calif.	60.6	10	10	89%	2,310	2.8	Yes	2	8	0.5%
29	New York-Presbyterian Hospital-Columbia and Cornell, N.Y.	60.3	10	10	89%	5,777	3.0	Yes	2	8	3.7%
30	University Hospitals Seidman Cancer Center, Cleveland	59.5	10	8	89%	1,864	2.6	Yes	2	8	0.8%
31	University of Chicago Medical Center	59.1	10	8	91%	2,151	2.3	Yes	2	8	3.5%
32	MUSC Health-University Medical Center, Charleston, S.C.	58.0	10	10	92%	1,397	2.0	Yes	2	8	0.4%
33	U. of Kentucky Albert B. Chandler Hospital, Lexington	57.9	10	10	90%	1,326	1.9	Yes	2	8	1.0%
34	U. of Michigan Hospitals-Michigan Medicine, Ann Arbor	57.7	9	10	91%	2,703	2.8	Yes	2	8	3.3%
35	Nebraska Medicine-Nebraska Medical Center, Omaha	57.5	10	9	90%	1,105	2.2	Yes	2	8	0.7%
36	Duncan Comp. Cancer Ctr. at Baylor St. Luke's Med. Ctr., Houston	57.0	10	10	87%	814	2.0	Yes	0	8	0.3%
37	Montefiore Medical Center, Bronx, N.Y.	56.9	10	9	84%	2,524	2.1	Yes	2	8	0.6%
37	UCHealth University of Colorado Hospital, Aurora	56.9	10	9	91%	2,227	2.0	Yes	2	8	1.4%
39	Houston Methodist Hospital	56.2	10	1	92%	2,151	2.0	No	2	8	0.7%
40	Duke University Hospital, Durham, N.C.	56.1	8	10	92%	2,864	2.1	Yes	2	8	5.1%
41	Emory University Hospital, Atlanta	56.0	9	10	92%	2,317	2.1	Yes	2	8	2.1%
42	UF Health Shands Hospital, Gainesville, Fla.	55.6	10	9	89%	1,687	2.0	No	2	8	0.9%
43	Mayo Clinic-Phoenix	55.4	9	5	96%	2,136	3.2	Yes	2	8	2.2%
43	University of Iowa Hospitals and Clinics, Iowa City	55.4	10	10	88%	1,692	1.9	Yes	2	8	1.1%
45	Smilow Cancer Hospital at Yale New Haven, Conn.	54.8	9	7	89%	3,024	2.0	Yes	2	8	2.5%
46	OHSU Hospital, Portland, Ore.	54.7	9	10	92%	2,216	2.1	Yes	2	8	1.1%
47	University of Kansas Hospital, Kansas City	54.3	10	8	93%	2,082	2.0	Yes	2	8	1.0%
48	OU Medical Center, Oklahoma City	54.1	10	10	87%	1,361	1.6	Yes	2	8	0.0%
48	University of Wisconsin Hospitals, Madison	54.1	10	7	93%	1,641	3.1	Yes	2	8	0.9%
50	University of Minnesota Medical Center, Fairview	53.8	10	9	89%	2,427	2.1	Yes	2	8	0.4%

Terms are explained on Page 118.

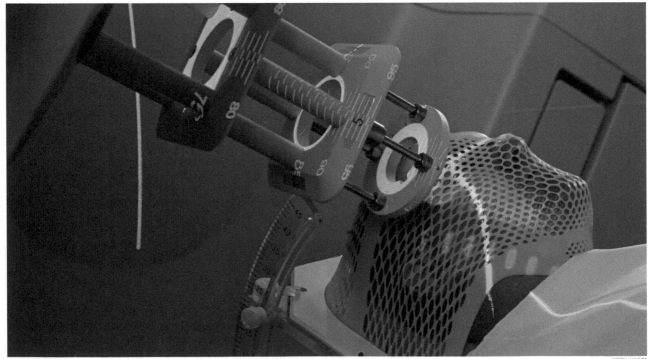

GETTY IMAGES

More @ usnews.com/besthospitals

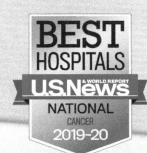

Cardiology & Heart Surgery

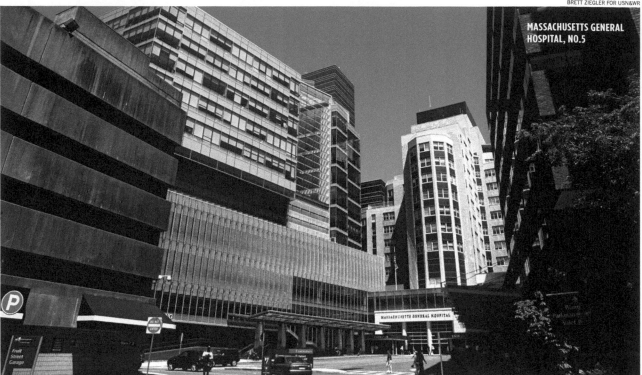

BRETT ZIEGLER FOR USN&WR

MASSACHUSETTS GENERAL HOSPITAL, NO.5

Rank	Hospital	U.S. News score	Survival score (10=best)	Discharge to home score (10=best)	Patient experience (% positive responses)	Trans-parency score (3=best)	Number of patients	Nurse staffing score (higher is better)	A Nurse Magnet hospital	Technology score (6=best)	Patient services score (7=best)	% of specialists recom-mending hospital
1	Cleveland Clinic	100.0	10	10	93%	3	16,592	2.5	Yes	6	7	40.1%
2	Mayo Clinic, Rochester, Minn.	91.9	10	9	94%	3	16,596	2.8	Yes	6	7	37.6%
3	Cedars-Sinai Medical Center, Los Angeles	82.4	10	10	92%	3	16,251	2.5	Yes	6	7	8.1%
4	New York-Presbyterian Hospital-Columbia and Cornell, N.Y.	79.7	10	10	89%	3	22,095	3.0	No	6	7	15.0%
5	Massachusetts General Hospital, Boston	77.9	10	9	93%	3	11,457	2.4	Yes	6	7	16.4%
6	Mount Sinai Hospital, New York	75.5	10	10	86%	3	13,644	2.0	Yes	6	7	4.7%
7	Northwestern Memorial Hospital, Chicago	70.0	10	10	92%	3	6,326	1.9	Yes	6	7	4.8%
8	UCLA Medical Center, Los Angeles	69.3	10	10	92%	3	7,256	3.1	Yes	6	7	3.4%
9	Brigham and Women's Hospital, Boston	69.0	10	9	92%	3	8,230	2.2	Yes	6	7	13.1%
10	Stanford Health Care-Stanford Hospital, Palo Alto, Calif.	68.8	10	10	90%	3	6,352	2.9	Yes	6	7	6.4%
11	Keck Hospital of USC, Los Angeles	67.4	10	10	91%	3	2,878	2.9	Yes	6	7	0.9%
12	Johns Hopkins Hospital, Baltimore	66.2	10	10	92%	3	5,071	2.2	Yes	6	7	10.4%
13	U. of Michigan Hospitals-Michigan Medicine, Ann Arbor	63.8	10	9	91%	3	7,201	2.8	Yes	6	7	4.2%
14	Minneapolis Heart Institute at Abbott Northwestern Hospital	63.4	10	9	91%	3	17,340	2.7	Yes	6	7	1.0%
15	NYU Langone Hospitals, New York, N.Y.	63.0	10	10	89%	3	9,365	2.3	Yes	5	7	4.2%
16	Houston Methodist Hospital	62.9	10	9	92%	3	10,188	2.0	Yes	6	7	5.6%
17	UC Davis Medical Center, Sacramento, Calif.	62.8	10	10	89%	3	5,629	2.8	Yes	5	7	0.2%
18	Hosps. of the U. of Pennsylvania-Penn Presby., Philadelphia	62.4	8	10	91%	3	13,332	2.5	Yes	6	7	8.8%
19	Beaumont Hospital-Royal Oak, Mich.	62.1	10	9	89%	3	12,086	1.9	Yes	5	7	1.1%
20	North Shore University Hospital, Manhasset, N.Y.	60.7	10	10	91%	3	9,378	2.1	Yes	5	7	1.6%
21	Texas Heart Inst. at Baylor St. Luke's Medical Ctr., Houston	60.2	10	10	87%	3	8,938	2.0	Yes	4	7	7.3%
22	Mayo Clinic-Phoenix	59.7	10	10	96%	3	4,900	3.2	Yes	6	7	1.8%
23	Duke University Hospital, Durham, N.C.	59.0	6	10	92%	3	8,510	2.1	Yes	6	7	10.4%
24	University Hospitals Cleveland Medical Center	58.9	10	8	89%	3	4,951	2.6	Yes	6	7	1.6%

(CONTINUED ON PAGE 128)

Terms are explained on Page 118.

More @ usnews.com/besthospitals

MORRISTOWN MEDICAL CENTER
#1 HOSPITAL IN NJ
(AGAIN!)

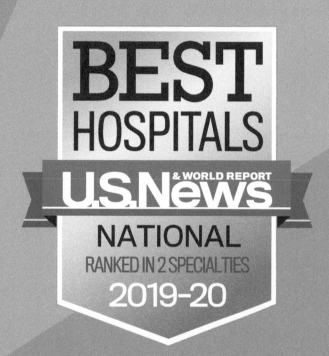

BEST
HOSPITALS

U.S.News & WORLD REPORT

NATIONAL
RANKED IN 2 SPECIALTIES
2019-20

With nationally recognized leadership in Cardiology & Heart Surgery and Orthopedics

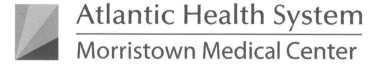

Atlantic Health System
Morristown Medical Center

To learn more visit **atlantichealth.org/usnews**

Cardiology & Heart Surgery (CONTINUED)

Rank	Hospital	U.S. News score	Survival score (10=best)	Discharge to home score (10=best)	Patient experience (% positive responses)	Trans-parency score (3=best)	Number of patients	Nurse staffing score (higher is better)	A Nurse Magnet hospital	Technology score (6=best)	Patient services score (7=best)	% of specialists recom-mending hospital
25	University of Wisconsin Hospitals, Madison	58.7	10	7	93%	3	4,718	3.1	Yes	6	7	0.5%
26	Morristown Medical Center, N.J.	58.1	10	7	90%	3	10,809	2.1	Yes	5	7	0.7%
27	Baylor Scott and White The Heart Hospital Plano, Texas	57.8	10	10	95%	3	6,481	2.3	Yes	5	7	1.5%
28	Barnes-Jewish Hospital, St. Louis	57.5	9	10	90%	3	9,271	2.2	Yes	6	7	2.1%
29	Scripps La Jolla Hospitals, La Jolla, Calif.	57.4	9	10	92%	3	7,139	3.0	Yes	5	7	1.4%
30	UCHealth University of Colorado Hospital, Aurora	57.1	10	10	91%	3	5,793	2.0	Yes	6	7	1.3%
31	Montefiore Medical Center, Bronx, N.Y.	56.9	10	9	84%	3	12,894	2.1	No	6	7	0.6%
32	University of Alabama at Birmingham Hospital	56.8	9	10	93%	3	7,017	1.9	Yes	6	7	2.2%
33	UPMC Presbyterian Shadyside, Pittsburgh	56.6	9	8	89%	3	11,827	2.1	Yes	6	7	1.7%
34	St. Francis Hospital-Roslyn, N.Y.	56.3	10	10	93%	3	11,681	1.7	Yes	4	7	1.0%
35	Vanderbilt University Medical Center, Nashville, Tenn.	55.9	9	9	91%	3	8,032	2.2	Yes	6	7	3.6%
36	Cleveland Clinic Fairview Hospital, Cleveland	55.6	10	6	90%	3	5,003	1.9	Yes	5	7	0.2%
36	UCSF Medical Center, San Francisco	55.6	9	10	93%	3	3,248	2.7	Yes	6	7	2.2%
38	Beaumont Hospital-Troy, Mich.	55.0	10	8	89%	3	7,842	1.9	Yes	5	7	0.3%
39	Loyola University Medical Center, Maywood, Ill.	54.8	10	8	88%	3	4,039	2.5	Yes	6	7	0.9%
40	OHSU Hospital, Portland, Ore.	54.6	10	10	92%	3	4,681	2.1	Yes	6	7	0.5%
41	MedStar Heart and Vascular Institute, Washington, D.C.	53.9	10	9	84%	3	11,135	1.9	No	6	7	1.4%
42	NYU Winthrop Hospital, Mineola, N.Y.	53.6	10	10	88%	3	7,009	2.0	Yes	5	7	0.7%
42	Saint Luke's Hospital of Kansas City, Mo.	53.6	10	9	92%	3	6,748	1.6	Yes	6	7	1.1%
44	Lenox Hill Hospital, New York	53.2	10	10	87%	3	5,794	2.5	No	5	7	0.9%
44	UC San Diego Health-Sulpizio Cardiovascular Center	53.2	9	10	92%	3	4,642	2.1	Yes	6	7	0.6%
46	Emory University Hospital, Atlanta	52.1	8	10	92%	3	5,146	2.1	Yes	6	7	3.8%
47	UT Southwestern Medical Center, Dallas	52.0	10	10	93%	2	3,811	2.1	Yes	6	7	1.4%
48	Jefferson Health-Thomas Jefferson U. Hospitals, Philadelphia	51.7	9	8	89%	3	5,208	2.0	Yes	6	7	0.8%
48	St. Cloud Hospital, St. Cloud, Minn.	51.7	9	7	91%	3	13,898	2.0	Yes	5	7	0.0%
48	Yale New Haven Hospital, Conn.	51.7	8	7	89%	3	12,882	2.0	Yes	6	7	1.3%

Terms are explained on Page 118.

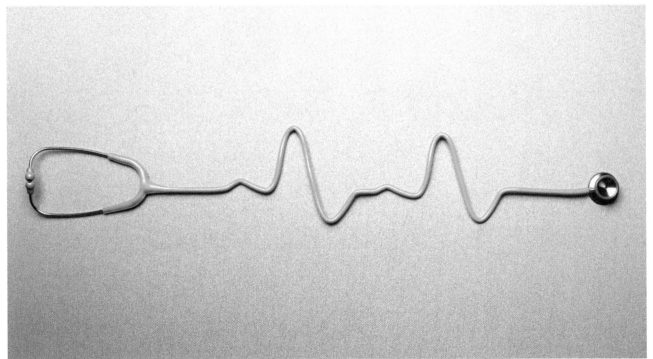

More @ usnews.com/besthospitals

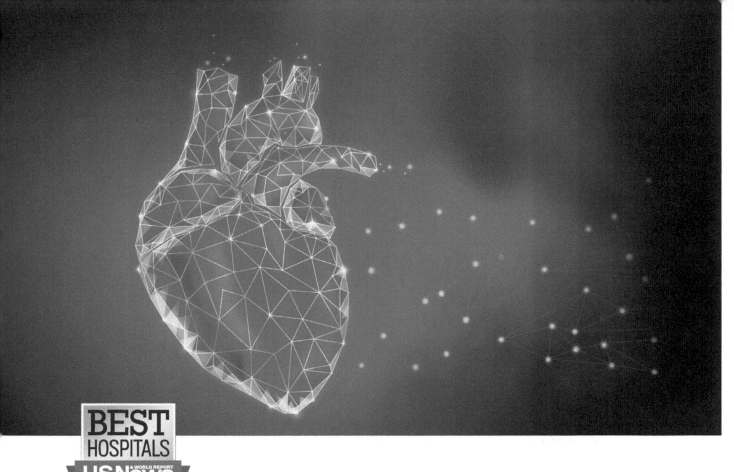
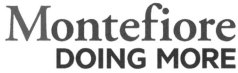

Diabetes & Endocrinology

Rank	Hospital	U.S. News score	Survival score (10=best)	Discharge to home score (10=best)	Patient experience (% positive responses)	Number of patients	Nurse staffing score (higher is better)	A Nurse Magnet hospital	Technology score (4=best)	Patient services score (8=best)	% of specialists recommending hospital
1	Mayo Clinic, Rochester, Minn.	100.0	10	10	94%	1,224	2.8	Yes	4	8	40.3%
2	Massachusetts General Hospital, Boston	81.0	7	9	93%	926	2.4	Yes	4	8	25.4%
3	UCSF Medical Center, San Francisco	78.6	10	10	93%	619	2.7	Yes	4	8	9.7%
4	UCLA Medical Center, Los Angeles	75.0	10	10	92%	958	3.1	Yes	4	8	5.3%
5	Johns Hopkins Hospital, Baltimore	72.9	8	9	92%	568	2.2	Yes	4	8	14.5%
6	New York-Presbyterian Hospital-Columbia and Cornell, N.Y.	70.9	8	8	89%	2,305	3.0	No	4	8	9.3%
7	Mount Sinai Hospital, New York	70.0	9	10	86%	1,008	2.0	Yes	4	8	5.4%
8	University of Washington Medical Center, Seattle	69.7	10	10	92%	258	2.1	Yes	4	8	6.4%
9	Lenox Hill Hospital, New York	68.7	10	10	87%	522	2.5	No	4	8	0.5%
10	UCHealth University of Colorado Hospital, Aurora	67.8	8	10	91%	861	2.0	Yes	4	8	7.4%
11	U. of Michigan Hospitals-Michigan Medicine, Ann Arbor	67.5	9	9	91%	606	2.8	Yes	4	8	5.2%
12	AdventHealth Orlando	66.9	10	9	90%	3,108	2.4	No	4	8	0.2%
13	Cleveland Clinic	66.7	3	4	93%	935	2.5	Yes	4	8	16.4%
14	Montefiore Medical Center, Bronx, N.Y.	65.4	10	10	84%	2,072	2.1	No	4	8	1.3%
15	North Shore University Hospital, Manhasset, N.Y.	65.2	10	10	91%	841	2.1	Yes	4	8	0.4%
16	Cedars-Sinai Medical Center, Los Angeles	65.1	8	10	92%	1,526	2.5	Yes	4	8	1.9%
17	NYU Langone Hospitals, New York, N.Y.	64.0	8	8	89%	1,076	2.3	Yes	4	8	4.2%
18	Beaumont Hospital-Royal Oak, Mich.	63.7	10	9	89%	1,385	1.9	Yes	4	8	0.1%
19	Beaumont Hospital-Grosse Pointe, Mich.	63.1	10	10	91%	503	1.5	Yes	4	8	0.0%
19	Brigham and Women's Hospital, Boston	63.1	3	9	92%	719	2.2	Yes	4	8	11.7%
19	Hosps. of the U. of Pennsylvania-Penn Presby., Philadelphia	63.1	6	7	91%	894	2.5	Yes	4	8	8.0%
22	Barnes-Jewish Hospital, St. Louis	62.7	4	10	90%	1,035	2.2	Yes	4	8	8.4%
23	Flagler Hospital, St. Augustine, Fla.	62.6	10	10	88%	366	1.9	Yes	3	6	0.0%
24	Yale New Haven Hospital, Conn.	62.4	8	6	89%	1,354	2.0	Yes	4	8	4.8%
25	Mount Sinai West and Mount Sinai St. Luke's Hosps., New York	61.8	10	10	85%	699	1.7	No	4	8	0.5%
26	Beaumont Hospital-Troy, Mich.	61.4	10	8	89%	865	1.9	Yes	4	8	0.0%
27	NYU Winthrop Hospital, Mineola, N.Y.	61.1	10	10	88%	542	2.0	Yes	4	8	1.0%
27	University of Wisconsin Hospitals, Madison	61.1	10	4	93%	450	3.1	Yes	4	8	1.1%
29	Mount Sinai Beth Israel, New York	60.8	10	10	84%	996	1.6	No	4	8	0.7%
30	Tampa General Hospital	60.4	10	9	90%	693	2.1	Yes	4	8	0.0%
31	Scripps La Jolla Hospitals, La Jolla, Calif.	59.8	9	7	92%	582	3.0	Yes	4	8	0.7%
32	Saint Barnabas Medical Center, Livingston, N.J.	59.7	10	7	89%	475	1.9	Yes	4	8	0.0%
33	Long Island Jewish Medical Center, New Hyde Park, N.Y.	59.6	9	9	86%	1,297	1.6	Yes	4	8	0.3%
33	UPMC Presbyterian Shadyside, Pittsburgh	59.6	7	7	89%	1,208	2.1	Yes	4	8	4.0%
35	Mission Hospitals, Mission Viejo and Laguna Beach, Calif.	59.5	9	10	91%	463	2.3	Yes	4	8	0.0%
36	Ohio State University Wexner Medical Center, Columbus	59.2	9	3	89%	843	2.1	Yes	4	7	2.1%
37	Northwestern Memorial Hospital, Chicago	59.1	6	10	92%	655	1.9	Yes	4	8	2.7%
38	Beth Israel Deaconess Medical Center, Boston	58.4	10	6	89%	561	1.6	No	4	8	3.0%
39	UT Southwestern Medical Center, Dallas	57.9	7	9	93%	595	2.1	Yes	4	8	2.8%
40	Lahey Hospital and Medical Center, Burlington, Mass.	57.7	10	8	91%	521	1.2	No	4	8	0.1%
40	Providence Tarzana Medical Center, Tarzana, Calif.	57.7	10	10	87%	440	2.4	No	4	8	0.1%
40	UF Health Shands Hospital, Gainesville, Fla.	57.7	9	9	89%	555	2.0	Yes	4	8	0.8%
43	Abbott Northwestern Hospital, Minneapolis	57.5	9	8	91%	758	2.7	Yes	4	8	0.1%
44	Emory University Hospital, Atlanta	57.1	6	10	92%	603	2.1	Yes	4	8	3.5%
45	Adventist Health-Glendale, Los Angeles	57.0	10	10	89%	552	1.7	No	4	8	0.0%
46	St. Luke's Regional Medical Center, Boise, Idaho	56.9	9	10	91%	664	2.8	Yes	4	6	0.0%
47	DMC Harper University Hospital, Detroit	56.8	10	10	87%	371	1.6	Yes	4	8	0.2%
48	Baptist Medical Center Jacksonville, Fla.	56.7	9	8	89%	1,108	1.7	Yes	4	8	0.0%
49	Houston Methodist Hospital	56.6	8	9	92%	939	2.0	Yes	4	8	0.5%
49	University of Kansas Hospital, Kansas City	56.6	9	6	93%	598	2.0	Yes	4	8	0.4%

Terms are explained on Page 118.

More @ usnews.com/besthospitals

Ear, Nose & Throat

Rank	Hospital	U.S. News score	Survival score (10=best)	Discharge to home score (10=best)	Patient experience (% positive responses)	Number of patients	Nurse staffing score (higher is better)	A Nurse Magnet hospital	Patient services score (8=best)	Trauma center	% of specialists recommending hospital
1	Mayo Clinic, Rochester, Minn.	100.0	10	9	94%	703	2.8	Yes	8	Yes	11.5%
2	Massachusetts Eye & Ear Infirmary, Mass. Gen. Hosp., Boston	94.9	10	4	93%	674	2.4	Yes	8	Yes	19.4%
3	Ohio State University Wexner Medical Center, Columbus	91.1	10	3	89%	677	2.1	Yes	7	Yes	6.1%
3	University of Texas MD Anderson Cancer Center, Houston	91.1	10	10	95%	1,007	1.8	Yes	8	No	10.2%
5	Memorial Sloan-Kettering Cancer Center, New York	87.5	10	10	93%	587	2.1	Yes	8	No	3.2%
6	University of Iowa Hospitals and Clinics, Iowa City	83.8	10	7	88%	318	1.9	Yes	8	Yes	11.0%
7	Hosps. of the U. of Pennsylvania-Penn Presby., Philadelphia	82.8	10	6	91%	640	2.5	Yes	8	Yes	10.2%
8	Stanford Health Care-Stanford Hospital, Palo Alto, Calif.	82.5	9	8	90%	550	2.9	Yes	8	Yes	10.0%
9	University of Miami Hospital and Clinics-UHealth Tower	81.9	10	10	NA	1,021	1.3	No	8	No	1.3%
10	University of Maryland Medical Center, Baltimore	80.1	10	7	88%	291	2.8	Yes	8	Yes	1.1%
11	UCLA Medical Center, Los Angeles	79.2	8	8	92%	880	3.1	Yes	8	Yes	7.3%
12	UC Davis Medical Center, Sacramento, Calif.	78.2	10	10	89%	360	2.8	Yes	8	Yes	2.0%
13	Johns Hopkins Hospital, Baltimore	76.6	7	9	92%	323	2.2	Yes	8	Yes	22.0%
13	UCSF Medical Center, San Francisco	76.6	9	6	93%	372	2.7	Yes	8	Yes	7.1%
15	University of Virginia Medical Center, Charlottesville	75.5	10	9	90%	183	2.0	Yes	8	Yes	3.6%
16	University of North Carolina Hospitals, Chapel Hill	74.3	10	9	92%	406	1.6	Yes	8	Yes	4.5%
17	New York-Presbyterian Hospital-Columbia and Cornell, N.Y.	73.9	10	8	89%	518	3.0	No	8	Yes	3.9%
18	Long Island Jewish Medical Center, New Hyde Park, N.Y.	73.6	10	10	86%	358	1.6	Yes	8	Yes	0.6%
19	Yale New Haven Hospital, Conn.	72.4	10	7	89%	565	2.0	Yes	8	Yes	1.3%
20	Vanderbilt University Medical Center, Nashville, Tenn.	71.2	8	6	91%	579	2.2	Yes	8	Yes	10.0%
21	Jefferson Health-Thomas Jefferson U. Hospitals, Philadelphia	70.9	9	6	89%	696	2.0	Yes	8	Yes	2.5%
22	U. of Michigan Hospitals-Michigan Medicine, Ann Arbor	70.6	7	5	91%	451	2.8	Yes	8	Yes	11.3%
23	MUSC Health-University Medical Center, Charleston, S.C.	69.7	7	10	92%	399	2.0	Yes	8	Yes	8.1%
24	Lenox Hill Hosp.-Manhattan Eye, Ear and Throat Inst., N.Y.	69.6	10	9	87%	218	2.5	No	8	No	1.3%
25	UPMC Presbyterian Shadyside, Pittsburgh	69.2	8	3	89%	796	2.1	Yes	8	Yes	7.9%
26	University of Alabama at Birmingham Hospital	68.9	8	10	93%	866	1.9	Yes	8	Yes	1.6%
27	Cleveland Clinic	68.2	9	3	93%	382	2.5	Yes	8	No	9.9%
28	Mount Sinai Hospital, New York	67.8	8	9	86%	583	2.0	Yes	8	Yes	4.6%
29	H. Lee Moffitt Cancer Center and Research Institute, Tampa	67.7	10	10	94%	322	1.3	Yes	7	No	0.2%
30	OHSU Hospital, Portland, Ore.	67.5	9	6	92%	506	2.1	Yes	8	Yes	2.9%
31	Northwestern Memorial Hospital, Chicago	66.2	9	10	92%	174	1.9	Yes	8	Yes	2.3%
32	Mayo Clinic-Phoenix	63.6	8	8	96%	369	3.2	Yes	8	No	1.9%
32	University of Kansas Hospital, Kansas City	63.6	9	3	93%	410	2.0	Yes	8	Yes	2.2%
34	Barnes-Jewish Hospital, St. Louis	62.9	6	10	90%	499	2.2	Yes	8	Yes	6.7%
35	NYU Langone Hospitals, New York, N.Y.	62.5	8	9	89%	252	2.3	Yes	8	Yes	2.5%
36	University of Chicago Medical Center	61.1	9	6	91%	253	2.3	Yes	8	Yes	1.2%
37	Vidant Medical Center, Greenville, N.C.	60.9	9	10	89%	165	1.6	Yes	8	Yes	0.1%
38	Cedars-Sinai Medical Center, Los Angeles	59.3	7	9	92%	320	2.5	Yes	8	Yes	0.9%
39	University Hospitals Cleveland Medical Center	58.7	9	1	89%	371	2.6	Yes	8	Yes	1.8%
40	Henry Ford Hospital, Detroit	57.4	9	7	89%	232	2.1	No	8	Yes	1.1%
41	UF Health Jacksonville, Fla.	56.5	9	6	88%	225	1.3	Yes	8	Yes	0.1%
42	U. of Arkansas for Med. Sciences, Little Rock, Ark.	56.2	9	9	89%	238	2.0	No	7	Yes	0.7%
43	Emory University Hospital Midtown, Atlanta	55.5	8	10	89%	523	1.5	No	8	No	2.0%
43	Sentara Norfolk General Hospital, Norfolk, Va.	55.5	8	7	90%	280	1.7	Yes	8	Yes	1.0%
45	Albany Medical Center, N.Y.	55.1	9	10	85%	227	1.9	No	7	Yes	0.3%
46	Beaumont Hospital-Troy, Mich.	54.9	8	7	89%	205	1.9	Yes	8	Yes	0.1%
47	University of Washington Medical Center, Seattle	54.7	7	6	92%	271	2.1	Yes	8	No	6.3%
48	Beaumont Hospital-Royal Oak, Mich.	54.0	7	7	89%	328	1.9	Yes	8	Yes	0.3%
49	University of Wisconsin Hospitals, Madison	53.9	7	6	93%	256	3.1	Yes	8	Yes	0.7%
50	UT Southwestern Medical Center, Dallas	53.8	7	6	93%	291	2.1	Yes	8	No	2.1%

NA=Not available. Terms are explained on Page 118.

Gastroenterology & GI Surgery

Rank	Hospital	U.S. News score	Survival score (10=best)	Discharge to home score (10=best)	Patient experience (% positive responses)	Number of patients	Nurse staffing score (higher is better)	A Nurse Magnet hospital	Technology score (7=best)	Patient services score (8=best)	Trauma center	% of specialists recommending hospital
1	Mayo Clinic, Rochester, Minn.	100.0	10	10	94%	9,872	2.8	Yes	7	8	Yes	39.2%
2	Cedars-Sinai Medical Center, Los Angeles	88.6	10	10	92%	9,655	2.5	Yes	7	8	Yes	8.7%
3	Johns Hopkins Hospital, Baltimore	86.8	10	10	92%	4,049	2.2	Yes	7	8	Yes	16.5%
4	Cleveland Clinic	84.7	10	9	93%	7,125	2.5	Yes	7	8	No	27.1%
5	Massachusetts General Hospital, Boston	75.8	10	10	93%	6,344	2.4	Yes	7	8	Yes	12.8%
6	UCLA Medical Center, Los Angeles	74.2	10	10	92%	5,438	3.1	Yes	7	8	Yes	9.4%
7	Mayo Clinic-Phoenix	71.3	10	10	96%	4,203	3.2	Yes	7	8	No	5.7%
8	UPMC Presbyterian Shadyside, Pittsburgh	71.0	10	8	89%	8,519	2.1	Yes	7	8	Yes	6.1%
9	Mount Sinai Hospital, New York	70.5	10	10	86%	5,665	2.0	Yes	7	8	Yes	10.8%
10	New York-Presbyterian Hospital-Columbia and Cornell, N.Y.	68.7	10	10	89%	11,207	3.0	No	7	8	Yes	8.3%
11	NYU Langone Hospitals, New York, N.Y.	67.7	10	10	89%	5,461	2.3	Yes	7	8	Yes	4.6%
11	UCSF Medical Center, San Francisco	67.7	10	10	93%	3,394	2.7	Yes	7	8	Yes	5.8%
13	Keck Hospital of USC, Los Angeles	66.9	10	10	91%	2,643	2.9	Yes	7	8	Yes	0.7%
14	Houston Methodist Hospital	66.5	10	9	92%	6,225	2.0	Yes	7	8	No	0.7%
15	Abbott Northwestern Hospital, Minneapolis	65.2	10	10	91%	5,746	2.7	Yes	6	8	No	0.1%
16	Jefferson Health-Thomas Jefferson U. Hospitals, Philadelphia	64.8	10	10	89%	5,235	2.0	Yes	7	8	Yes	2.1%
17	Cleveland Clinic Florida, Weston	64.7	10	10	92%	2,960	2.5	No	7	8	No	3.3%
18	AdventHealth Orlando	64.0	10	9	90%	15,559	2.4	No	7	8	No	1.1%
19	Hosps. of the U. of Pennsylvania-Penn Presby., Philadelphia	63.9	10	9	91%	5,053	2.5	Yes	7	8	Yes	5.9%
20	Northwestern Memorial Hospital, Chicago	63.4	10	10	92%	3,809	1.9	Yes	7	8	Yes	4.5%
20	U. of Michigan Hospitals-Michigan Medicine, Ann Arbor	63.4	9	9	91%	4,764	2.8	Yes	7	8	Yes	6.6%
22	Baylor St. Luke's Medical Center, Houston	63.0	10	10	87%	3,362	2.0	Yes	7	8	No	1.1%
22	Tampa General Hospital	63.0	10	9	90%	3,528	2.1	Yes	7	8	Yes	1.2%
22	University of Chicago Medical Center	63.0	9	10	91%	2,743	2.3	Yes	7	8	Yes	7.5%
25	Scripps La Jolla Hospitals, La Jolla, Calif.	62.5	10	10	92%	3,909	3.0	Yes	7	8	Yes	0.2%
26	University of Wisconsin Hospitals, Madison	62.0	10	9	93%	3,533	3.1	Yes	7	8	Yes	0.6%
27	Memorial Sloan-Kettering Cancer Center, New York	61.7	10	10	93%	7,443	2.1	Yes	6	8	No	2.1%
28	University Hospitals Cleveland Medical Center	61.3	10	10	89%	3,225	2.6	Yes	7	8	Yes	1.3%
29	Beth Israel Deaconess Medical Center, Boston	60.9	10	8	89%	4,234	1.6	No	7	8	Yes	1.8%
30	Barnes-Jewish Hospital, St. Louis	60.8	9	10	90%	6,348	2.2	Yes	7	8	Yes	4.0%
31	Beaumont Hospital-Royal Oak, Mich.	60.3	10	9	89%	7,039	1.9	Yes	7	8	Yes	0.5%
32	Lahey Hospital and Medical Center, Burlington, Mass.	60.2	10	9	91%	4,009	1.2	No	7	8	Yes	1.6%
33	Loyola University Medical Center, Maywood, Ill.	60.1	10	10	88%	2,641	2.5	Yes	7	8	Yes	0.3%
33	North Shore University Hospital, Manhasset, N.Y.	60.1	10	10	91%	5,251	2.1	Yes	6	8	Yes	0.7%
35	University of Virginia Medical Center, Charlottesville	60.0	10	10	90%	2,773	2.0	Yes	7	8	Yes	1.4%
36	St. Francis Hospital-Roslyn, N.Y.	59.9	10	10	93%	3,148	1.7	Yes	6	8	No	0.1%
36	UCI Medical Center, Orange, Calif.	59.9	10	10	90%	2,809	2.0	Yes	6	7	Yes	2.0%
38	California Pacific Medical Center, San Francisco	59.7	10	10	87%	3,435	2.0	No	7	8	No	0.3%
39	Virginia Mason Medical Center, Seattle	59.4	10	10	92%	3,295	1.7	No	5	8	No	1.1%
40	NYU Winthrop Hospital, Mineola, N.Y.	59.3	10	9	88%	3,408	2.0	Yes	6	8	Yes	1.0%
40	UF Health Shands Hospital, Gainesville, Fla.	59.3	10	9	89%	2,744	2.0	Yes	7	8	Yes	2.0%
42	University of North Carolina Hospitals, Chapel Hill	59.2	10	9	92%	3,231	1.6	Yes	7	8	Yes	4.2%
43	Ochsner Medical Center, New Orleans	58.7	10	10	88%	5,547	1.6	Yes	7	8	Yes	1.3%
44	Emory University Hospital, Atlanta	58.4	10	10	92%	3,216	2.1	Yes	7	8	No	1.5%
45	Duke University Hospital, Durham, N.C.	58.2	8	10	92%	4,118	2.1	Yes	7	8	Yes	5.4%
45	Yale New Haven Hospital, Conn.	58.2	9	7	89%	6,964	2.0	Yes	7	8	Yes	1.7%
47	Cleveland Clinic Hillcrest Hospital, Cleveland	58.1	10	6	89%	3,393	1.7	Yes	6	8	Trauma	0.3%
48	Brigham and Women's Hospital, Boston	58.0	8	10	92%	5,173	2.2	Yes	6	8	Yes	4.4%
48	Hoag Memorial Hospital Presbyterian, Newport Beach, Calif.	58.0	10	10	94%	6,044	2.4	Yes	6	8	No	0.2%
50	Huntington Memorial Hospital, Pasadena, Calif.	57.4	10	9	93%	3,066	1.5	Yes	6	8	Yes	0.0%
50	Montefiore Medical Center, Bronx, N.Y.	57.4	10	7	84%	7,108	2.1	No	7	8	Yes	0.5%
50	St. Cloud Hospital, St. Cloud, Minn.	57.4	10	8	91%	5,933	2.0	Yes	5	8	Yes	0.0%

Terms are explained on Page 118.

More @ usnews.com/besthospitals

Geriatrics

Rank	Hospital	U.S. News score	Survival score (10=best)	Discharge to home score (10=best)	Patient experience (% positive responses)	Number of patients	Nurse staffing score (higher is better)	A Nurse Magnet hospital	NIA Alzheimer's center	Patient services score (9=best)	% of specialists recommending hospital
1	Johns Hopkins Hospital, Baltimore	100.0	10	10	92%	12,111	2.2	Yes	Yes	9	16.7%
2	Mayo Clinic, Rochester, Minn.	98.9	10	8	94%	45,186	2.8	Yes	Yes	9	10.4%
3	Mount Sinai Hospital, New York	98.6	10	10	86%	30,699	2.0	Yes	Yes	9	23.5%
4	UCLA Medical Center, Los Angeles	97.5	10	10	92%	28,458	3.1	Yes	No	9	23.6%
5	UCSF Medical Center, San Francisco	94.7	10	10	93%	13,452	2.7	Yes	Yes	9	11.8%
6	Keck Hospital of USC, Los Angeles	92.7	10	10	91%	8,441	2.9	Yes	Yes	9	0.5%
7	Northwestern Memorial Hospital, Chicago	89.3	10	10	92%	16,964	1.9	Yes	Yes	9	2.3%
8	Cleveland Clinic	88.9	10	9	93%	25,727	2.5	Yes	No	9	8.3%
9	New York-Presbyterian Hospital-Columbia and Cornell, N.Y.	87.5	10	9	89%	70,688	3.0	No	Yes	9	5.1%
9	NYU Langone Hospitals, New York, N.Y.	87.5	10	10	89%	35,080	2.3	Yes	Yes	9	3.8%
11	Massachusetts General Hospital, Boston	86.9	10	9	93%	32,488	2.4	Yes	Yes	9	4.3%
12	Cedars-Sinai Medical Center, Los Angeles	86.4	10	10	92%	54,772	2.5	Yes	No	8	0.2%
13	UPMC Presbyterian Shadyside, Pittsburgh	86.0	10	8	89%	36,081	2.1	Yes	Yes	9	7.3%
14	Mayo Clinic-Phoenix	85.9	10	10	96%	17,685	3.2	Yes	Yes	8	0.9%
15	U. of Michigan Hospitals-Michigan Medicine, Ann Arbor	85.3	10	8	91%	16,347	2.8	Yes	Yes	9	6.2%
16	Yale New Haven Hospital, Conn.	83.1	9	6	89%	40,940	2.0	Yes	Yes	9	5.8%
17	Stanford Health Care-Stanford Hospital, Palo Alto, Calif.	82.1	10	9	90%	21,061	2.9	Yes	Yes	9	0.8%
18	UC Davis Medical Center, Sacramento, Calif.	81.7	10	10	89%	16,557	2.8	Yes	Yes	9	0.7%
19	Rush University Medical Center, Chicago	81.1	10	10	91%	12,391	1.6	Yes	Yes	8	2.4%
20	UT Southwestern Medical Center, Dallas	80.7	10	9	93%	11,802	2.1	Yes	Yes	9	0.6%
21	University of Wisconsin Hospitals, Madison	80.6	10	6	93%	14,180	3.1	Yes	Yes	9	1.3%
22	Barnes-Jewish Hospital, St. Louis	79.9	9	10	90%	23,564	2.2	Yes	Yes	9	2.7%
22	Emory University Hospital at Wesley Woods, Atlanta	79.9	10	10	92%	14,020	2.1	Yes	Yes	9	1.7%
24	Brigham and Women's Hospital, Boston	79.8	10	9	92%	21,309	2.2	Yes	Yes	9	0.9%
25	OHSU Hospital, Portland, Ore.	79.6	10	9	92%	11,384	2.1	Yes	Yes	9	0.5%
26	University of Kansas Hospital, Kansas City	79.1	10	8	93%	14,305	2.0	Yes	Yes	9	0.8%
27	Hosps. of the U. of Pennsylvania-Penn Presby., Philadelphia	78.7	9	7	91%	22,488	2.5	Yes	Yes	9	2.5%
28	Beaumont Hospital-Royal Oak, Mich.	77.7	10	9	89%	46,668	1.9	Yes	No	9	1.0%
29	UC San Diego Health-Jacobs Medical Center	77.5	9	10	92%	13,642	2.1	Yes	Yes	9	1.7%
29	University of Washington Medical Center, Seattle	77.5	10	10	92%	6,926	2.1	Yes	Yes	9	2.0%
31	Mayo Clinic-Jacksonville, Fla.	76.9	9	9	96%	11,642	2.5	Yes	Yes	8	2.3%
32	Oroville Hospital, Calif.	76.8	10	10	82%	7,268	1.4	No	No	8	0.0%
33	Abbott Northwestern Hospital, Minneapolis	76.7	10	8	91%	37,177	2.7	Yes	No	9	0.1%
34	Houston Methodist Hospital	76.4	10	9	92%	29,490	2.0	Yes	No	9	0.9%
35	North Shore University Hospital, Manhasset, N.Y.	76.1	10	10	91%	36,427	2.1	Yes	No	9	1.6%
36	Scripps La Jolla Hospitals, La Jolla, Calif.	75.5	10	9	92%	23,269	3.0	Yes	NIA	8	0.4%
37	UF Health Shands Hospital, Gainesville, Fla.	75.1	9	8	89%	14,470	2.0	Yes	Yes	9	1.6%
38	Jefferson Health-Thomas Jefferson U. Hospitals, Philadelphia	73.8	10	9	89%	23,018	2.0	Yes	No	9	2.2%
39	AdventHealth Orlando	73.5	10	9	90%	94,815	2.4	No	No	9	0.7%
39	DMC Harper University Hospital, Detroit	73.5	10	10	87%	7,922	1.6	Yes	No	8	0.0%
41	Banner University Medical Center Phoenix	72.9	9	9	88%	10,081	2.3	Yes	Yes	9	0.4%
42	Beth Israel Deaconess Medical Center, Boston	72.8	10	6	89%	20,134	1.6	No	Yes	9	2.2%
42	UCI Medical Center, Orange, Calif.	72.8	9	10	90%	10,891	2.0	Yes	Yes	7	0.7%
44	St. Francis Hospital-Roslyn, N.Y.	72.7	10	10	93%	22,710	1.7	Yes	No	8	0.6%
45	Indiana University Health Medical Center, Indianapolis	72.5	8	6	87%	16,335	2.0	Yes	Yes	9	2.7%
45	University Hospitals Cleveland Medical Center	72.5	10	7	89%	14,641	2.6	Yes	No	9	0.6%
47	Beaumont Hospital-Grosse Pointe, Mich.	72.3	10	10	91%	11,801	1.5	Yes	No	8	0.0%
48	Montefiore Medical Center, Bronx, N.Y.	72.1	10	9	84%	45,502	2.1	No	No	9	1.6%
49	Lenox Hill Hospital, New York	72.0	10	10	87%	18,307	2.5	No	No	9	0.5%
50	St. Cloud Hospital, St. Cloud, Minn.	71.8	10	6	91%	36,871	2.0	Yes	No	8	0.0%

Terms are explained on Page 118.

Gynecology

Rank	Hospital	U.S. News score	Survival score (10=best)	Discharge to home score (10=best)	Patient experience (% positive responses)	Number of patients	Nurse staffing score (higher is better)	A Nurse Magnet hospital	Technology score (5=best)	Patient services score (9=best)	% of specialists recom- mending hospital
1	Memorial Sloan-Kettering Cancer Center, New York	100.0	10	10	93%	827	2.1	Yes	5	8	6.3%
2	Mayo Clinic, Rochester, Minn.	99.0	10	7	94%	728	2.8	Yes	5	9	12.6%
3	Cleveland Clinic	92.4	10	3	93%	343	2.5	Yes	5	9	10.9%
4	New York-Presbyterian Hospital-Columbia and Cornell, N.Y.	92.1	10	9	89%	581	3.0	No	5	9	7.4%
5	Brigham and Women's Hospital, Boston	87.7	10	9	92%	448	2.2	Yes	5	9	11.3%
6	Massachusetts General Hospital, Boston	82.5	10	8	93%	377	2.4	Yes	5	9	6.2%
7	Johns Hopkins Hospital, Baltimore	81.6	9	10	92%	225	2.2	Yes	5	9	10.2%
8	Cedars-Sinai Medical Center, Los Angeles	79.0	10	10	92%	630	2.5	Yes	5	9	1.5%
9	Stanford Health Care-Stanford Hospital, Palo Alto, Calif.	78.9	10	9	90%	405	2.9	Yes	5	9	3.0%
10	Beaumont Hospital-Royal Oak, Mich.	78.6	10	10	89%	358	1.9	Yes	5	9	0.4%
11	Hosps. of the U. of Pennsylvania-Penn Presby., Philadelphia	78.5	10	6	91%	320	2.5	Yes	5	9	3.5%
12	University of Wisconsin Hospitals, Madison	78.3	10	4	93%	501	3.1	Yes	5	9	1.0%
13	Inova Fairfax Hospital, Falls Church, Va.	77.8	10	10	91%	669	1.8	No	5	9	0.6%
14	Rush University Medical Center, Chicago	76.7	10	9	91%	344	1.6	Yes	5	9	0.5%
15	Barnes-Jewish Hospital, St. Louis	75.7	8	6	90%	784	2.2	Yes	5	9	4.4%
16	UC Davis Medical Center, Sacramento, Calif.	74.1	10	9	89%	412	2.8	Yes	5	9	0.7%
17	U. of Michigan Hospitals-Michigan Medicine, Ann Arbor	73.5	9	7	91%	289	2.8	Yes	5	9	5.0%
18	Mount Sinai Hospital, New York	73.2	9	10	86%	482	2.0	Yes	5	9	3.3%
19	University of Iowa Hospitals and Clinics, Iowa City	72.8	10	2	88%	332	1.9	Yes	5	9	1.3%
20	UCI Medical Center, Orange, Calif.	71.8	10	6	90%	297	2.0	Yes	5	7	1.2%
21	Long Island Jewish Medical Center, New Hyde Park, N.Y.	71.4	10	9	86%	463	1.6	Yes	5	9	0.8%
22	Scripps La Jolla Hospitals, La Jolla, Calif.	70.4	9	8	92%	354	3.0	Yes	5	9	1.3%
22	White Plains Hospital, N.Y.	70.4	10	10	91%	163	1.1	Yes	5	9	0.0%
24	Christiana Care Hospitals, Newark, Del.	69.8	9	9	89%	593	2.1	Yes	5	8	0.4%
25	Saint Barnabas Medical Center, Livingston, N.J.	69.7	10	8	89%	348	1.9	Yes	5	9	0.3%
26	AdventHealth Orlando	69.5	10	5	90%	824	2.4	No	5	8	0.7%
26	Emory University Hospital, Atlanta	69.5	9	10	92%	195	2.1	Yes	5	9	2.2%
28	Baptist Medical Center Jacksonville, Fla.	69.3	9	8	89%	440	1.7	Yes	5	9	0.3%
29	St. Peter's Hospital-Albany, N.Y.	67.7	10	8	89%	368	1.0	Yes	5	6	0.0%
29	University of North Carolina Hospitals, Chapel Hill	67.7	8	9	92%	363	1.6	Yes	5	9	4.3%
31	ProMedica Toledo Hospital, Ohio	67.6	10	5	88%	454	1.8	No	5	8	0.0%
32	University of Texas MD Anderson Cancer Center, Houston	66.7	3	10	95%	689	1.8	Yes	5	8	7.3%
33	OSF HealthCare St. Francis Medical Center, Peoria, Ill.	65.9	9	3	89%	334	2.2	Yes	5	9	0.0%
34	Maine Medical Center, Portland	65.5	9	6	90%	371	2.2	Yes	5	9	0.1%
34	NYU Langone Hospitals, New York, N.Y.	65.5	6	10	89%	288	2.3	Yes	5	9	4.5%
34	University of Chicago Medical Center	65.5	9	3	91%	222	2.3	Yes	5	9	2.3%
37	NorthShore University HealthSystem-Metro Chicago	65.2	10	3	90%	303	1.4	Yes	5	8	0.1%
37	University of Washington Medical Center, Seattle	65.2	8	6	92%	317	2.1	Yes	5	9	2.1%
39	Avera McKennan Hosp. and U. Hlth. Ctr., Sioux Falls, S.D.	65.1	9	6	88%	286	2.6	Yes	5	8	0.1%
39	Yale New Haven Hospital, Conn.	65.1	8	3	89%	448	2.0	Yes	5	9	2.0%
41	Hoag Memorial Hospital Presbyterian, Newport Beach, Calif.	64.5	7	10	94%	390	2.4	Yes	5	9	0.1%
42	Loma Linda University Medical Center, Calif.	64.4	10	9	90%	269	2.5	No	5	8	0.2%
43	H. Lee Moffitt Cancer Center and Research Institute, Tampa	64.2	8	10	94%	402	1.3	Yes	5	8	0.2%
43	Pennsylvania Hospital, Philadelphia	64.2	9	9	90%	216	2.2	Yes	5	9	0.8%
45	Baylor University Medical Center, Dallas	64.1	8	8	93%	359	1.7	Yes	5	9	0.8%
46	UCSF Medical Center, San Francisco	64.0	7	2	93%	175	2.7	Yes	5	9	6.0%
47	Beth Israel Deaconess Medical Center, Boston	63.7	10	10	89%	240	1.6	No	5	9	0.9%
47	University of Alabama at Birmingham Hospital	63.7	5	9	93%	582	1.9	Yes	5	9	3.0%
49	Vidant Medical Center, Greenville, N.C.	63.6	8	10	89%	210	1.6	Yes	5	9	0.1%
50	Montefiore Medical Center, Bronx, N.Y.	63.1	10	9	84%	361	2.1	No	5	9	0.2%
50	Prisma Health Greenville Memorial Hospital, S.C.	63.1	9	8	88%	293	1.4	Yes	5	9	0.2%

Terms are explained on Page 118.

More @ usnews.com/besthospitals

Nephrology

Rank	Hospital	U.S. News score	Survival score (10=best)	Discharge to home score (10=best)	Patient experience (% positive responses)	Number of patients	Nurse staffing score (higher is better)	A Nurse Magnet hospital	Technology score (7=best)	Patient services score (8=best)	% of specialists recom-mending hospital
1	Mayo Clinic, Rochester, Minn.	100.0	10	10	94%	2,706	2.8	Yes	7	8	25.3%
2	Johns Hopkins Hospital, Baltimore	92.6	10	10	92%	1,431	2.2	Yes	7	8	15.0%
3	UCLA Medical Center, Los Angeles	91.1	10	10	92%	1,686	3.1	Yes	7	8	9.1%
4	Cleveland Clinic	89.5	10	10	93%	2,395	2.5	Yes	7	8	17.0%
5	New York-Presbyterian Hospital-Columbia and Cornell, N.Y.	87.7	10	9	89%	4,002	3.0	No	7	8	17.9%
6	UCSF Medical Center, San Francisco	83.8	10	10	93%	1,349	2.7	Yes	7	8	9.1%
7	Massachusetts General Hospital, Boston	80.8	10	10	93%	1,877	2.4	Yes	7	8	12.8%
8	Brigham and Women's Hospital, Boston	77.0	9	10	92%	1,420	2.2	Yes	7	8	12.5%
9	Vanderbilt University Medical Center, Nashville, Tenn.	73.1	9	10	91%	1,809	2.2	Yes	7	8	10.2%
10	Cedars-Sinai Medical Center, Los Angeles	72.9	10	10	92%	2,929	2.5	Yes	7	8	4.1%
11	Mount Sinai Hospital, New York	69.5	10	10	86%	1,785	2.0	Yes	7	8	4.1%
12	NYU Langone Hospitals, New York, N.Y.	69.2	10	10	89%	1,989	2.3	Yes	7	8	2.3%
13	Keck Hospital of USC, Los Angeles	66.2	10	10	91%	1,820	2.9	Yes	7	8	2.3%
14	DMC Harper University Hospital, Detroit	65.3	10	10	87%	885	1.6	Yes	7	8	0.0%
15	Houston Methodist Hospital	64.8	10	10	92%	2,016	2.0	Yes	7	8	1.3%
16	Barnes-Jewish Hospital, St. Louis	63.8	9	10	90%	2,148	2.2	Yes	7	8	4.8%
17	Stanford Health Care-Stanford Hospital, Palo Alto, Calif.	63.6	9	9	90%	1,325	2.9	Yes	7	8	4.8%
18	University of Alabama at Birmingham Hospital	63.4	8	10	93%	1,434	1.9	Yes	7	8	5.9%
19	AdventHealth Orlando	62.7	10	10	90%	6,819	2.4	No	7	8	0.1%
20	Yale New Haven Hospital, Conn.	62.5	9	7	89%	2,821	2.0	Yes	7	8	3.3%
21	Duke University Hospital, Durham, N.C.	62.2	7	9	92%	1,505	2.1	Yes	7	8	6.7%
22	Hosps. of the U. of Pennsylvania-Penn Presby., Philadelphia	62.1	7	7	91%	1,580	2.5	Yes	7	8	7.4%
23	Mount Sinai West and Mount Sinai St. Luke's Hosps., New York	61.6	10	10	85%	1,084	1.7	No	7	8	0.7%
24	UF Health Shands Hospital, Gainesville, Fla.	61.5	10	9	89%	1,354	2.0	Yes	7	8	1.6%
25	Northwestern Memorial Hospital, Chicago	61.4	9	10	92%	1,791	1.9	Yes	7	8	2.6%
26	UC Davis Medical Center, Sacramento, Calif.	60.8	10	10	89%	1,461	2.8	Yes	7	8	1.1%
27	Montefiore Medical Center, Bronx, N.Y.	60.5	10	7	84%	2,740	2.1	No	7	8	0.6%
28	Emory University Hospital, Atlanta	59.8	10	10	92%	1,527	2.1	Yes	7	8	2.3%
29	University of North Carolina Hospitals, Chapel Hill	59.2	8	10	92%	1,125	1.6	Yes	7	8	5.2%
30	Tampa General Hospital	58.8	10	8	90%	1,737	2.1	Yes	7	8	1.0%
31	University of Chicago Medical Center	58.2	9	10	91%	1,115	2.3	Yes	7	8	2.5%
32	U. of Michigan Hospitals-Michigan Medicine, Ann Arbor	58.1	8	9	91%	1,550	2.8	Yes	7	8	3.3%
33	University of Kansas Hospital, Kansas City	57.9	10	9	93%	1,487	2.0	Yes	7	8	0.7%
34	University Hospitals Cleveland Medical Center	57.8	10	6	89%	1,039	2.6	Yes	7	8	1.9%
35	Beaumont Hospital-Royal Oak, Mich.	57.3	10	10	89%	2,548	1.9	Yes	7	8	0.1%
35	Long Island Jewish Medical Center, New Hyde Park, N.Y.	57.3	10	9	86%	1,753	1.6	Yes	7	8	0.4%
37	UT Southwestern Medical Center, Dallas	56.6	9	10	93%	1,683	2.1	A Nurse	7	8	1.9%
38	Lenox Hill Hospital, New York	56.5	10	9	87%	711	2.5	No	6	8	0.5%
39	Avera McKennan Hosp. and U. Hlth. Ctr., Sioux Falls, S.D.	56.1	10	8	88%	897	2.6	Yes	7	8	0.0%
40	Ohio State University Wexner Medical Center, Columbus	55.5	8	7	89%	1,884	2.1	Yes	7	7	3.2%
41	John Muir Health-Walnut Creek Med. Ctr., Walnut Creek, Calif.	55.1	10	10	91%	941	2.1	Yes	6	8	0.0%
41	Providence Tarzana Medical Center, Tarzana, Calif.	55.1	10	10	87%	1,219	2.4	No	6	8	0.0%
41	UCHealth University of Colorado Hospital, Aurora	55.1	8	9	91%	1,431	2.0	Yes	7	8	2.5%
44	Staten Island University Hospital, New York	54.9	10	9	84%	1,175	1.6	No	6	8	0.1%
45	UF Health Jacksonville, Fla.	54.8	10	10	88%	746	1.3	Yes	6	8	0.2%
46	North Shore University Hospital, Manhasset, N.Y.	54.6	9	10	91%	1,416	2.1	Yes	7	8	0.7%
47	NYU Winthrop Hospital, Mineola, N.Y.	54.4	10	9	88%	954	2.0	Yes	6	8	0.6%
47	AMITA Saints Mary and Elizabeth Medical Center Chicago	54.4	10	9	89%	622	0.8	Yes	5	8	0.2%
49	Rush University Medical Center, Chicago	54.2	9	10	91%	973	1.6	Yes	7	8	1.5%
50	Beaumont Hospital-Grosse Pointe, Mich.	53.9	10	10	91%	715	1.5	Yes	6	8	0.0%
50	University of Wisconsin Hospitals, Madison	53.9	9	8	93%	1,248	3.1	Yes	7	8	0.5%

Terms are explained on Page 118.

Neurology & Neurosurgery

Rank	Hospital	U.S. News score	Survival score (10=best)	Discharge to home score (10=best)	Patient experience (% positive responses)	Number of patients	Nurse staffing score (higher is better)	A Nurse Magnet hospital	NAEC epilepsy center	Technology score (5=best)	Patient services score (9=best)	% of specialists recommending hospital
1	Johns Hopkins Hospital, Baltimore	100.0	10	10	92%	3,006	2.2	Yes	Yes	5	9	25.6%
2	Mayo Clinic, Rochester, Minn.	92.9	10	9	94%	6,291	2.8	Yes	Yes	5	9	36.3%
3	UCSF Medical Center, San Francisco	92.1	10	10	93%	3,160	2.7	Yes	Yes	5	9	22.0%
4	New York-Presbyterian Hospital-Columbia and Cornell, N.Y.	90.3	10	10	89%	9,729	3.0	No	Yes	5	9	15.5%
5	Northwestern Memorial Hospital, Chicago	88.3	10	10	92%	3,110	1.9	Yes	Yes	5	9	2.9%
6	UCLA Medical Center, Los Angeles	86.9	10	10	92%	4,378	3.1	Yes	Yes	5	9	10.0%
7	NYU Langone Hospitals, New York, N.Y.	85.2	10	9	89%	4,656	2.3	Yes	Yes	5	9	4.9%
8	Rush University Medical Center, Chicago	82.0	10	10	91%	3,008	1.6	Yes	Yes	5	9	2.7%
9	Stanford Health Care-Stanford Hospital, Palo Alto, Calif.	81.9	10	10	90%	3,676	2.9	Yes	Yes	5	9	6.8%
10	Cleveland Clinic	81.0	10	10	93%	4,616	2.5	Yes	Yes	5	9	17.7%
11	St. Joseph's Hospital and Medical Center, Phoenix	79.4	10	10	90%	5,637	2.1	No	Yes	5	9	7.2%
12	Cedars-Sinai Medical Center, Los Angeles	79.2	10	10	92%	6,597	2.5	Yes	Yes	5	9	1.7%
13	Massachusetts General Hospital, Boston	78.7	7	9	93%	5,834	2.4	Yes	Yes	5	9	22.8%
14	Mount Sinai Hospital, New York	75.3	10	9	86%	3,569	2.0	Yes	Yes	5	9	2.7%
15	UT Southwestern Medical Center, Dallas	73.4	10	10	93%	2,785	2.1	Yes	Yes	5	9	2.6%
16	Keck Hospital of USC, Los Angeles	73.0	10	10	91%	1,342	2.9	Yes	Yes	5	9	1.6%
17	Brigham and Women's Hospital, Boston	71.7	9	10	92%	4,433	2.2	Yes	Yes	5	9	5.5%
18	Baylor St. Luke's Medical Center, Houston	69.9	10	10	87%	2,761	2.0	Yes	Yes	5	8	2.6%
19	U. of Michigan Hospitals-Michigan Medicine, Ann Arbor	69.6	9	8	91%	2,958	2.8	Yes	Yes	5	9	5.1%
20	Barnes-Jewish Hospital, St. Louis	69.0	8	9	90%	5,854	2.2	Yes	Yes	5	9	8.0%
21	Jefferson Health-Thomas Jefferson U. Hospitals, Philadelphia	68.9	10	9	89%	6,018	2.0	Yes	Yes	5	9	2.4%
22	University Hospitals Cleveland Medical Center	67.3	10	6	89%	3,470	2.6	Yes	Yes	5	9	1.7%
23	Duke University Hospital, Durham, N.C.	66.2	9	10	92%	3,609	2.1	Yes	Yes	5	9	4.9%
23	UPMC Presbyterian Shadyside, Pittsburgh	66.2	8	7	89%	9,032	2.1	Yes	Yes	5	9	3.5%
25	Hosps. of the U. of Pennsylvania-Penn Presby., Philadelphia	65.2	7	2	91%	4,631	2.5	Yes	Yes	5	9	9.0%
26	Huntington Memorial Hospital, Pasadena, Calif.	65.0	10	10	93%	2,804	1.5	Yes	No	5	9	0.4%
27	University of Kansas Hospital, Kansas City	64.6	10	9	93%	3,007	2.0	Yes	Yes	5	9	1.0%
28	Loyola University Medical Center, Maywood, Ill.	64.5	10	9	88%	1,900	2.5	Yes	Yes	5	9	1.1%
29	Montefiore Medical Center, Bronx, N.Y.	63.6	10	8	84%	5,253	2.1	No	Yes	5	9	0.3%
30	UC Davis Medical Center, Sacramento, Calif.	63.3	8	10	89%	2,985	2.8	Yes	Yes	5	9	0.9%
31	North Shore University Hospital, Manhasset, N.Y.	63.2	10	9	91%	3,939	2.1	Yes	Yes	5	9	1.0%
31	Pennsylvania Hospital, Philadelphia	63.2	10	10	90%	1,083	2.2	Yes	No	5	9	0.5%
33	Abbott Northwestern Hospital, Minneapolis	63.0	10	9	91%	5,910	2.7	Yes	Yes	5	9	0.4%
34	Beaumont Hospital-Royal Oak, Mich.	62.7	10	9	89%	5,820	1.9	Yes	Yes	5	9	0.1%
34	Houston Methodist Hospital	62.7	10	9	92%	4,985	2.0	Yes	Yes	5	9	2.5%
36	Emory University Hospital, Atlanta	62.2	8	10	92%	3,028	2.1	Yes	Yes	5	9	3.1%
37	Hoag Memorial Hospital Presbyterian, Newport Beach, Calif.	61.7	10	10	94%	4,457	2.4	Yes	Yes	5	9	0.2%
38	Yale New Haven Hospital, Conn.	61.5	8	7	89%	5,514	2.0	Yes	Yes	5	9	1.9%
39	AdventHealth Orlando	60.9	10	10	90%	11,905	2.4	No	Yes	5	9	0.1%
40	UC San Diego Health-Jacobs Medical Center	60.3	7	10	92%	2,229	2.1	Yes	Yes	5	9	1.7%
41	Mayo Clinic-Jacksonville, Fla.	60.2	7	10	96%	2,084	2.5	Yes	Yes	5	9	4.1%
42	DMC Harper University Hospital, Detroit	60.1	10	10	87%	826	1.6	Yes	Yes	5	8	0.1%
42	Henry Ford Hospital, Detroit	60.1	10	8	89%	2,910	2.1	No	Yes	5	9	1.0%
44	OHSU Hospital, Portland, Ore.	60.0	7	10	92%	3,459	2.1	Yes	Yes	5	9	1.2%
45	UCHealth University of Colorado Hospital, Aurora	59.6	9	10	91%	3,004	2.0	Yes	Yes	5	9	0.9%
46	Beaumont Hospital-Troy, Mich.	59.3	10	8	89%	3,730	1.9	Yes	No	5	9	0.0%
47	University of Wisconsin Hospitals, Madison	59.2	8	6	93%	3,111	3.1	Yes	Yes	5	9	0.3%
48	Scripps La Jolla Hospitals, La Jolla, Calif.	58.9	10	10	92%	3,243	3.0	Yes	No	5	8	0.1%
49	Saint Luke's Hospital of Kansas City, Mo.	58.6	9	9	92%	4,339	1.6	Yes	Yes	5	9	0.6%
50	Ochsner Medical Center, New Orleans	58.2	9	10	88%	4,825	1.6	Yes	Yes	5	9	0.5%

Terms are explained on Page 118.

More @ usnews.com/besthospitals

HOSPITAL DATA **INSIGHTS** | ADULT

U.S.News & WORLD REPORT

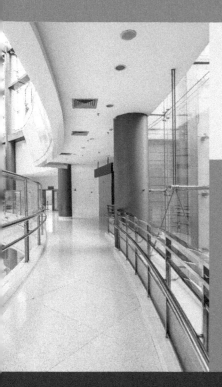

Your Hospital by the Numbers

U.S. News Hospital Data Insights is a new analytics platform from U.S. News & World Report based on the data underpinning the Best Hospitals rankings.

Why Hospital Data Insights?

- Best-in-class analytics
- Superior peer benchmarking
- Extract charts and graphs easily for detailed analysis
- Study year on year data trends to drive clinical improvements

2,700+
HOSPITALS

2,500+
METRICS

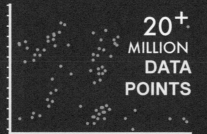

20+
MILLION
DATA
POINTS

EXCLUSIVE, UNPUBLISHED

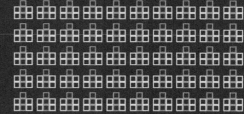

DATA POINTS
& RANKINGS

UNLIMITED PEER GROUPS

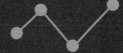

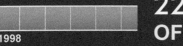

22 YEARS
OF DATA

1998   2019

To request a demo, contact us   **hdi.usnews.com**

 hdi@usnews.com
 202.955.2171

Orthopedics

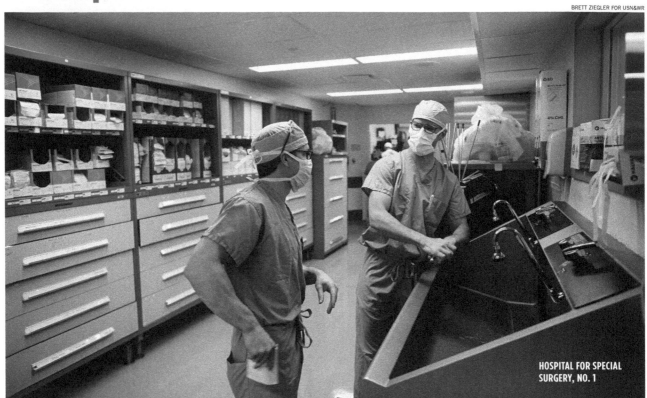

BRETT ZIEGLER FOR USN&WR

HOSPITAL FOR SPECIAL
SURGERY, NO. 1

Rank	Hospital	U.S. News score	Survival score (10=best)	Discharge to home score (10=best)	Patient experience (% positive responses)	Number of patients	Nurse staffing score (higher is better)	A Nurse Magnet hospital	Technology score (2=best)	Patient services score (7=best)	% of specialists recommending hospital
1	Hospital for Special Surgery, New York	100.0	10	7	95%	8,955	3.7	Yes	2	7	29.5%
2	Mayo Clinic, Rochester, Minn.	80.0	10	5	94%	8,970	2.8	Yes	2	7	26.6%
3	Cedars-Sinai Medical Center, Los Angeles	78.5	10	10	92%	7,939	2.5	Yes	2	7	2.1%
4	UCSF Medical Center, San Francisco	67.4	10	6	93%	3,651	2.7	Yes	2	7	3.4%
5	NYU Langone Orthopedic Hospital, New York	66.0	10	8	89%	5,689	2.3	Yes	2	7	8.0%
6	Massachusetts General Hospital, Boston	64.7	10	5	93%	4,063	2.4	Yes	2	7	9.5%
7	Rush University Medical Center, Chicago	62.7	10	7	91%	3,054	1.6	Yes	2	7	8.2%
8	UCLA Medical Center, Los Angeles	61.8	10	6	92%	2,567	3.1	Yes	2	7	2.9%
9	Stanford Health Care-Stanford Hospital, Palo Alto, Calif.	61.2	10	5	90%	5,124	2.9	Yes	2	7	3.5%
10	Rothman Institute at Thomas Jefferson U. Hosp., Philadelphia	60.2	9	6	89%	6,557	2.0	Yes	2	7	7.4%
11	North Shore University Hospital, Manhasset, N.Y.	60.0	10	5	91%	3,300	2.1	Yes	2	7	0.4%
11	Scripps La Jolla Hospitals, La Jolla, Calif.	60.0	10	8	92%	5,330	3.0	Yes	2	7	0.7%
13	New York-Presbyterian Hospital-Columbia and Cornell, N.Y.	59.7	10	5	89%	6,129	3.0	No	2	7	2.3%
14	Houston Methodist Hospital	58.8	10	7	92%	4,342	2.0	Yes	2	7	1.9%
15	Beaumont Hospital-Royal Oak, Mich.	57.5	10	5	89%	5,658	1.9	Yes	2	7	1.3%
16	Tampa General Hospital	56.3	10	7	90%	3,284	2.1	Yes	2	6	1.3%
17	Cleveland Clinic	56.2	6	3	93%	3,582	2.5	Yes	2	7	15.1%
18	Mount Sinai Hospital, New York	56.0	10	7	86%	2,911	2.0	Yes	2	7	1.0%
19	New England Baptist Hospital, Boston	55.8	10	3	94%	3,504	2.6	No	2	7	1.7%
19	University of Wisconsin Hospitals, Madison	55.8	10	6	93%	2,319	3.1	Yes	2	7	1.0%
21	Huntington Memorial Hospital, Pasadena, Calif.	55.7	10	9	93%	3,432	1.5	Yes	1	7	0.0%
22	Johns Hopkins Hospital, Baltimore	55.4	9	6	92%	1,869	2.2	Yes	2	7	6.1%
23	Mayo Clinic-Phoenix	55.0	10	8	96%	2,414	3.2	Yes	2	7	1.9%
24	Long Island Jewish Medical Center, New Hyde Park, N.Y.	54.6	10	5	86%	1,792	1.6	Yes	2	7	0.4%

(CONTINUED ON PAGE 140)

Terms are explained on Page 118.

More @ usnews.com/besthospitals

WE CELEBRATE HOW YOU MOVE AND BEING U.S. #1 FOR 10 STRAIGHT YEARS.

As the nation's #1 orthopedic hospital for 10 straight years, we've had hundreds of thousands of successful outcomes—a testament to our unique focus on how you move. Our world-class physicians will always be dedicated to giving our patients the most personalized care and innovative treatment options.

We're proud to have been top ranked in orthopedics and rheumatology for 28 straight years. Visit us at one of our convenient locations or online at HSS.edu.

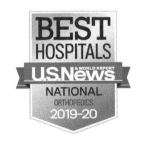

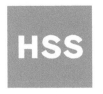

HOSPITAL FOR SPECIAL SURGERY

Orthopedics (CONTINUED)

Rank	Hospital	U.S. News score	Survival score (10=best)	Discharge to home score (10=best)	Patient experience (% positive responses)	Number of patients	Nurse staffing score (higher is better)	A Nurse Magnet hospital	Technology score (2=best)	Patient services score (7=best)	% of specialists recommending hospital
25	Duke University Hospital, Durham, N.C.	54.4	8	6	92%	2,837	2.1	Yes	2	7	5.6%
26	Northwestern Memorial Hospital, Chicago	54.2	10	4	92%	2,256	1.9	Yes	2	7	3.2%
27	University of Iowa Hospitals and Clinics, Iowa City	53.9	9	4	88%	1,942	1.9	Yes	2	7	4.5%
28	Cleveland Clinic Hillcrest Hospital, Cleveland	53.8	10	2	89%	1,860	1.7	Yes	2	7	0.2%
29	UPMC Presbyterian Shadyside, Pittsburgh	53.7	6	6	89%	5,759	2.1	Yes	2	7	5.0%
30	Abbott Northwestern Hospital, Minneapolis	53.6	9	4	91%	8,232	2.7	Yes	2	7	0.1%
30	UCHealth University of Colorado Hospital, Aurora	53.6	10	5	91%	3,063	2.0	Yes	2	7	1.7%
32	Northwestern Medicine Central DuPage Hosp., Winfield, Ill.	53.2	10	2	93%	1,639	2.1	Yes	2	7	0.2%
32	NYU Winthrop Hospital, Mineola, N.Y.	53.2	10	4	88%	1,527	2.0	Yes	2	7	0.3%
34	Morristown Medical Center, N.J.	52.5	10	2	90%	3,224	2.1	Yes	2	7	0.6%
35	Cleveland Clinic Fairview Hospital, Cleveland	52.0	10	1	90%	1,154	1.9	Yes	2	7	0.1%
35	Lehigh Valley Hospital, Allentown, Pa.	52.0	10	3	90%	3,501	1.7	Yes	2	7	0.0%
37	UC Davis Medical Center, Sacramento, Calif.	51.9	9	7	89%	2,795	2.8	Yes	2	7	0.9%
38	Penn State Health Milton S. Hershey Medical Ctr., Hershey, Pa.	51.8	10	6	90%	2,087	1.8	Yes	2	7	0.5%
39	Jersey Shore University Medical Center, Neptune, N.J.	51.7	10	1	88%	1,645	2.3	Yes	2	7	0.3%
40	Stony Brook University Hospital, Stony Brook, N.Y.	50.5	10	7	87%	2,100	2.0	No	2	7	0.5%
41	Hoag Orthopedic Institute, Irvine, Calif.	50.1	8	9	94%	5,423	2.4	Yes	2	7	0.8%
42	Torrance Memorial Medical Center, Torrance, Calif.	49.8	9	10	93%	2,199	2.5	Yes	2	7	0.1%
43	Memorial Hermann-Texas Medical Center, Houston	49.6	7	10	91%	2,837	2.6	Yes	2	7	1.0%
43	St. Jude Medical Center, Fullerton, Calif.	49.6	10	6	92%	1,457	1.5	Yes	2	7	0.5%
45	MemorialCare Saddleback Medical Center, Laguna Hills, Calif.	49.4	10	7	89%	1,285	2.2	Yes	2	7	0.0%
46	Miami Orthopedics & Sports Medicine Inst. at Baptist Hosp. of Miami	49.3	10	8	88%	2,451	1.7	Yes	2	6	0.0%
47	Penn Medicine Lancaster General Hospital, Pa.	49.2	9	6	89%	3,617	1.6	Yes	2	6	0.0%
48	Huntington Hospital, Huntington, N.Y.	49.1	10	4	89%	1,468	1.8	Yes	2	7	0.1%
48	John Muir Health-Walnut Creek Med. Ctr., Walnut Creek, Calif.	49.1	9	5	91%	2,932	2.1	Yes	2	6	0.1%
50	U. of Michigan Hospitals-Michigan Medicine, Ann Arbor	48.9	8	4	91%	1,958	2.8	Yes	2	7	1.1%
50	University of Utah Hospital, Salt Lake City	48.9	9	4	93%	2,777	1.9	No	2	7	3.1%

Terms are explained on Page 118.

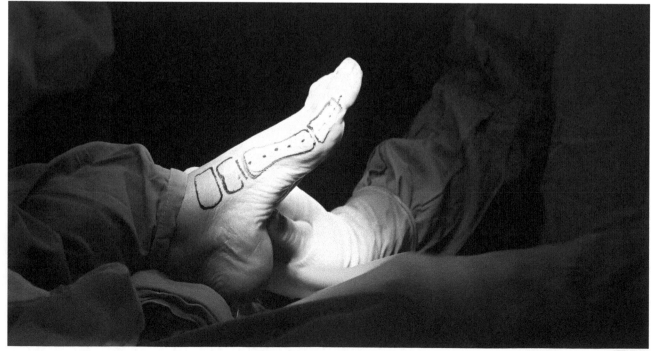

GETTY IMAGES

More @ usnews.com/besthospitals

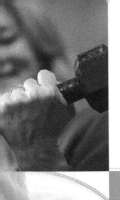

OUTSTANDING HOSPITALS DON'T SIMPLY TREAT FRAGILITY FRACTURES—
THEY PREVENT FRACTURES FROM RECURRING

THE BEST HOSPITALS AND PRACTICES OWN THE BONE

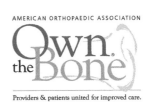

AMERICAN ORTHOPAEDIC ASSOCIATION

Own the Bone

Providers & patients united for improved care.

The American Orthopaedic Association applauds the following institutions for their achievements and participation in the Own the Bone® quality improvement program:

STAR PERFORMERS

Institutions are recognized for at least 75% compliance on at least 5 of the 10 recommended secondary fracture prevention measures over the last year.

Advent Health Orlando - Winter Park, FL

Allegheny Health Network (AHN) - Jefferson Hospital - Pittsburgh, PA

Ascension Sacred Heart - Pensacola, FL

Anne Arundel Medical Group Orthopedics and Sports Medicine Specialists - Annapolis, MD

Berkshire Medical Center - Pittsfield, MA

The Bone and Joint Center at AdventHealth Zephyrhills - Zephyrhills, FL

^Christiana Care Health Systems, Christiana Hospital - Greenville, DE

^Christiana Care Health Systems, Wilmington Hospital - Wilmington, DE

Coastal Fracture Prevention Center - Sebastian, FL

Colorado Spine Institute PLLC - Johnstown, CO

Concord Hospital - Concord, NH

The CORE Institute - Arizona - Phoenix, AZ

Forsyth Medical Center - Winston-Salem, NC

Froedtert & the Medical College of Wisconsin - Milwaukee, WI

Henry Ford Hospital - Detroit, MI

Hoag Orthopedic Institute - Irvine, CA

Huntington Hospital - Northwell Health - Huntington, NY

Illinois Bone & Joint Institute, LLC - Morton Grove, IL

JPS Health Network - Fort Worth, TX

Lahey Hospital and Medical Center - Burlington, MA

Lenox Hill Hospital Northwell Health - Manhasset, NY

LewisGale Medical Center - Salem, VA

MaineGeneral Medical Center - Augusta, ME

Marshfield Clinic Health System - Marshfield, WI

Medical City Arlington - Arlington, TX

Medical University of South Carolina - Charleston, SC

Memorial Regional Hospital - Hollywood , FL

Mercy Health – Orthopedics and Sports Medicine - Toledo - Toledo, OH

Mercy Regional Medical Center - Durango, CO

Methodist Hospitals Spine Care Center - Merrillville, IN

Michigan Medicine, University of Michigan - Ann Arbor, MI

Mission Hospital - Asheville, NC

Mission Trail Baptist Hospital - San Antonio, TX

Newton Medical Center - Newton, KS

Norton Women's and Children's Hospital - Louisville, KY

NYU Langone Health - New York, NY

NYU Winthrop Hospital - Mineola, NY

OhioHealth Grant Medical Center - Columbus, OH

OHSU Department of Orthopaedics & Rehabilitation - Portland, OR

Orthopaedic Associates of Michigan - Grand Rapids, MI

Paramount Health Care - Maumee, OH

^Park Nicollet Methodist Hospital/TRIA Orthopaedic Center - Minneapolis, MN

Peninsula Regional Medical Center - Salisbury, MD

^Penrose-St. Francis Health Services - Colorado Springs, CO

^Prisma Health-Upstate - Greenville, SC

ProMedica Toledo Hospital - Toledo, OH

Regions Hospital - Minneapolis, MN

^Sanford Medical Center – Fargo - Fargo, ND

SIH Herrin Hospital - Herrin, IL

Southeast Georgia Health System - Brunswick, GA

St. Francis Orthopaedic Institute - Columbus, GA

St. Luke's Health System Osteoporosis and Bone Health Program - Boise, ID

St. Luke's University Hospital and Health Network - Bethlehem, PA

St. Vincent's Medical Center - Bridgeport, CT

Tahoe Forest Health System - Truckee, CA

Tallahassee Memorial Health Care - Tallahassee, FL

University Hospital - San Antonio, TX

University of Wisconsin Hospitals and Clinics - Madison, WI

UT Health East Texas Orthopedic Institute - Tyler, TX

Wake Forest Baptist Medical Center - Winston-Salem, NC

^WVU Medicine Department of Orthopedics - Morgantown, WV

UW Medicine/Northwest Hospital and Medical Center - Seattle, WA

^The University of Vermont Health Network - Central Vermont Medical Center - Berlin, VT

NEWLY ENROLLED INSTITUTIONS

Baptist Health - Northeast Baptist Hospital - San Antonio, TX

*Bryan Health - Lincoln, NE

Centers for Advanced Orthopaedics, Orthopaedic Associates of Central Maryland Division - Catonsville, MD

^Center for Musculoskeletal Care, Yale New Haven Hospital - New Haven, CT

Centura Orthopaedics & Spine Meridian - Parker, CO

Colquitt Regional Medical Center - Moultrie, GA

Greater Baltimore Medical Center - Baltimore, MD

Miami Valley Hospital - Dayton, OH

*Penn Medicine Princeton Medical Center - Plainsboro, NJ

*Sonoran Orthopedics - Scottsdale, AZ

South Texas Fracture Prevention Clinic - San Antonio, TX

Sunrise Hospital and Medical Center - Las Vegas, NV

*Unity Point Health Central Illinois & Midwest Orthopedic Center - Peoria, IL

University of Alabama Health Services Foundation P.C. - Birmingham, AL

Own the Bone is a national quality improvement initiative that provides tools and a web-based registry to ensure fragility fracture patients receive bone health care to prevent future fractures.

www.ownthebone.org

AOA
Own the Bone®
EDUCATIONAL
ALLIANCE

The AOA recognizes **Amgen** and **DePuy Synthes** for their 2019 Educational Alliance support.

^First in State to enroll in Own the Bone®
*Also a Star Performer

Pulmonology & Lung Surgery

Rank	Hospital	U.S. News score	Survival score (10=best)	Discharge to home score (10=best)	Patient experience (% positive responses)	Number of patients	Nurse staffing score (higher is better)	A Nurse Magnet hospital	Technology score (6=best)	Patient services score (8=best)	% of specialists recommending hospital
1	National Jewish Health, Denver-U. of Colorado Hosp., Aurora	100.0	10	10	91%	5,851	2.0	Yes	6	8	40.2%
2	Mayo Clinic, Rochester, Minn.	97.1	10	9	94%	10,904	2.8	Yes	6	8	24.3%
3	UCLA Medical Center, Los Angeles	88.0	10	10	92%	9,439	3.1	Yes	6	8	7.9%
4	Cedars-Sinai Medical Center, Los Angeles	87.3	10	10	92%	14,776	2.5	Yes	6	8	1.9%
5	Massachusetts General Hospital, Boston	85.3	10	9	93%	8,256	2.4	Yes	6	8	12.2%
6	Mayo Clinic-Phoenix	84.3	10	10	96%	6,275	3.2	Yes	5	8	3.2%
7	Cleveland Clinic	83.7	9	9	93%	6,154	2.5	Yes	6	8	21.8%
8	UCSF Medical Center, San Francisco	82.0	9	10	93%	4,407	2.7	Yes	6	8	10.1%
9	Johns Hopkins Hospital, Baltimore	81.8	8	10	92%	3,524	2.2	Yes	6	8	16.0%
10	U. of Michigan Hospitals-Michigan Medicine, Ann Arbor	80.4	10	8	91%	4,927	2.8	Yes	6	8	6.4%
11	Kaiser Permanente Anaheim & Irvine Med. Ctrs., Anaheim, Calif.	79.2	10	10	92%	6,499	1.4	Yes	5	8	0.6%
12	Scripps La Jolla Hospitals, La Jolla, Calif.	78.4	10	9	92%	5,386	3.0	Yes	5	8	0.2%
12	St. Cloud Hospital, St. Cloud, Minn.	78.4	10	8	91%	10,386	2.0	Yes	4	8	0.0%
14	Abbott Northwestern Hospital, Minneapolis	78.3	10	9	91%	8,169	2.7	Yes	5	8	0.1%
14	UC San Diego Health-Jacobs Medical Center	78.3	9	10	92%	4,896	2.1	Yes	6	8	6.7%
16	Yale New Haven Hospital, Conn.	78.1	10	7	89%	13,176	2.0	Yes	5	8	3.0%
17	Northwestern Memorial Hospital, Chicago	77.4	10	10	92%	5,023	1.9	Yes	6	8	2.3%
18	Beaumont Hospital-Royal Oak, Mich.	77.3	10	9	89%	11,426	1.9	Yes	5	8	0.8%
18	OHSU Hospital, Portland, Ore.	77.3	10	10	92%	3,276	2.1	Yes	5	8	0.2%
18	UPMC Presbyterian Shadyside, Pittsburgh	77.3	8	7	89%	9,429	2.1	Yes	6	8	8.6%
21	Mercy Hospital-Coon Rapids, Minn.	77.1	10	9	88%	12,380	2.3	No	4	8	0.0%
21	North Shore University Hospital, Manhasset, N.Y.	77.1	10	10	91%	9,338	2.1	Yes	5	8	1.0%
23	Avera McKennan Hosp. and U. Hlth. Ctr., Sioux Falls, S.D.	76.8	10	8	88%	4,294	2.6	Yes	5	8	0.0%
24	Houston Methodist Hospital	76.7	10	8	92%	8,126	2.0	Yes	6	8	0.9%
25	St. Luke's Regional Medical Center, Boise, Idaho	76.6	10	10	91%	7,035	2.8	Yes	5	6	0.0%
26	NYU Langone Hospitals, New York, N.Y.	76.5	9	9	89%	10,117	2.3	Yes	5	8	3.2%
27	University of Iowa Hospitals and Clinics, Iowa City	76.3	10	9	88%	3,305	1.9	Yes	6	8	1.5%
28	Brigham and Women's Hospital, Boston	75.8	8	9	92%	6,348	2.2	Yes	6	8	7.5%
28	Hosps. of the U. of Pennsylvania-Penn Presby., Philadelphia	75.8	7	8	91%	7,337	2.5	Yes	6	8	9.9%
30	New York-Presbyterian Hospital-Columbia and Cornell, N.Y.	75.4	7	9	89%	17,333	3.0	No	6	8	9.1%
31	Stanford Health Care-Stanford Hospital, Palo Alto, Calif.	74.8	8	10	90%	5,866	2.9	Yes	6	8	4.2%
32	Barnes-Jewish Hospital, St. Louis	74.4	6	10	90%	6,944	2.2	Yes	6	8	9.3%
33	Keck Hospital of USC, Los Angeles	74.3	9	10	91%	1,507	2.9	Yes	6	8	1.5%
34	University of Wisconsin Hospitals, Madison	74.2	9	8	93%	4,150	3.1	Yes	6	8	2.3%
35	Intermountain Medical Center, Murray, Utah	73.8	10	10	89%	5,368	2.6	No	5	8	0.7%
35	Reading Hospital, West Reading, Pa.	73.8	10	7	90%	7,791	1.3	Yes	5	7	0.0%
35	St. Joseph's Hospital-West Bend, Wis.	73.8	10	9	91%	1,856	1.5	No	5	8	0.0%
38	Vanderbilt University Medical Center, Nashville, Tenn.	73.6	6	10	91%	5,830	2.2	Yes	6	8	7.5%
39	UC Davis Medical Center, Sacramento, Calif.	73.1	9	10	89%	6,081	2.8	Yes	5	8	0.7%
40	University of Alabama at Birmingham Hospital	73.0	8	10	93%	6,959	1.9	Yes	6	8	2.7%
41	Fairview Ridges Hospital, Burnsville, Minn.	72.9	10	10	90%	4,668	2.1	No	5	8	0.0%
42	Duke University Hospital, Durham, N.C.	72.8	5	9	92%	5,723	2.1	Yes	6	8	9.6%
43	Parker Adventist Hospital, Colo.	72.7	10	7	90%	1,658	2.1	Yes	5	8	0.0%
44	Beaumont Hospital-Grosse Pointe, Mich.	72.5	10	10	91%	3,333	1.5	Yes	5	8	0.0%
44	UF Health Shands Hospital, Gainesville, Fla.	72.5	9	8	89%	5,174	2.0	Yes	6	8	1.8%
46	UPMC Pinnacle, Harrisburg, Pa.	71.8	10	7	89%	8,104	1.5	Yes	5	8	0.0%
47	Park Nicollet Methodist Hospital, St. Louis Park, Minn.	71.6	10	7	90%	10,507	1.9	No	5	8	0.0%
48	Sky Ridge Medical Center, Lone Tree, Colo.	71.4	10	9	89%	2,176	1.8	No	4	8	0.0%
49	University of Kansas Hospital, Kansas City	71.3	9	9	93%	4,839	2.0	Yes	5	8	1.2%
50	John Muir Health-Walnut Creek Med. Ctr., Walnut Creek, Calif.	71.2	9	9	91%	7,053	2.1	Yes	5	8	0.0%
50	Mission Hospitals, Mission Viejo and Laguna Beach, Calif.	71.2	9	10	91%	6,355	2.3	Yes	5	8	0.0%
50	St. Patrick Hospital, Missoula, Mont.	71.2	10	10	92%	2,360	1.3	Yes	5	8	0.0%

Terms are explained on Page 118.

More @ usnews.com/besthospitals

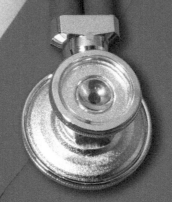
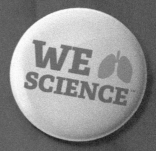

Breathing Science is Life.®

It's easy to take breathing for granted — until you can't.
At National Jewish Health in Denver, the nation's leading
respiratory hospital, we help people who struggle to
breathe get back to living the life they enjoy. For 120 years,
our groundbreaking research and personalized care have
transformed millions of lives. We breathe science, so you can
breathe life. **To make an appointment, call 800.621.0505
or visit njhealth.org.**

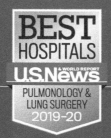

BEST
HOSPITALS
U.S.News & WORLD REPORT
PULMONOLOGY &
LUNG SURGERY
2019–20

National Jewish
Health®

#1 in Respiratory Care

Urology

Rank	Hospital	U.S. News score	Survival score (10=best)	Discharge to home score (10=best)	Patient experience (% positive responses)	Number of patients	Nurse staffing score (higher is better)	A Nurse Magnet hospital	Technology score (6=best)	Patient services score (9=best)	% of specialists recommending hospital
1	Mayo Clinic, Rochester, Minn.	100.0	10	10	94%	2,497	2.8	Yes	6	9	23.1%
2	Johns Hopkins Hospital, Baltimore	99.1	10	10	92%	1,407	2.2	Yes	6	9	25.9%
3	UCSF Medical Center, San Francisco	91.2	10	10	93%	1,315	2.7	Yes	6	9	8.8%
4	Cleveland Clinic	85.3	10	9	93%	1,657	2.5	Yes	6	9	33.1%
4	Keck Hospital of USC, Los Angeles	85.3	10	10	91%	2,169	2.9	Yes	6	9	8.1%
6	Memorial Sloan-Kettering Cancer Center, New York	84.3	10	10	93%	1,469	2.1	Yes	6	8	8.3%
7	University of Texas MD Anderson Cancer Center, Houston	83.6	10	10	95%	2,206	1.8	Yes	6	8	9.3%
8	U. of Michigan Hospitals-Michigan Medicine, Ann Arbor	82.2	10	7	91%	1,152	2.8	Yes	6	9	6.7%
9	New York-Presbyterian Hospital-Columbia and Cornell, N.Y.	81.7	10	10	89%	2,121	3.0	No	6	9	6.9%
10	UCLA Medical Center, Los Angeles	78.4	10	10	92%	1,126	3.1	Yes	6	9	12.1%
11	Massachusetts General Hospital, Boston	77.7	10	8	93%	1,267	2.4	Yes	6	9	4.5%
12	Cedars-Sinai Medical Center, Los Angeles	72.5	10	10	92%	2,101	2.5	Yes	6	9	0.9%
13	Northwestern Memorial Hospital, Chicago	72.3	10	10	92%	1,194	1.9	Yes	6	9	4.6%
14	University of Wisconsin Hospitals, Madison	72.0	10	8	93%	746	3.1	Yes	6	9	2.4%
15	Montefiore Medical Center, Bronx, N.Y.	71.5	10	9	84%	1,112	2.1	No	6	9	0.4%
16	UPMC Presbyterian Shadyside, Pittsburgh	70.3	10	7	89%	1,354	2.1	Yes	6	9	3.0%
17	NYU Langone Hospitals, New York, N.Y.	70.1	10	10	89%	1,124	2.3	Yes	6	9	5.1%
18	Vanderbilt University Medical Center, Nashville, Tenn.	69.7	9	10	91%	1,413	2.2	Yes	6	9	9.2%
19	University of Kansas Hospital, Kansas City	68.8	10	8	93%	875	2.0	Yes	6	9	1.7%
20	AdventHealth Orlando	67.3	10	9	90%	4,654	2.4	No	6	8	1.1%
20	Mayo Clinic-Phoenix	67.3	10	10	96%	1,358	3.2	Yes	6	8	3.3%
22	Beaumont Hospital-Royal Oak, Mich.	67.1	10	9	89%	1,240	1.9	Yes	6	9	1.8%
22	NYU Winthrop Hospital, Mineola, N.Y.	67.1	10	9	88%	564	2.0	Yes	6	9	0.5%
24	Abbott Northwestern Hospital, Minneapolis	66.5	10	7	91%	838	2.7	Yes	6	9	0.1%
24	UF Health Shands Hospital, Gainesville, Fla.	66.5	10	10	89%	646	2.0	Yes	6	9	1.1%
26	University Hospitals Cleveland Medical Center	66.4	10	7	89%	598	2.6	Yes	6	9	2.0%
27	Miriam Hospital, Providence, R.I.	65.5	10	9	93%	618	1.4	Yes	6	7	0.3%
28	Emory University Hospital, Atlanta	64.9	10	10	92%	716	2.1	Yes	6	9	2.2%
29	H. Lee Moffitt Cancer Center and Research Institute, Tampa	64.3	10	10	94%	1,037	1.3	Yes	6	8	0.6%
30	Yale New Haven Hospital, Conn.	63.7	10	6	89%	1,396	2.0	Yes	6	9	0.9%
31	Long Island Jewish Medical Center, New Hyde Park, N.Y.	63.5	10	9	86%	1,056	1.6	Yes	6	9	1.0%
32	Lenox Hill Hospital, New York	63.3	10	10	87%	1,077	2.5	No	6	9	0.5%
32	Stanford Health Care-Stanford Hospital, Palo Alto, Calif.	63.3	8	10	90%	1,057	2.9	Yes	6	9	3.4%
32	University of Chicago Medical Center	63.3	9	9	91%	984	2.3	Yes	6	9	3.4%
35	Huntington Memorial Hospital, Pasadena, Calif.	63.2	10	9	93%	624	1.5	Yes	6	9	0.2%
35	South Nassau Communities Hospital, Oceanside, N.Y.	63.2	10	10	86%	329	1.4	A Nurse Magnet	6	8	0.1%
37	West Virginia University Hospitals, Morgantown, W.Va.	63.1	10	10	90%	335	2.3	Yes	6	9	0.8%
38	North Shore University Hospital, Manhasset, N.Y.	63.0	10	10	91%	871	2.1	Yes	6	9	0.7%
39	UC Davis Medical Center, Sacramento, Calif.	62.9	9	10	89%	968	2.8	Yes	6	9	0.8%
40	Hosps. of the U. of Pennsylvania-Penn Presby., Philadelphia	62.8	8	7	91%	1,493	2.5	Yes	6	9	3.4%
41	Brigham and Women's Hospital, Boston	62.5	9	10	92%	971	2.2	Yes	6	9	2.9%
41	Duke University Hospital, Durham, N.C.	62.5	7	8	92%	1,082	2.1	Yes	6	9	6.6%
41	Loyola University Medical Center, Maywood, Ill.	62.5	10	10	88%	616	2.5	Yes	6	8	1.5%
44	Tampa General Hospital	62.4	10	9	90%	813	2.1	Yes	6	9	0.8%
45	UT Southwestern Medical Center, Dallas	62.3	9	10	93%	1,430	2.1	Yes	6	9	3.7%
46	Moses H. Cone Memorial Hospital, Greensboro, N.C.	62.1	10	5	89%	593	1.6	Yes	6	8	0.1%
47	Miami Valley Hospital, Dayton, Ohio	62.0	10	8	89%	532	2.3	Yes	6	8	0.0%
48	Mayo Clinic-Jacksonville, Fla.	61.9	9	10	96%	691	2.5	Yes	6	8	2.3%
49	Penn State Health Milton S. Hershey Medical Ctr., Hershey, Pa.	61.8	10	8	90%	558	1.8	Yes	6	9	0.7%
50	NorthShore University HealthSystem-Metro Chicago	61.7	10	4	90%	1,199	1.4	Yes	6	8	0.0%

Terms are explained on Page 118.

More @ usnews.com/besthospitals

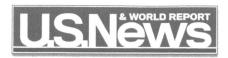
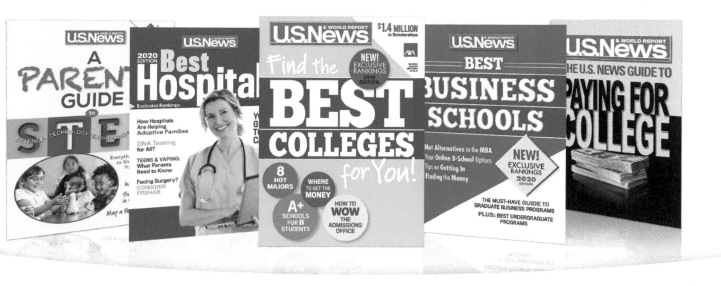
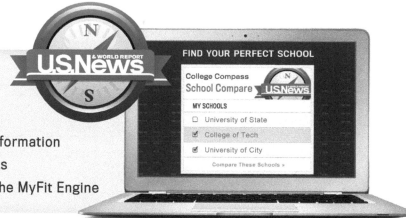

These hospitals are among the best in their specialty

for particularly challenging patients, in the view of at least 5% of medical specialists surveyed by U.S. News over the past three years.

Ophthalmology

Rank	Hospital	% of specialists recommending hospital
1	Bascom Palmer Eye Institute-U. of Miami Hospital and Clinics	52.3%
2	Wills Eye Hosp., Thomas Jefferson U. Hosp., Philadelphia	47.5%
3	Wilmer Eye Institute, Johns Hopkins Hospital, Baltimore	36.8%
4	Massachusetts Eye & Ear Infirmary, Mass. Gen. Hosp., Boston	24.2%
5	Stein and Doheny Eye Institutes, UCLA Med. Ctr., Los Angeles	22.6%
6	University of Iowa Hospitals and Clinics, Iowa City	14.0%
7	Duke University Hospital, Durham, N.C.	13.0%
8	U. of Michigan Hospitals-Michigan Medicine, Ann Arbor	9.3%
9	UCSF Medical Center, San Francisco	8.3%
10	Cole Eye Institute, Cleveland Clinic	8.2%
11	USC Roski Eye Institute, Los Angeles	6.6%
12	New York Eye and Ear Infirmary of Mount Sinai, N.Y.	6.5%

Psychiatry

Rank	Hospital	% of specialists recommending hospital
1	Massachusetts General Hospital, Boston	21.8%
2	McLean Hospital, Belmont, Mass.	19.7%
3	Johns Hopkins Hospital, Baltimore	18.6%
4	New York-Presbyterian Hospital-Columbia and Cornell, N.Y.	15.8%
5	Menninger Clinic, Houston	12.6%
6	Mayo Clinic, Rochester, Minn.	11.7%
7	Sheppard Pratt Hospital, Baltimore	11.4%
8	Resnick Neuropsychiatric Hospital at UCLA, Los Angeles	10.2%
9	UCSF Medical Center, San Francisco	6.3%
9	Yale New Haven Hospital, Conn.	6.3%
11	Cleveland Clinic	5.0%

Rehabilitation

Rank	Hospital	% of specialists recommending hospital
1	Shirley Ryan AbilityLab, Chicago	32.1%
2	Kessler Institute for Rehabilitation, West Orange, N.J.	18.9%
3	Spaulding Rehab. Hosp., Massachusetts Gen. Hosp., Boston	18.6%
4	TIRR Memorial Hermann, Houston	16.7%
5	University of Washington Medical Center, Seattle	14.4%
6	Mayo Clinic, Rochester, Minn.	13.1%
7	Rusk Rehabilitation at NYU Langone Hospitals, New York	12.2%
8	Craig Hospital, Englewood, Colo.	11.1%
9	Shepherd Center, Atlanta	9.9%
10	MossRehab, Elkins Park, Pa.	7.2%
11	New York-Presbyterian Hospital-Columbia and Cornell, N.Y.	6.9%
12	UPMC Presbyterian Shadyside, Pittsburgh	5.0%

Rheumatology

Rank	Hospital	% of specialists recommending hospital
1	Johns Hopkins Hospital, Baltimore	42.2%
2	Cleveland Clinic	41.3%
3	Hosp. for Special Surgery, New York-Presbyterian Hosp., N.Y.	34.7%
4	Mayo Clinic, Rochester, Minn.	30.4%
5	Brigham and Women's Hospital, Boston	21.4%
6	Massachusetts General Hospital, Boston	15.6%
7	UCSF Medical Center, San Francisco	15.1%
8	NYU Langone Hospitals, New York	12.3%
9	UCLA Medical Center, Los Angeles	11.6%
10	University of Alabama at Birmingham Hospital	9.2%
11	Duke University Hospital, Durham, N.C.	5.9%
12	U. of Michigan Hospitals-Michigan Medicine, Ann Arbor	5.6%
13	MUSC Health-University Medical Center, Charleston, S.C.	5.5%
14	Northwestern Memorial Hospital, Chicago	5.0%

More @ usnews.com/besthospitals

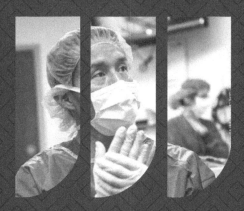

IF YOU'RE SEARCHING FOR ANSWERS, FIND THEM **HERE.**

Since 1832, Wills Eye Hospital has led the way in eye care.
Here, the largest medical staff in the United States comes together
as a single team to solve what often seems unsolvable.
The extraordinary happens every day.

Cataract • Comprehensive Ophthalmology • Cornea • Glaucoma
Neuro-Ophthalmology • Ocular Genetics • Ocular Oncology • Ocular Pathology
Oculoplastic and Orbital Surgery • Pediatric Ophthalmology
Refractive Surgery • Retina

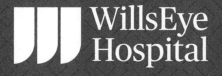

WillsEye Hospital

Believing is Seeing

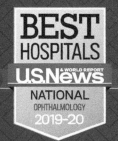

BEST HOSPITALS
U.S.News & WORLD REPORT
NATIONAL
OPHTHALMOLOGY
2019-20

PATIENT NAVIGATOR PROGRAM: FOCUS MI
The Team That Navigates Your Patients Home

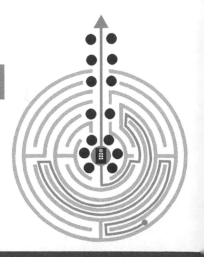

CONGRATULATIONS

to the Patient Navigator Program: Focus MI participants for their dedication to improving the care and outcomes of myocardial infarction patients.

Advocate Sherman Hospital* *Elgin, IL*	**North Vista Hospital North** *Las Vegas, NV*
Alamance Regional Medical Center *Burlington, NC*	**OakBend Medical Center** *Richmond, TX*
Atrium Health's Carolinas Medical Center *Charlotte, NC*	**Olathe Medical Center*** *Olathe, KS*
Atrium Medical Center *Middletown, OH*	**OSF HealthCare Saint Francis Medical Center** *Peoria, IL*
Aurora BayCare Medical Center* *Green Bay, WI*	**OSF Saint Anthony Medical Center** *Rockford, IL*
Barnes Jewish Hospital/Washington University* *Saint Louis, MO*	**Presbyterian Healthcare Services** *Albuquerque, NM*
Baylor Jack and Jane Hamilton Heart and Vascular Hospital *Dallas, TX*	**Providence Medford Medical Center** *Medford, OR*
Baylor Scott & White Medical Center-Temple* *Temple, TX*	**Saint Luke's East Hospital Lee's** *Summit, MO*
California Pacific Medical Center* *San Francisco, CA*	**Saint Luke's Hospital of Kansas City** *Kansas City, MO*
Capital Health Medical Center - Hopewell *Pennington, NJ*	**Saint Luke's North Hospital - Barry Road** *Kansas City, MO*
Centra Lynchburg General Hospital* *Lynchburg, VA*	**San Juan Regional Medical Center** *Farmington, NM*
DLP Conemaugh Memorial Medical Center, LLC *Johnstown, PA*	**Sanford Medical Center Bismarck** *Bismarck, ND*
Doylestown Hospital *Doylestown, PA*	**Self Regional Healthcare** *Greenwood, SC*
El Camino Hospital *Mountain View, CA*	**Seton Medical Center Austin** *Austin, TX*
Galesburg Cottage Hospital *Galesburg, IL*	**South GA Medical Center** *Valdosta, GA*
Hardin Memorial Hospital *Elizabethtown, KY*	**SOVAH Health - Danville** *Danville, VA*
Hays Medical Center *Hays, KS*	**SSM Health St. Mary's Hospital - Madison** *Madison, WI*
Houston Methodist West Hospital *Houston, TX*	**St. Anthony Hospital** *Lakewood, CO*
Indian River Medical Center* *Vero Beach, FL*	**St. Elizabeth Medical Center** *Utica, NY*
Indiana University Health Methodist Hospital* *Indianapolis, IN*	**St. Rose Hospital** *Hayward, CA*
Inova Fairfax Hospital/Inova Heart & Vascular Institute *Falls Church, VA*	**St. Vincent's Medical Center*** *Bridgeport, CT*
Jackson Madison County General Hospital *Jackson, TN*	**Summa Health System - Akron Campus** *Akron, OH*
Jewish Hospital *Louisville, KY*	**Tabba Heart Institute** *Karachi/Gulberg*
Littleton Adventist Hospital *Littleton, CO*	**The Brooklyn Hospital Center** *Brooklyn, NY*
McAllen Heart Hospital *McAllen, TX*	**The MetroHealth System** *Cleveland, OH*
McLeod Regional Medical Center *Florence, SC*	**The Toledo Hospital** *Toledo, OH*
Mease Countryside Hospital *Safety Harbor, FL*	**Trident Medical Center*** *Charleston, SC*
Menorah Medical Center *Overland Park, KS*	**UCH-Memorial Hospital** *Colorado Springs, CO*
Mercy Hospital Joplin *Joplin, MO*	**Unity Health White County Medical Center** *Searcy, AR*
Mercy Medical Center *Canton, OH*	**University of Kentucky** *Lexington, KY*
MercyOne Des Moines Medical Center *Des Moines, IA*	**University of Texas Southwestern Medical Center*** *Dallas, TX*
Meriter Hospital *Madison, WI*	**University of Wisconsin Hospital & Clinics** *Madison, WI*
Mon Health Medical Center *Morgantown, WV*	**Vanderbilt University Medical Center** *Nashville, TN*
Moses H. Cone Memorial Hospital *Greensboro, NC*	**WakeMed Raleigh Campus*** *Raleigh, NC*
MountainView Hospital *Las Vegas, NV*	**Western Maryland Health System Regional Medical Center*** *Cumberland, MD*
MultiCare Tacoma General Hospital* *Tacoma, WA*	**Wise Health System** *Decatur, TX*
North Memorial Medical Center *Robbinsdale, MN*	

*Diplomat Hospital

Founding Sponsor:

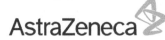
AstraZeneca

CVQuality.ACC.org/PatientNavigator

REDUCE THE RISK:
PCI BLEED
Anticipate. Prepare. Save Lives.

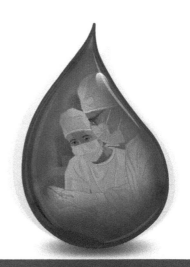

CONGRATULATIONS

to the first 50 hospitals that joined Reduce the Risk: PCI Bleed to minimize PCI-associated bleeding risks through widespread adoption of evidence-based best practices.*

AdvocateTrinity Hospital *Chicago, IL*
Aurora St Luke's Medical Center *Milwaukee, WI*
Bayfront Health Saint Petersburg *St. Petersburg, FL*
Community Memorial Hospital *Menomonee Falls, WI*
Doctors Hospital *Columbus, OH*
Fort Hamilton Hospital *Ross, OH*
Froedtert Hospital *Milwaukee, WI*
Good Samaritan Heart Center *Vincennes, IN*
Grandview Medical Center *Dayton, OH*
Grant Medical Center *Columbus, OH*
Harlingen Medical Center *Harlington, TX*
Henry Ford Macomb Hospital *Clinton Township, MI*
Houston Healthcare Southeast *Pasadena, TX*
Houston Healthcare West *Houston, TX*
Inova Alexandria Hospital *Alexandria, VA*
Inova Fairfax Hospital/Inova Heart & Vascular Institute *Falls Church, VA*
Jamaica Hospital Medical Center *Jamaica, NY*
Jewish Hospital *Louisville, KY*
Kettering Medical Center *Centerville, OH*
LE Cox Medical Centers *Springfield, MO*
Lee's Summit Medical Center *Lee's Summit, MO*
Lima Memorial Health System *Lima, OH*
Medical Center of Aurora *Aurora, CO*
Mercy Hospital Jefferson *Crystal City, MO*
Mercy Hospital South *St. Louis, MO*
Mercy Hospital St. Louis *St. Louis, MO*

Mon Health Medical Center *Morgantown, WV*
Nash UNC Health Care *Wesleyan College, NC*
Northeast Methodist Hospital *San Antonio, TX*
Norwegian American Hospital *Chicago, IL*
Novant Health Presbyterian Medical Center *Matthews, NC*
OhioHealth Marion General Hospital *Marion, OH*
Oklahoma Heart Hospital South *Oklahoma City, OK*
OSF HealthCare Saint Francis Medical Center *Peoria, IL*
Our Lady of The Lake Regional Medical Ctr *Baton Rouge, LA*
PeaceHealth Southwest Medical Center *Vancouver, WA*
Piedmont Hospital *Atlanta, GA*
Rex Hospital *Raleigh, NC*
Riverside Methodist Hospital *Columbus, OH*
Sacred Heart Medical Center *Springfield, OR*
Saint Lukes Hospital *Cedar Rapids, IA*
Soin Medical Center *Dayton, OH*
SouthView Hosptial *Centerville, OH*
Spectrum Health *Grand Rapids, MI*
Swedish Medical Center *Englewood, CO*
The Cleveland Clinic Foundation *Independence, OH*
The Heart Hospital Baylor Plano *Plano, TX*
Um Upper Chesapeake Medical Center, Inc *Bel Air, MD*
University of Missouri Hospital and Clinics *Columbia, MO*
York Hospital *York, PA*

* The 50 hospitals listed above joined the Reduce the Risk: PCI Bleed campaign between August and September 2018. Since then, 113 more hospitals have joined. For the full list, visit: CVQuality.ACC.org/ReduceRiskParticipants.

CVQuality.ACC.org/ReduceRisk

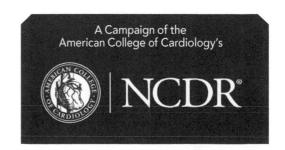

A Campaign of the
American College of Cardiology's

NCDR®

Once again ranked in all 10 specialties

BEST CHILDREN'S HOSPITALS
U.S.News & WORLD REPORT
RANKED IN
10 SPECIALTIES
2019-20

We're honored to be recognized for the 15th consecutive year by U.S. News & World Report as one of the best children's hospitals in the nation, affirming the exceptional quality of care that our physicians and staff provide to patients and families. With over 60 Bay Area locations, world-class pediatric care is close to home. Learn more at stanfordchildrens.org

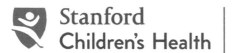

Stanford Children's Health | Lucile Packard Children's Hospital Stanford

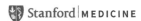

Stanford MEDICINE

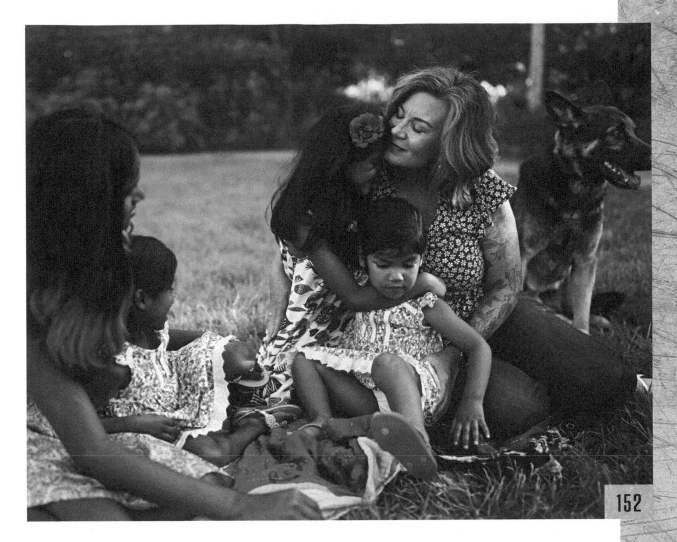

152

Children's Health

Helping
Forever
Families

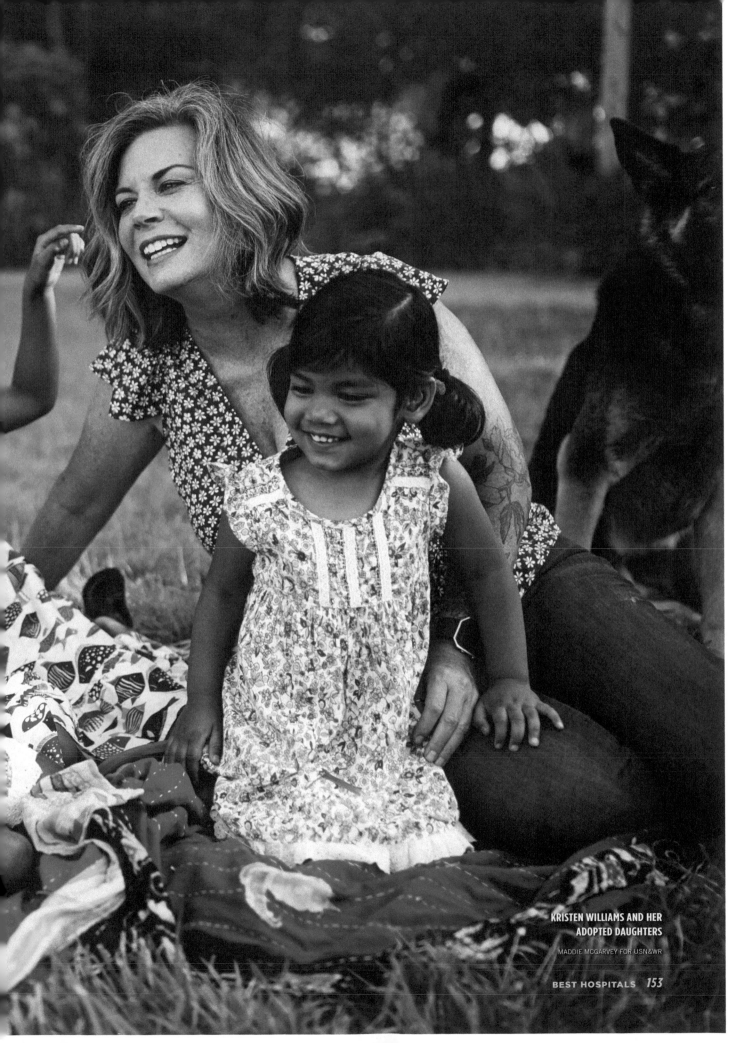

KRISTEN WILLIAMS AND HER
ADOPTED DAUGHTERS

MADDIE MCGARVEY FOR USN&WR

Adoption medicine clinics help parents cope with complex needs

by **Beth Howard**

WHEN KRISTEN WILLIAMS brought her newly adopted daughter, Munni, home to Ohio from a crowded Indian orphanage in 2013, she had no idea what to expect. Within days, the girl, then 7, developed a badly irritated eye that baffled the local urgent care clinic. So Williams called the International Adoption Center at Cincinnati Children's Hospital Medical Center.

Mary Staat, an infectious disease physician and adoption clinic director, tapped the hospital's network of specialists. With the help of her colleague, a corneal expert, they identified the culprit: ocular tuberculosis, a condition rarely seen in the U.S. The TB "was so deep in her eye that it risked infiltrating her brain," Williams says. Blood tests and X-rays revealed other serious infections, too.

Treatment began immediately, but it took a year for Munni to recover. "The clinic was relentless in finding out all that was wrong with her and coordinating her care," says Williams, who feels fortunate to have found help in time and hopes to alert other families that these programs exist.

Adoption medicine clinics – which aim to address the complex medical, developmental, psychological, and social needs of adopted children – have emerged around the country in response to shifting societal trends. Typically housed in major medical centers and children's hospitals, they got their start in the 1990s, when international adoptions were on the rise. "In the past 20 to 30 years, tens of thousands of kids were coming from other countries to the U.S.," says pediatrician Judith Eckerle, director of the Adoption Medicine Clinic at the University of Minnesota, who herself was adopted from South Korea.

While international adoptions have dropped by over 80% since their height in 2004, owing in large part to policy changes in placing and receiving countries, clinics are seeing an influx of patients from domestic adoptions, driven largely by the unrelenting opioid epidemic, declared a public health emergency in 2017. Families across the country are responding by offering permanent homes to help kids whose lives have been devastated by parental addiction, says neonatologist Dana Johnson, co-founder of the Adoption Medicine Clinic at UMN. Indeed, the number of kids entering foster care rose 8% between 2011 and 2017, and foster care adoptions are up some 60% from 20 years ago, Johnson says. Regardless of a child's birthplace, the need for specialized medical care for these kids remains strong. "In the old days, a college-age woman got pregnant and decided to relinquish her healthy baby," says Jerri Ann Jenista, a pediatrician with St. Joseph Mercy Ann Arbor Hospital in Michigan and adoptive mother of five. "That rarely happens anymore," she says. "These days nearly 100% of [adoptive] children have special needs," be it a disability, rare disease or a history of neglect, abuse or other trauma, Eckerle adds. Consequently, the American Academy of Pediatrics has issued new guidelines calling for all children to receive a thorough medical evaluation prior to adoption.

"We can make a profound difference with a family that's open to and takes advantage of all the services we offer," says pediatric nurse Karen Belcher, clinical program coordinator for the UAB International Adoption Clinic at Children's of Alabama.

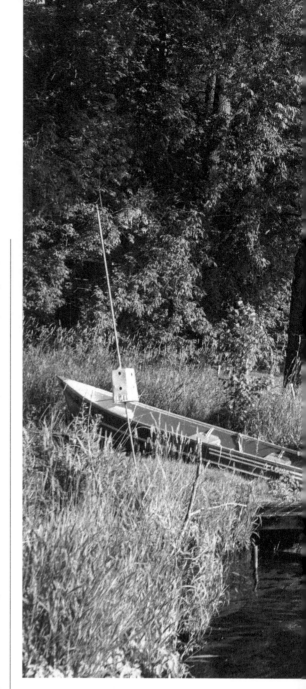

Because of their affiliation with major medical centers, adoption medicine clinics can often draw on myriad medical specialties, with doctors, social workers, psychologists, physical therapists, surgeons and others all joining forces to help kids and "forever families" thrive. Many of the clinics are staffed by providers who have adopted children or are themselves adoptees, bringing lived experience to the exam room.

Pre-adoption help. Adoptive parents typically contact adoption medicine centers after they've begun working with an adoption agency and have received a file on a child – what's known about his or her medical and social history – and want help making sense of it. "We go through them with the parent and highlight any red flags – for example, if the child had some type of congenital heart condition," says Theresa Fiorito, a pediatric infectious disease physician who practices adoption medicine

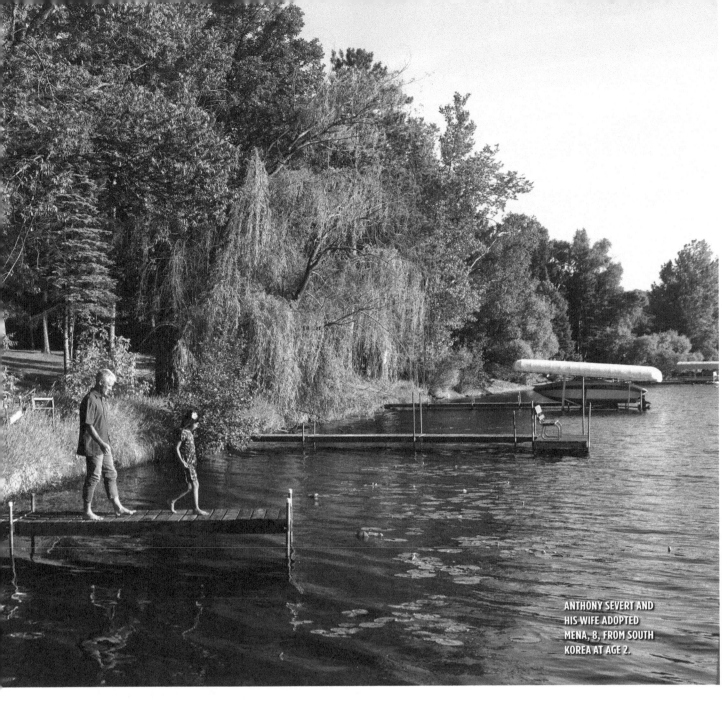

ANTHONY SEVERT AND HIS WIFE ADOPTED MENA, 8, FROM SOUTH KOREA AT AGE 2.

at NYU Winthrop Hospital in Mineola, New York. "We also look at growth parameters and developmental milestones and might ask parents to go back to the orphanage with additional questions."

Katie Severt of Minneapolis felt overwhelmed by the information she received on a girl from South Korea. Even though her husband is a physician, "when you're welcoming a child into your own family, you don't want to be the only eyes on the information," she says, adding that much of their paperwork was in Korean. They had the girl's file reviewed by the UMN clinic and ultimately decided to adopt Mena when she was 2, after the clinic eased their minds about her health status.

This review process helps match families to children whose health needs they are best suited to support. These can range from correctable conditions such as a malformed limb that could benefit from surgery to those requiring long-term treatments, like a cleft lip and palate. "A child from China may have their lip repaired already, but they don't always correct the palate," says Staat, who has three adult children adopted from other countries. "The palate will be repaired here, but then usually around 4, 5 or 6 years of age, the child will need another corrective surgery to make the back of the throat a little more anatomically correct." Additional surgeries, orthodontia treatment and speech therapy may also be on the horizon, she adds.

In addition, adoption medicine programs help families think through their resources, insurance policies and access to care. "If you're in rural Alaska, you don't want to take on a kid who may need a lot of medical intervention," says Julia Bledsoe, director of the Center for Adoption Medicine at the Pediatric Care Center at University of Washington Medical Center, who adopted two children from South Korea.

Addressing emotional needs. Prospective parents also learn about the mental and behavioral health issues that arise from living through adverse childhood circumstances or other trauma, or being exposed to drugs or alcohol in the womb.

"We know that these children have had a little rockier start in life than the average person," Eckerle says. "Most of the time, love is not enough." They may need ongoing therapy or specialized training, for example.

In trying conditions like extreme poverty, people produce high levels of the stress hormone cortisol, Belcher says. "If you are a pregnant mom and you are living with an elevated cortisol level, your baby's brain is taking a bath in cortisol," which can negatively impact brain development, she says. Add to that disruptions like housing instability, neglect, malnutrition and lack of early parent-child bonding and there can be steep consequences, such as anxiety, trouble self-regulating and learning challenges that should be addressed to help the child succeed.

"Kids with these prenatal exposures are at risk for learning disabilities and attention deficit disorder," Bledsoe says. "And if you're taken into foster care because of birth parent addiction, then there is also a risk that you have experienced neglect or witnessed violence, sexual abuse or emotional abuse. Those things, too, can influence both brain development and attachment to a primary caregiver."

The pre-adoption review can result in parents deciding

'The opioid epidemic is fueling U.S. adoptions.'

against adopting a particular child if the long-term picture seems too overwhelming. A youngster with complex special needs should be adopted "by a family who really can go to bat for them," Bledsoe says. "It doesn't do anybody any good to adopt a child that they're woefully unprepared to take care of. It may ruin the family or disrupt the adoption down the road." Reversals of adoptions are rare, but they do happen. However, says Bledsoe: "Studies show some 93% of adoptive families feel like they are with the kid they're supposed to be with. There's a feeling of destiny, like 'I was really supposed to parent this kid,' even when the outcomes are sometimes really hard."

Post-adoption care. When an adoption goes forward, clinic staff will offer advice and even be available on call in case issues arise when parents are physically united with their adoptive children. "We'll give them some do's and don'ts for the country they're in, if it's an international adoption, and alert them to behaviors to watch for," such as not eating or gorging on food (common among kids who have faced food insecurity or are experiencing extreme anxiety), Belcher says.

Once home, adoptees typically spend a day at the clinic, where they are assessed by a team of specialists and receive blood tests and radiologic imaging, if needed. Clinic staff also evaluate children for developmental delays and make referrals to other specialists when appropriate. "Parents will have heard, 'Kids in orphanage care are delayed' or 'Kids are delayed if they come from neglect or abuse,' and to some extent that's true," Eckerle

says. "But we look at that child and say, 'Yes, this is a typical delay. This looks like the 99% of kids who just pick up and start running when they get into a good home versus a child who is really far behind.'"

That's largely been the case for Anne and Olivia Bryson Doyle of Seattle, whose family includes eight children, ages 10 to 18 – seven of whom were adopted from foster care and several after exposure to methamphetamines or opioids. Early on, their first adopted son had developmental delays that they chalked up to neglect in his troubled childhood. But after evaluating him, Bledsoe suspected autism and referred him to a specialist. "She told us, 'This is not an adoption issue,'" Anne recalls. Their son now attends a special school and is doing well. "My kids are thriving, and I believe it's because we've gotten such good guidance."

Parents leave adoption medicine clinics armed with strategies for making the transition as smooth as possible. For instance: "General pediatrics would tell a family most of the time that kids should sleep in their own room. We say bring them into your room – they need safety, nurturing and connection," Belcher says. This may impact how readily a child attaches to adoptive parents, which "can be life-changing."

Parents may also be advised to limit the number of people involved in the child's care until the child has a sense of security and attachment to the adoptive parents.

For families whose kids have ongoing medical needs, the adoption clinic can be a lifeline. That's been true for Kristen Williams. After adopting Munni, the single mom went on to adopt three more girls from India: Roopa, Mohini and Sonali. Between her four daughters, the family has weathered, among other challenges, meningitis, hearing loss, tuberculosis, hepatitis A, microcephaly, anxiety, cerebral palsy, speech delays, and facial disfiguration – Roopa was found abandoned and is believed to have been attacked by an animal. "Because we're getting care through the hospital, we're able to get referrals to all the departments and it has been seamless," she says. "When your children have multiple needs, it's convenient to have a home base." Despite their rocky beginnings, she says, her girls are blossoming.

"I'm routinely shocked at how much we can do for kids," Eckerle says, "and how much progress they can make in a family once we clear the path for them and get them into a loving, stable environment." •

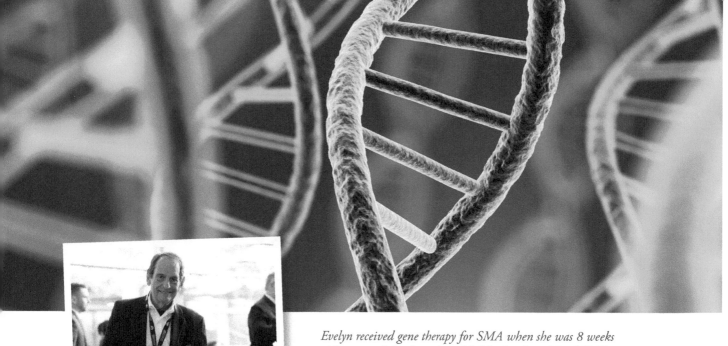

Evelyn received gene therapy for SMA when she was 8 weeks old as part of the clinical trial led by Dr. Jerry Mendell. She is now walking, running and dancing at age 4, surpassing all expectations associated with SMA.

Delivering Hope Through Gene Therapy

Children with devastating neuromuscular disorders are finding hope through precise gene-based therapies.

A case in point: Dr. Jerry Mendell's gene replacement therapy for spinal muscular atrophy type 1, a progressive muscle-weakening disease that typically results in death by age 2.

The SMA gene therapy, developed at Nationwide Children's, harnesses the ability of a viral vector to deliver missing genetic material to a cell. Remarkable outcomes from clinical trials have resulted in FDA approval of this therapy – only the second approval for gene therapy in the United States.

Learn more about this landmark therapy at NationwideChildrens.org/SMA-approval

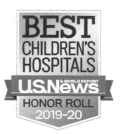

BEST
CHILDREN'S
HOSPITALS
U.S.News & WORLD REPORT
HONOR ROLL
2019–20

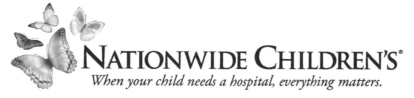

NATIONWIDE CHILDREN'S®
When your child needs a hospital, everything matters.

Spare the Rod

Research shows that spanking and other forms of harsh punishment can have lasting effects

by **K. Aleisha Fetters**

SPANKING IS NOT ONLY PASSÉ – it should never be used. The American Academy of Pediatrics and American Psychological Association recently became the latest public health organizations to publicly assert that spanking and other types of physical punishment are ineffective and potentially damaging to children. A 2016 analysis of more than 160,000 kids showed a link between spanking and increased aggression and defiance. At the same time, data suggest that two-thirds of young children in the United States have been spanked by their parents.

More than 50 other countries, including France, Sweden and Argentina, outlaw corporal punishment of children of any kind. The push for the shift in the U.S. is borne out of accumulating evidence that spanking is not only ineffectual – interrupting children's undesired behaviors without teaching them the desired behaviors – but also comes with potentially harmful and long-lasting effects, says Robert D. Sege, a pediatrician at Floating Hospital for Children in Boston and co-lead author of the AAP's recent statement on the practice, the association's first updated stance on child discipline in more than 20 years.

Indeed, spanking may be extremely distressing for children, and could potentially even alter their brain development. A 2009 study from Harvard Medical School revealed that children who were regularly spanked had less gray matter, or neuron-rich tissue, in areas of the brain associated with addiction and post-traumatic stress disorder than those who were not regularly spanked. It also found "significant correlations" between lower levels of gray matter and poor performance on IQ tests. Researchers say such changes in gray matter may help explain why

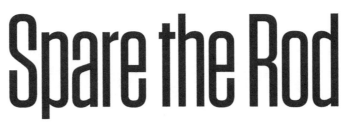

U.S.News
HOSPITAL DATA **INSIGHTS** | PEDIATRICS

hdi.usnews.com | An Analytics Platform from *U.S. News & World Report*

125+
HOSPITALS

1,800+
METRICS

1,000,000+
DATA POINTS

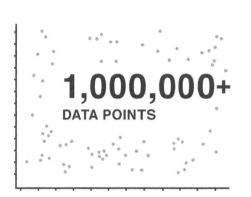

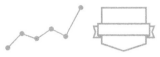

**EXCLUSIVE, UNPUBLISHED
DATA POINTS & RANKINGS**

UNLIMITED PEER GROUPS

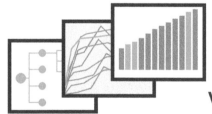

6
**CUSTOM
VISUALIZATIONS**

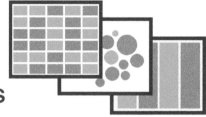

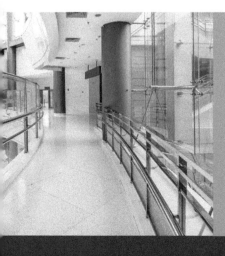

Why Hospital Data Insights Pediatrics?

- Best-in-class analytics
- Superior benchmarking
- Extract charts and graphs easily for detailed analysis
- Study year on year data trends to drive clinical improvements

For more information or to request a demo, contact us at

hdi.usnews.com

✉ hdi@usnews.com
✆ 202.955.2171

those who are regularly spanked in childhood are more likely to suffer mental health problems later in life. Unrelated prior research has linked depression and schizophrenia with gray matter loss in certain brain regions.

Spanking is a "toxic stressor," notes Ann M. Lagges, a pediatric psychologist with Riley Children's Health in Indianapolis. Exposure to toxic stressors, like living in poverty or an unsafe neighborhood, may impact brain development by chronically affecting levels of the stress hormone cortisol. This can play out by making kids grow up distrustful, looking for potential threats in their environment, and may place them in more danger, either as violence victims or aggressors, Sege explains.

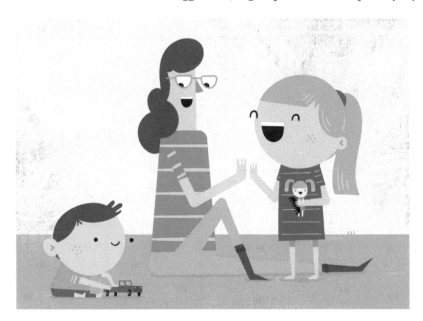

Indeed, one 2019 JAMA Network Open study of more than 36,000 adults found that those who experienced some type of harsh physical punishment as a child were more likely to exhibit antisocial behaviors such as breaking the law, lying, impulsivity, aggression, recklessness, an inability to hold down a job or pay bills, and a lack of remorse for physically or emotionally hurting others.

Pediatricians say spanking and even harsh verbal punishment should be replaced with techniques that teach kids right from wrong in healthier ways. Here are some tactics to try, even in moments of sheer exasperation and depleted patience.

Catch your kids behaving. Very young children crave attention, so make a point to give kudos for good behavior, Sege advises. Say, for example, "I love how you're playing with your indoor voice. You're doing such a great job." Give a thumbs up or high-five. Over time, this will reinforce the behaviors you want and encourage a nurturing relationship.

Frame rules in the "positive." It's a subtle switch, but you'll get further using guidance like "Keep your hands and feet to yourself" than "No hitting," Lagges says. By highlighting what to do, rather than what not to do, you more clearly establish your expectations and cut the risk of, "Ugh, I can't do anything" sentiments.

Implement one new rule at a time. Small change is the name of the game. Start with anything high priority (think: safety or preventing destruction of property) before expending energy on annoying habits like a whiny voice, Lagges recommends. Once your child masters a new good behavior, move on to the next one.

Learn "active ignoring." Say your child is banging on the bathroom door while you're in the shower, Lagges says. Respond by saying, "I'll talk to you when you knock on the door nicely" and then say nothing – nothing – until your child "gets with the program." Once you hear a more polite knock, give praise and engage: "Thank you for knocking on the door nicely. Now what do you need?"

Count to 10. When disciplining, it's important to be "calm and rational rather than upset and uncontrolled," counsels Elizabeth Gershoff, professor of human development and family sciences at The University of Texas–Austin. Of course, staying calm when your walls are lined with permanent marker is easier said than done. Take a deep breath and explain to your kids that what they did was a bad choice (and why). This also models how your children should approach conflicts with others, she says.

Rework time-outs. If time-outs don't seem to stick in your house, chances are your kids are still getting some sort of attention during the process. "Time-out is supposed to be a time in which they get no attention," Lagges says. "It's a time of absolutely nothing." She recommends doling out one minute of time-out for every year of a child's age. If there is any misstep once kiddos get the green-light to emerge, right back into time-out they go.

Teach natural consequences. With older children and teens, parents have the opportunity to use misbehavior as a teaching moment. "My oldest son used to like to play softball," Sege says. "When he broke a window of the house with a softball, I had him to go the hardware store with me, pay for the materials with his allowance and sit with me for an hour while I fixed the window. Afterward, he and his friends reconfigured the softball field so that they never again broke a window."

Get help. If nothing seems to work, it may be time to bring up your concerns to a pediatrician, Sege says. Pediatricians can help you problem-solve or determine if your child should be evaluated for issues such as autism spectrum disorder or attention deficit hyperactivity disorder, Sege says. They can also point you to parenting classes or other resources, such as the "Ask the Pediatrician" tool at healthychildren.org, powered by the AAP. ●

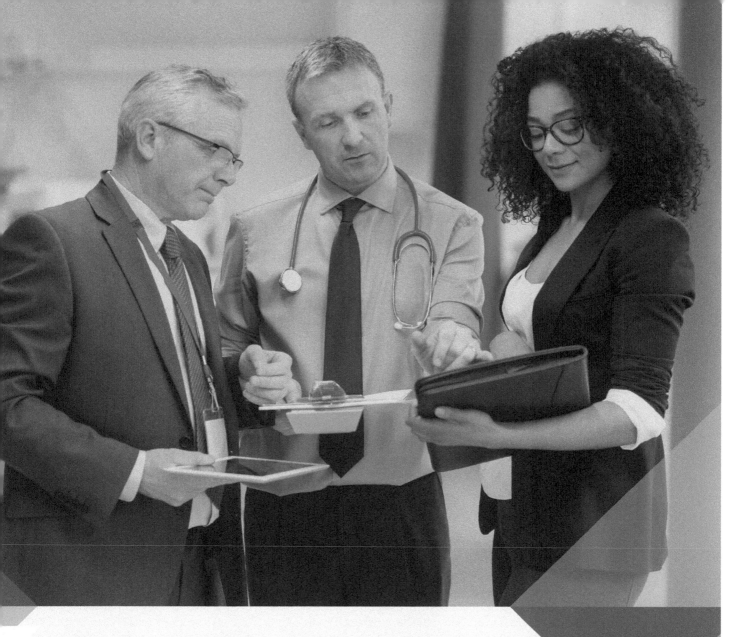

ENGAGE WITH THE BEST

U.S. News & World Report brings its legacy of health care reporting, analysis and industry insights to life in this seventh annual leadership forum. **Healthcare of Tomorrow** unites a community of forward-thinking executives to exchange ideas, share best practices and set new standards for patient care.

Exclusive offer for Best Hospitals readers:

Register at www.USNewsHoT.com using code **BEST50** to receive a **50% discount.**

U.S.News BEST HOSPITALS PRESENTS
HEALTHCARE OF **TOMORROW**
NOV. 17-19, 2019 | WASHINGTON, D.C.

Making the Right

Some common treatments and diagnostic tests for kids are overused and may do more harm than good

by **Linda Marsa**

KIAN YAZDANI was always an active boy, but it wasn't until second grade that he started having meltdowns nearly every day. "It seemed like the least little thing would set off a temper tantrum," says his mom, Melody, a 35-year-old photographer and mother of four who lives in Vienna, Virginia. Kian also had a persistent cough and severe headaches, so his doctors loaded him up with antibiotics and steroid inhalers to control his postnasal drip. At the same time, a psychologist believed his agitation, trouble focusing and anxiety suggested he should be tested for attention deficit hyperactivity disorder.

The testing showed Kian was gifted but had a severe processing speed deficit that caused him problems with his focus and impulse control. Yet a trip to the dentist's office revealed that Kian had a very different problem than ADHD. The dental exam showed that the boy's teeth were ground almost halfway down – a telltale symptom of sleep apnea, a disorder in which breathing stops and starts often during sleep. Movement of the lower jaw can apply pressure, cutting off the airway, and the body must push the jaw forward to reopen it, causing the teeth grinding. A sleep study revealed that Kian was waking up dozens of times an hour gasping for air, so he was getting none of the restorative REM sleep. His sinuses were almost completely blocked and his adenoids were so swollen he was breathing through his mouth. Kian, now 8, has since had his adenoids and tonsils removed and can sleep through the night. After surgery, his tantrums ceased. "He's a completely different kid," Melody says. "He's calm, and he's not having behavioral problems."

For Kian, the real culprit was identified. But mistaking sleep apnea for another condition is just one way children can be misdiagnosed, given the wrong treatments, or subjected to diagnostic tests that may be doing more harm than good, experts say. What follows are some of the major offenders and what parents need to know to ensure kids get the right treatment.

ADHD misdiagnoses

Despite diagnostic guidelines from the American Psychiatric Association, experts believe there is an epidemic of misdiagnosis of ADHD. More than 1 in 10 school-age children – and up to 20% of high school boys – do meet the criteria. However, a recent study of 50 pediatric practices found that only half of the physicians surveyed followed these established protocols to determine whether ADHD or another condition was causing symptoms. Yet nearly all of them – a whopping 93% – immediately prescribed medications to treat it. "That means many children are misdiagnosed" and are taking pills they don't need, says Michael Manos, head of the Center for Pediatric Behavioral Health at Cleveland Clinic Children's Hospital.

Part of the problem is that other ills that plague children – bipolar disorder, depression, anxiety, trauma, seizure disorders, learning disabilities, vision or hearing difficulties, and chronic sleep deprivation, as was the case with Kian – share many characteristics with ADHD.

Parents should keep in mind a few key points when dealing with a potential ADHD diagnosis. It typically begins before adolescence, and more than one observer – teacher, parent, athletic coach – should be able to document a persistent pattern of inattention or hyperactivity severe enough to interfere with how kids develop and function day to day in at least two or more settings – at home, in school and in social situations. In addition, other conditions should be ruled out before treatment begins. Pediatricians must do a systematic evaluation, Manos says; that means questioning children

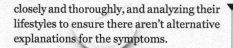

Call

closely and thoroughly, and analyzing their lifestyles to ensure there aren't alternative explanations for the symptoms.

Unnecessary CT scans

Roughly half a million children arrive in emergency rooms each year with head injuries, and about half will receive a CT scan (a diagnostic procedure also used for other conditions, including spinal and stomach injuries, and abdominal pain). Yet a landmark study published in The Lancet in 2009 noted that only 5% of CT scans flagged potential trouble in kids with minor head trauma, and a mere 0.1% of those kids needed neurosurgery. And CT scans aren't risk-free: One head scan can emit 100 to 200 times more radiation than an X-ray, and estimates suggest an additional 1 in 5,000 kids may go on to develop cancer from that exposure. This radiation risk may seem minimal, but experts believe it outweighs the smaller likelihood that the scan will uncover significant brain trauma, particularly since doctors have other tools they can use to detect trouble. In the case of a head injury, unless a child has two or more potential indicators of trauma, such as evidence of a skull fracture or a scalp hematoma; or the child lost consciousness (even momentarily), seems disoriented, has a severe headache, or is vomiting, then experts suggest parents can generally skip a head CT.

With suspected cases of appendicitis, CT scans are also often used as diagnostic aids. Yet blood tests, an ultrasound and an evaluation of symptoms are just as good at identifying trouble. "There are millions of CT scans done on children," says Nathan Kuppermann, a professor of emergency medicine and pediatrics at the University

of California–Davis School of Medicine and lead author of The Lancet study. "If we could eliminate a big percentage of them, thousands of children's lives would be saved from cancer. That's why parents need to talk to doctors and share in the decision-making."

Antibiotic overload

Family doctors and pediatricians write more than 50 million prescriptions for antibiotics every year, even though roughly 30% are unnecessary. Despite more than a decade of public health campaigns, the rate of inappropriate prescribing of these potent pills remains too high. That worrisome trend is contributing to the problem of drug-resistant infections that kill 23,000 people annually. Physicians often cave in to pressure from parents, who want their ailing kids treated, and end up sending families home with antibiotic prescriptions even for ills that don't respond to antibiotics, evidence suggests. "There is a culture of expectation – when a doctor thinks that a parent wants an antibiotic, they are 23 times more likely to prescribe one," says Nicole Poole, a pediatric infectious disease specialist at Seattle Children's Hospital.

Antibiotics can also have nasty side effects, like diarrhea, rashes and yeast infections. Moreover "antibiotic exposure changes the intestinal bacteria, and those changes may promote the development of certain autoimmune diseases," says Mary Anne Jackson, a pediatrician and interim dean of the University of Missouri–Kansas City School of Medicine (story, Page 73). Before filling a prescription, parents should confirm that their child has a bacterial infection; antibiotics are useless against viruses, the germs that cause common colds and some sore throats, most cases of acute bronchitis, and many sinus and ear infections. "Find out if there are any tests to confirm the presence of bacteria," Jackson says.

If antibiotics are a must, kids tend to do better with narrow-spectrum varieties – amoxicillin – than with broad-spectrum ones (azithromycin), since they cause fewer side effects. Watchful waiting may be best, although it may take a week or two for kids to feel better; some 80% of ear infections resolve on their own. Humidifiers can help clear out sinuses and help sickly children breathe better, over-the-counter remedies like acetaminophen and ibuprofen can rein in fevers and the inflammation of an ear infection, and a spoonful of honey can soothe coughs and sore throats, Poole says. "These small things won't decrease how long a kid is going to be sick, but they can provide temporary relief."

Dangerous opioid exposure

Despite strenuous efforts to curb the opioid epidemic, millions of youth are still being prescribed narcotic painkillers. A recent Harvard study

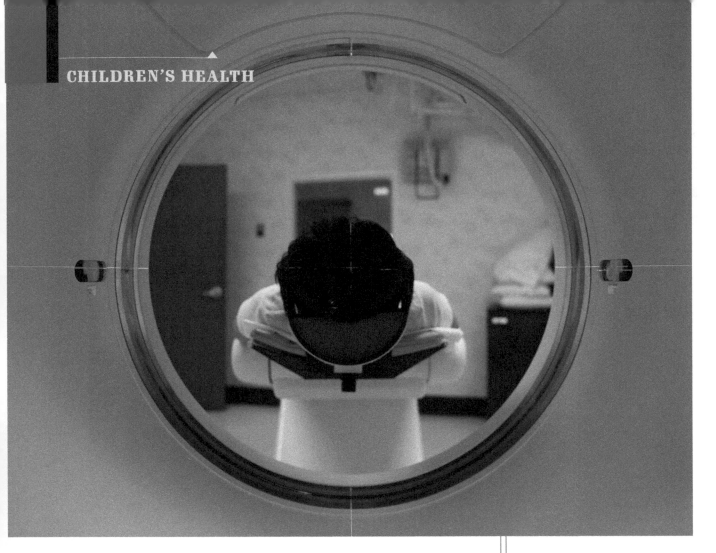

examining prescribing patterns in the nation's ERs from 2005 to 2015 found that nearly 57 million ER visits – of which about 15% were made by adolescents and young adults (ages 13 to 22) – resulted in a prescription for these painkillers. Collarbone and ankle fractures were treated most frequently with opioids, but even 60% of teens with dental complaints left with a prescription. What shocked the Harvard researchers most was that kids were leaving with opioid scripts for headaches, sore throats and urinary tract infections.

This is happening despite research consistently showing how dangerous this can be for teens: Many young people are particularly susceptible to becoming addicted after being given an opioid for medical conditions, especially for wisdom tooth extraction. Parents "need to recognize the power of simple exposure to an opioid and how it might change an adolescent's risk profile if they're exposed while their brains are still forming," says Andrew Herring, an emergency room doctor at Alameda Health System-Highland Hospital in Oakland and a researcher at the University of California–San Francisco.

When Tim Rabolt was a freshman in high school, he had his wisdom teeth extracted and left the dentist's office with prescriptions for two potent opioids, Demerol and Vicodin. "When my prescription ran out, I bought them from friends who had similar surgeries, and we were taking them like candy," he recalls. Within

A 2009 STUDY FOUND THAT ONLY 5% OF PEDIATRIC CT SCANS FOR MINOR HEAD TRAUMA REVEALED SIGNS OF TROUBLE.

a year, he was swallowing these painkillers every day and was, he says, "one step away from buying heroin on the street."

In his senior year, Rabolt got clean. Today, it's "absolutely worrisome that a high school student can get prescribed such strong drugs," Rabolt says. The 27-year-old is now executive director of The Association of Recovery in Higher Education in Minneapolis. He uses his own experience to help college students in recovery programs nationwide.

There are plenty of alternatives to opioids, including non-narcotic pain relievers that may work just as well, like acetaminophen, naproxen sodium and ibuprofen. Physical therapy, massage and nerve blocks (pain-relieving injections) can also ease pain. If narcotics are the only meds that will do the trick, find out how many days they will be needed. Usually, taking them for three to five days should be enough. And safe storage and disposal is critical, too. Two-thirds of teens who have reported misusing prescription medications got them from friends, family and acquaintances, says Pat Aussem, director of clinical content and development at the Center on Addiction, a national nonprofit that conducts research to identify the most effective strategies to combat addiction. So properly securing and disposing of unneeded

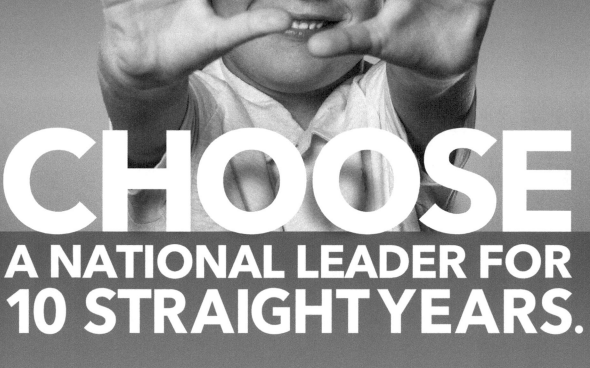
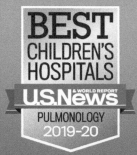
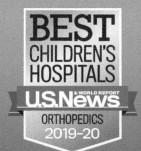
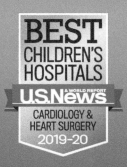
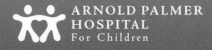

meds is essential. "You can dispose of unused pills at your local pharmacy and some police stations," she says.

Excessive use of acid blockers

New parents tend to fret when their infant is spitting up and crying, and want to do everything possible to make their babies feel better. As a result, "Pediatricians prescribe acid blockers quite often," says Paul Kaplowitz, a pediatric endocrinologist and

'Acid blockers can pose risks for infants.'

the American Academy of Pediatrics' "physician champion" for Choosing Wisely, a nationwide initiative that identifies unnecessary medical tests, treatments and procedures. These prescriptions can include liquid versions of acid-blocking medications called proton pump inhibitors, although PPIs aren't approved by the Food and Drug Administration for infants under age 1.

Yet stomach distress at this age is often not a cause for concern. In their first six to 12 months, some 40% to 70% of babies spit up at least once daily for various reasons. Many may also cry and be irritable, but with thriving babies, the irritability generally resolves by six months of age, notes Eric Hassall, a pediatric gastroenterologist in San Francisco. However, infants with these symptoms can often be misdiagnosed with gastroesophageal reflux disease. And acid blockers, if prescribed, can be problematic, especially if unnecessary.

Stomach acids are the first line of defense against infection and aid in the absorption of key nutrients babies need to thrive. Not only can acid blockers remove that defense, but they may also cause gastrointestinal and respiratory infections, impaired bone health and possibly food allergies, among other issues. Experts say these medications may only be helpful if a baby shows signs of more serious trouble. Spitting up frequently when combined with symptoms like not gaining weight, prolonged coughing episodes and irritability may be signs of GE reflux disease and warrant further evaluation. For other kids, you probably don't need medication, says Kaplowitz: "Just keep an eye on the child and make sure they're growing and are breathing normally." ●

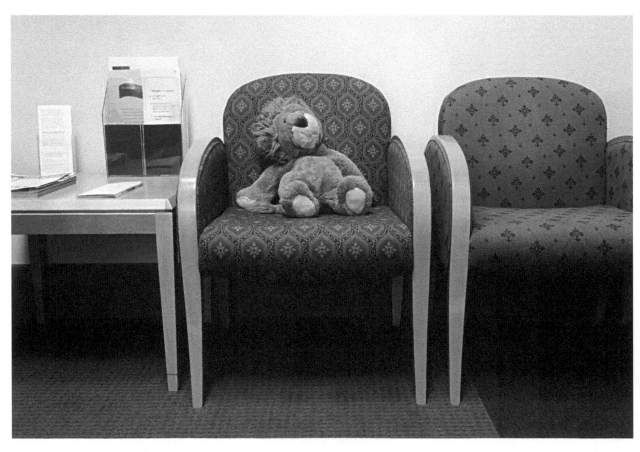

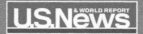

Connect with Patients Seeking the Right Specialists

U.S. News and Doximity have joined together to provide Patient Connect, a tool to reach consumers seeking a new healthcare provider during the critical decision-making process. With patients connected to existing scheduling channels, Patient Connect is a quick, turnkey solution.

7M+
Visitors per month

77%
Visitors are looking for a specialist

8%
Click or call to schedule an appointment

To learn more about Patient Connect, email: patientconnect@doximity.com

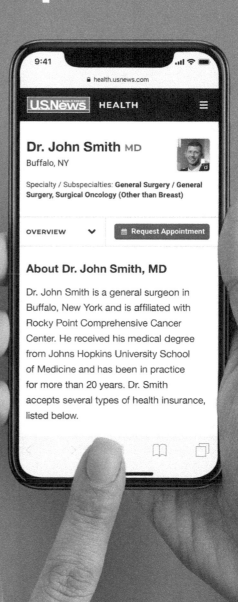

Trying to Curb a Teen Epidemic

Millions of young people have turned to **vaping**, a risky alternative to cigarettes

by **Barbara Sadick**

MEREDITH BERKMAN, a New York City mother of four, began to suspect something was amiss when more than once her teenage son Caleb Mintz had friends over and she heard the "ping" of his bedroom window alarm, signaling it was being opened. When she entered Caleb's room one day without knocking, she found a group of polite, smiling kids and didn't notice anything awry. When asked about the window, Caleb said they were just hot. Puzzled, she let it go, but around that time, the mother of another teen happened to mention finding what looked like USB flash drives lying around the house. "Like me, other parents hadn't yet grasped the problem," Berkman says. She and her friends realized their kids were vaping – using e-cigarettes or similar electronic devices that mimic the experience of smoking – and began to do some research.

According to both the U.S. surgeon general and the Food and Drug Administration, vaping has reached epidemic proportions among young people. And data from the 2018 National Youth Tobacco Survey showed that over 3.6 million American middle and high school students used e-cigarettes at least once in 2018. Michael Blaha, director of clinical research at the Ciccarone Center for the Prevention of Cardiovascular Disease at Johns Hopkins Medicine, says e-cigarettes originally came on the U.S. market over a decade ago as a nicotine delivery system for smoking cessation. They were marketed as being safer than cigarettes, which they were designed to look like. Today, e-cigarettes are sleek, well-designed, high-tech-looking devices also referred to as "e-cigs," "vapes," "e-hookahs," "vape pens," "juuls" (named after a popular brand from JUUL Labs) and "electronic nicotine delivery systems" that allow users to inhale aerosol produced from a heated liquid pod that typically contains nicotine, flavorings and other addictive substances.

Early research has highlighted the possible health risks and addictive potential of these devices. Stanton Glantz, professor of tobacco control and a professor of medicine at the University of California–San Francisco, says that in terms of heart disease, e-cigarettes approach the risks of traditional cigarettes – and for lung diseases they may be worse. While studies have not yet shown an association between e-cigarettes and lung cancer, evidence does point to one between vaping and other lung issues such as asthma and chronic obstructive pulmonary disease.

The JUUL Labs e-cigarette brand delivers in one 5% pod roughly as much nicotine as a whole pack of "full flavor," or regular, cigarettes. (JUUL also sells 3% pods.) Research presented at the Society for Research on Nicotine and Tobacco in 2019 by Bonnie Halpern-Felsher, professor of pediatrics at Stanford University, indicates that young adults tend to have trouble determining how quickly they use up a pod; for some it might be a day, a week or more. But of particular concern to experts are studies showing that young people who vape are two to four times more likely to smoke cigarettes a year after they begin vaping than those who don't use e-cigarettes, undercutting arguments that the devices serve as effective smoking cessation aids or that youth begin tobacco use solely through cigarettes.

Peak vulnerability. "Nicotine is one of the most addictive substances that exists," says Linda Richter, director of policy research and analysis at the nonprofit Center on Addiction (which recently merged with the Partnership for Drug-Free Kids). It "affects concentration, attention and mood." Young people are particularly at risk, she says, because a person's peak vulnerability to addiction is during adolescence, when the brain is still engaged in intense change and development.

Alarmed by the research, Berkman finally raised the subject with

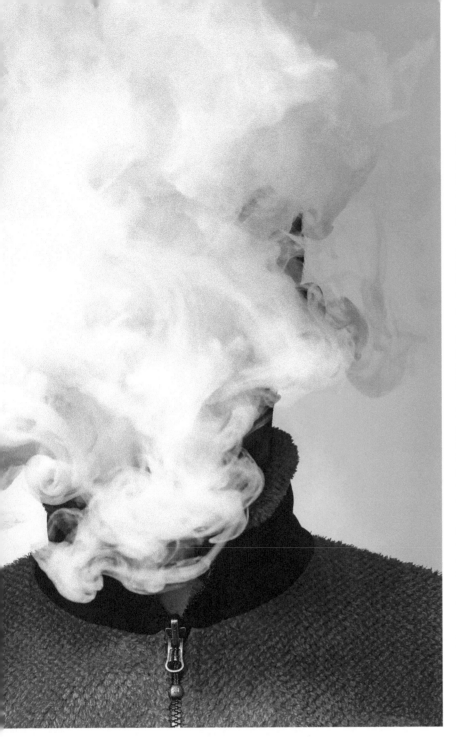

them online. It has also created a web tool for adults to anonymously register serial numbers of confiscated devices to identify retailers selling to minors without proper ID.) According to Kwong, all of JUUL's U.S. Facebook and Instagram accounts have also been discontinued.

Playing catch-up. Public health experts and parents concerned by the spread of vaping among young people are trying to get the word out. Berkman teamed up with two other mothers, Dina Alessi and Dorian Fuhrman, to form Parents Against Vaping E-cigarettes or PAVe. Caleb, now 17, has also pitched in with his friends Phillip Fuhrman, 16, and Luke Alessi, 16, who all spoke at a private FDA listening session.

Caleb believes many teens have no idea how addictive e-cigarettes are. He suspects they crave the intense, quick head rush or the pleasant disoriented feeling they get, he says. But he's also seen them become irritable and moody, which Richter says can be signs of nicotine withdrawal.

The FDA now regulates electronic smoking devices like other tobacco products and bans sales to minors. It also requires warning labels on packaging and in advertising. In March 2019, the FDA announced a proposal to require vendors to limit sales of flavored e-cigarette products by enforcing age verification. Glantz says cities and states are also taking proactive steps by integrating e-cigarettes into their clean indoor air laws and banning the sale of flavored tobacco products.

For families seeking more information, parentsagainstvaping.org, PAVe's website, provides educational resources while also advocating for regulatory and legislative action. Stanford's Tobacco Prevention Toolkit (med. stanford.edu/tobaccopreventiontoolkit) offers resources on e-cigarettes as well as other tobacco and nicotine products.

The health community is also trying to help. Jonathan Avery, director of addiction psychiatry at New York-Presbyterian Hospital's Weill Cornell Medical Center, says that like other hospitals, NYP/WCMC is training doctors how to screen teens for vaping. "Rather than simply asking young people if they smoke or use nicotine, the medical staff specifically asks if they use e-cigarettes or are juuling," says Avery, "because many have never associated these new devices with using nicotine." The hospital is also exploring new strategies and alternate behavior modification techniques to help young people resist peer pressure to vape. "This epidemic of adolescent nicotine use came so quickly out of nowhere that we're working to catch up," Avery says. ●

Caleb, who admitted vaping occasionally. But her son had already started doing his own research. His understanding of the health consequences combined with his anger that the initial marketing campaigns by JUUL Labs seemed to be targeting and profiting off of teens, prompted him to quit.

Ted Kwong, a spokesman for the company, told U.S. News by email that JUUL's mission is to offer adult smokers an alternative to combustible cigarettes. "As a young company, innovating a new category, we learned from our experiences," he wrote. Of JUUL's marketing initiatives, he noted: "Our current efforts feature only adult smokers who switched from combustible cigarettes with JUUL and we are ensuring this campaign is targeted at adult smokers age 35 and up." (JUUL has stopped selling its fruity-flavored pods, so appealing to many young people, in retail outlets, though it will continue to offer

Your priority.
Our specialty.

Your child is your number one priority. We understand. Your child is important to us too. In fact, this isn't our job, it's our calling.

From urgent care, to cancer care, Cincinnati Children's is changing the outcome for patients and families.

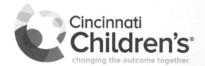

Cincinnati Children's
changing the outcome together

If illness or injury impacts your child, turn to us. At Cincinnati Children's, your child is our specialty.

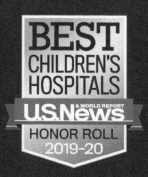

BEST
CHILDREN'S
HOSPITALS
U.S.News & WORLD REPORT
HONOR ROLL
2019-20

CHAPTER 5

BEST CHILDREN'S HOSPITALS
U.S.News & WORLD REPORT
2019-20

Best Children's Hospitals

Best Children's Hospitals
HONOR ROLL

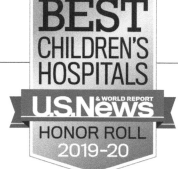

This elite list showcases hospitals with unusual breadth of excellence in pediatric specialty care. For each specialty, each hospital that ranked among the top 50 earned points toward the Honor Roll: 25 points for ranking No. 1, 24 points for No. 2 and so on; hospitals ranked 21-50 received 5 points. The hospitals with the most points defined the Honor Roll.

1 Boston Children's Hospital
239 points

2 Children's Hospital of Philadelphia
228 points

3* Cincinnati Children's Hospital Medical Center
217 points

3* Texas Children's Hospital
Houston, 217 points

5 Children's Hospital Los Angeles
168 points

6 Children's National Medical Center
Washington, D.C.
147 points

7 Nationwide Children's Hospital
Columbus, Ohio
146 points

8 UPMC Children's Hospital of Pittsburgh
137 points

9 Johns Hopkins Children's Center
Baltimore, 135 points

10* Children's Hospital Colorado
Aurora, 129 points

10* Seattle Children's Hospital
129 points

*Denotes a tie

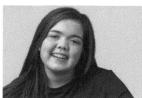
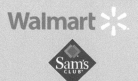

A Key to the Rankings

How we identified 84 outstanding pediatric hospitals

by **Ben Harder** ▶

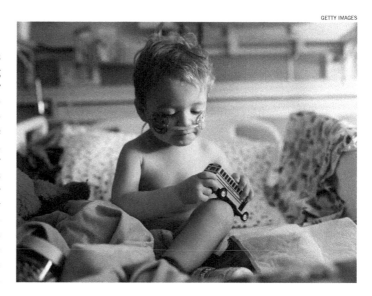

GETTY IMAGES

HERE SHOULD anxious parents take a newborn with a life-threatening heart defect, or find ongoing care for a child with failing kidneys or lung-clogging cystic fibrosis? A local hospital's pediatric department might be perfectly capable of managing ear infections, allergies, flu and other common childhood ailments. But it may not have the expertise to treat severely ill kids. That's where children's hospitals come in. There are fewer than 200 hospitals in the country that either exclusively treat pediatric patients or possess a pediatric department that functions like a self-contained children's hospital. Even within that group, some centers are better than others. U.S. News created the Best Children's Hospitals rankings to help parents, in consultation with their doctors, find those best suited to their child.

The 2019-20 rankings highlight top children's centers in 10 specialties: cancer, cardiology and heart surgery, diabetes and endocrinology, gastroenterology and GI surgery, neonatology, nephrology, neurology and neurosurgery, orthopedics, pulmonology and lung surgery, and urology. This year, 84 hospitals ranked in at least one specialty. The 2019-20 Honor Roll recognizes the standouts that scored near the top in all or most specialties.

Rich data. Judging the excellence of children's hospitals is challenging, and no single metric or ranking should be viewed as a definitive guide. U.S. News gathers more than 1,000 data points on hospitals to determine their strengths and weaknesses. Many summary measures appear in the tables in the following pages, and more are available at usnews.com/childrenshospitals, which also features data on dozens of additional children's hospitals.

Almost all of the medical data used in these rankings were obtained by asking hospitals to complete a lengthy online data-collection form. This year, 125 of nearly 200 hospitals surveyed by U.S. News provided enough data to be evaluated in at least one specialty. Most surveyed hospitals are members of the Children's Hospital Association.

This year's data-collection instrument was updated with the help of 160 medical directors, clinical specialists and other pediatric experts who served as advisers in 12 U.S. News pediatric working groups. RTI International, a North Carolina-based research and consulting firm, oversaw data collection and analyzed the findings.

Whether and how high an institution was ranked depended on three elements: its clinical outcomes (such as survival and surgical complications), its delivery of care (how well a hospital synchronizes all that must be done to treat patients effectively and keep them safe), and its resources (such as staffing and technol-

IT'S ONE THING TO PROVIDE CARE.

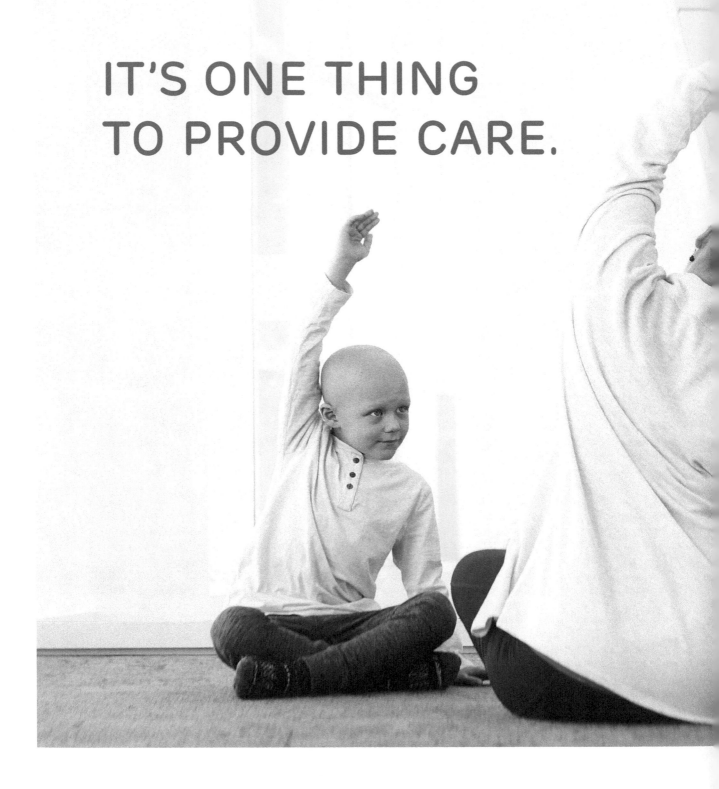

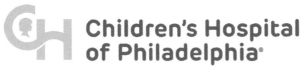

Children's Hospital of Philadelphia®

Breakthroughs.
Every day.

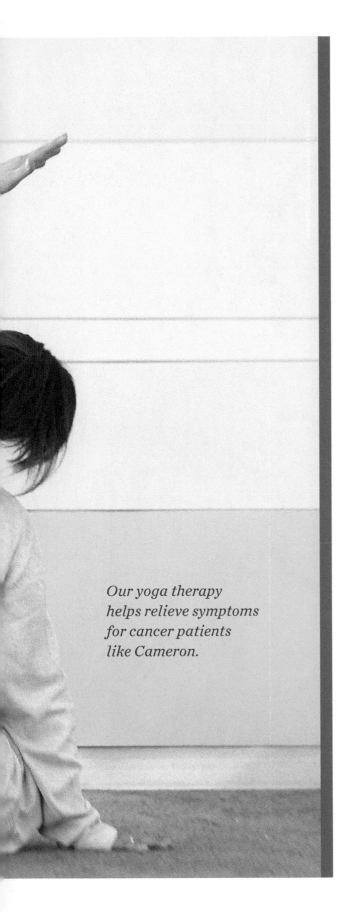

*Our yoga therapy
helps relieve symptoms
for cancer patients
like Cameron.*

IT'S ANOTHER
TO DEFINE IT.

At Children's Hospital of Philadelphia,
our robust clinical programs are
complemented by brilliant researchers
who are pioneering new advances in
children's health at an astonishing pace.
As a result, we are able to provide
answers often not available anywhere
else in the world for rare conditions
and chronic, debilitating diseases.

We set the standard for cutting-edge
clinical care for kids like Cameron.

chop.edu

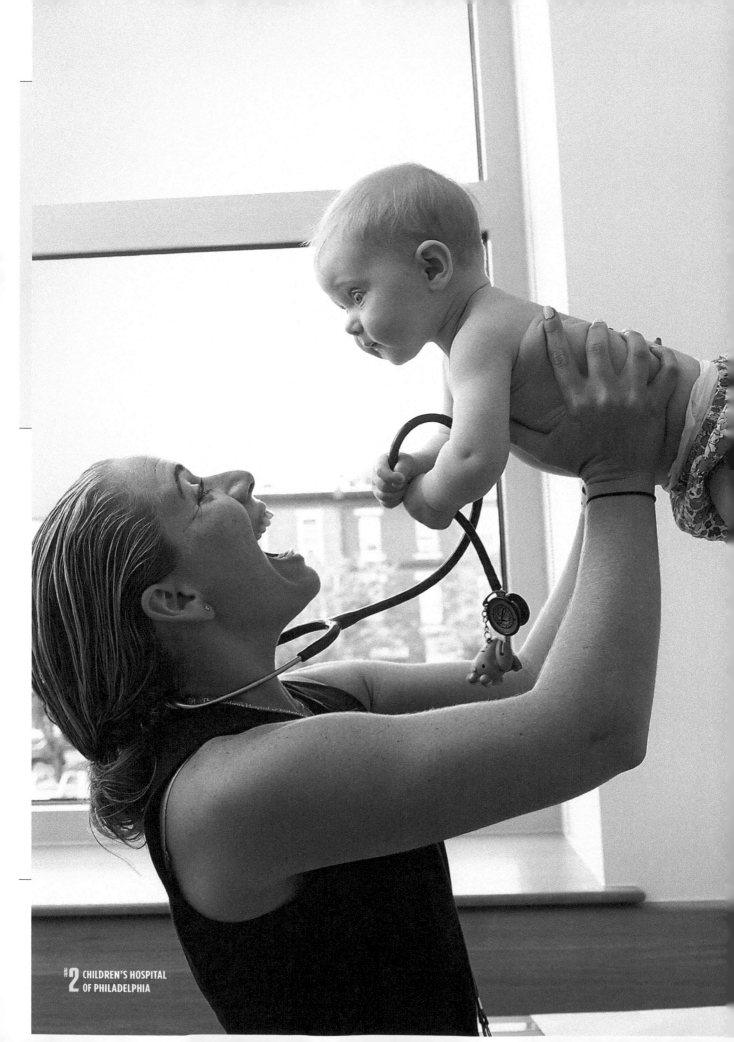

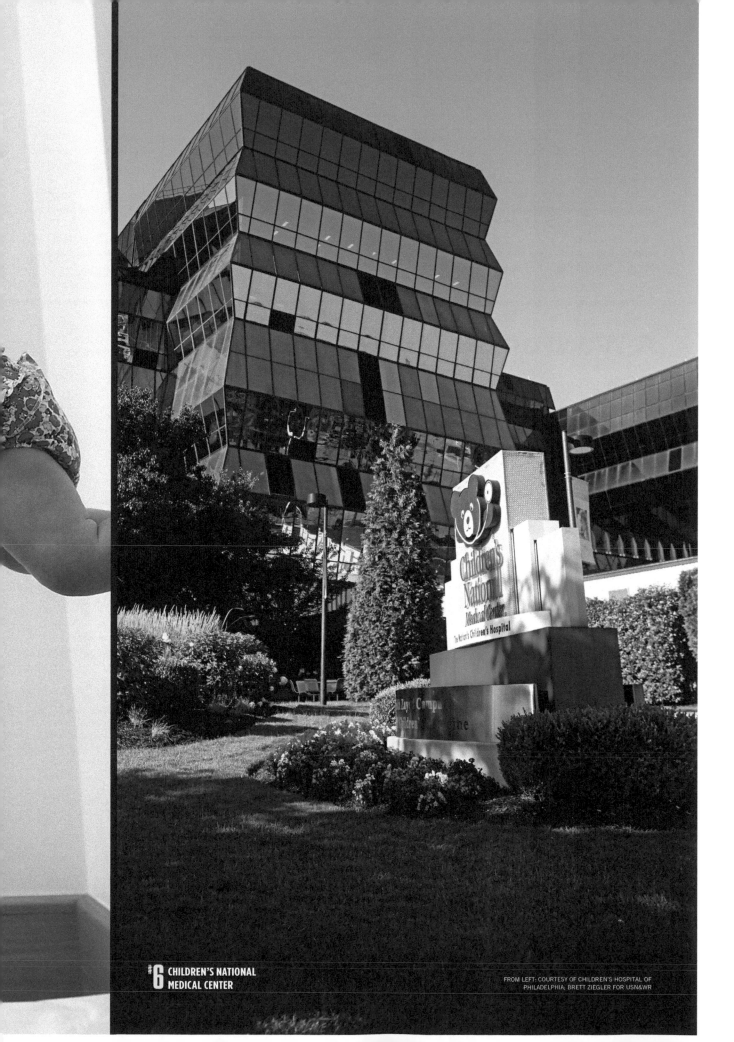

ogy). A detailed FAQ about the rankings is available at usnews.com/aboutchildrens. Each element contributed one-third of a hospital's overall score in most specialties. Here are the basics:

Clinical outcomes. These reveal a hospital's success at keeping kids alive after their treatment or surgery, protecting them from infections and complications, and improving their quality of life. Though tough to measure, outcomes often matter most to families and doctors alike.

Delivery of care. How well a hospital handles day-to-day care was determined in part by compliance with accepted "best practices," such as having a full-time infection preventionist and holding regular conferences to discuss unexpected deaths and complications. U.S. News also surveyed pediatric specialists, asking them to identify up to 10 hospitals they consider best in their area of expertise for children with serious or difficult medical problems, ignoring distance and cost.

Resources. Surgical volume, nurse-patient ratio, clinics and programs for conditions such as asthma, and dozens of other measures were considered. ●

A Word on the Terms

USED IN MORE THAN ONE SPECIALTY

A Nurse Magnet hospital: hospital recognized by American Nurses Credentialing Center as meeting standards for nursing excellence.
Infection prevention score, ICU: ability to prevent central-line bloodstream infections in intensive care units.
Infection prevention score, overall: ability to prevent infections through measures such as hand hygiene and vaccination.
No. of best practices: how well hospital adheres to recommended ways of diagnosing and treating patients, such as documenting blood sugar levels for a high percentage of outpatients (diabetes & endocrinology) and conducting hip exams with ultrasound specialists (orthopedics).
Nurse-patient ratio: balance of full-time registered nurses to inpatients.
Patient volume score: relative number of patients in past year with specified disorders.
% of specialists recommending hospital: percentage of physician specialists surveyed in 2017, 2018 and 2019 who named hospital among best for very challenging patients.
Procedure volume score: relative number of tests and nonsurgical procedures in past one, two or three years, such as implanting radioactive seeds in a cancerous thyroid (diabetes & endocrinology) and using an endoscope for diagnosis (gastroenterology). Surgical procedures are included in orthopedics.

Surgery volume score: relative number of patients who had specified surgical procedures in past year.
Surgical complications prevention score: ability to prevent surgery-related complications and readmissions within 30 days (neurology & neurosurgery, orthopedics, urology).
U.S. News score: 0 to 100 summary of overall performance in specialty.
NA: not applicable; service not provided by hospital.
NR: data not reported or unavailable.

USED IN ONE SPECIALTY

CANCER
Bone marrow transplant survival score: survival of stem cell recipients at 100 days.
Five-year survival score: survival five years after treatment for acute lymphoblastic leukemia, acute myeloid leukemia, and neuroblastoma.
Palliative care score: how well program meets specified training and staffing standards for children with terminal or life-limiting conditions, and number of cancer patients referred to program.

CARDIOLOGY & HEART SURGERY
Catheter procedure volume score: relative number of specified catheter-based procedures in past year, such as inserting stents and treating heart rhythm problems.
Norwood/hybrid surgery survival score: survival at one year after the first in a series of reconstructive surgeries,

evaluated over past four years.
Risk-adjusted surgical survival score: survival in the hospital and 30 days from discharge after congenital heart surgery, adjusted for operative and patient risk, evaluated over past four years.

DIABETES & ENDOCRINOLOGY
Diabetes management score: ability to prevent serious problems in children with Type 1 diabetes and to keep blood sugar levels in check.
Hypothyroid management score: relative proportions of children treated for underactive thyroid who test normal and of infants who begin treatment by 3 weeks of age.

GASTROENTEROLOGY & GI SURGERY
Liver transplant survival score: One- and three-year survival after liver transplant.
Nonsurgical procedure volume score: relative number of tests and noninvasive procedures.
Selected treatments success score: shown, for example, by high remission rates for inflammatory bowel disease and few complications from endoscopic procedures.

NEONATOLOGY
Infection prevention score, NICU: ability to prevent central-line bloodstream infections in neonatal ICU.
Leaves NICU on breast milk score: relative percentage of infants discharged from NICU receiving some nutrition from breast milk.
Keeping breathing tube in place score: ability to minimize inappropriate breathing-tube removal in intubated infants.

NEPHROLOGY
Biopsy complications prevention score: ability to minimize

complications after kidney biopsy.
Dialysis management score: relative proportion of dialysis patients in past two years who tested normal.
Infection prevention score, dialysis: ability to minimize dialysis-related infection.
Kidney transplant survival score: based on patient survival and functioning kidney at one and three years.

NEUROLOGY & NEUROSURGERY
Epilepsy management score: ability to treat children with epilepsy.
Surgical survival score: survival at 30 days after complex surgery and procedures, such as those involving brain tumors, epilepsy and head trauma.

ORTHOPEDICS
Fracture repair score: ability to treat complex leg and forearm fractures efficiently.

PULMONOLOGY & LUNG SURGERY
Asthma inpatient care score: ability to minimize asthmatic children's asthma-related deaths, length of stay and readmissions.
Cystic fibrosis management score: ability to improve lung function and nutritional status.
Lung transplant survival score: reflects number of transplants in past two years, one-year survival, and recognition by United Network for Organ Sharing.

UROLOGY
Minimally invasive volume score: relative number of patients in past year who had specified nonsurgical procedures.
Testicular torsion care score: promptness of emergency surgery to correct twisted spermatic cord.

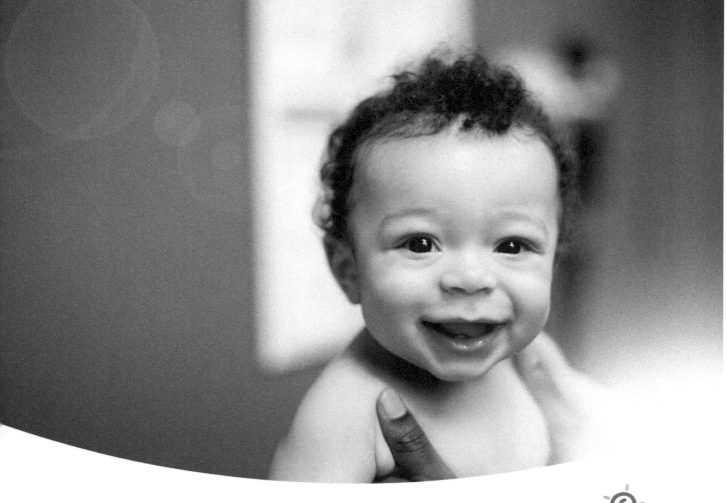

Children's
HOSPITAL & MEDICAL CENTER
OMAHA

When children are your everything, Anything can be.

At Children's Hospital & Medical Center, science and heart lead us to even greater pediatric breakthroughs. We give all we have to advance research, educate tomorrow's experts, advocate for children, families and communities, and provide the best pediatric specialty care. This commitment to improve the life of every child and the future of medicine once again led *U.S. News & World Report* to name us as one of the Best Children's Hospitals in the country for Cardiology & Heart Surgery, Diabetes & Endocrinology, Gastroenterology & GI Surgery, Orthopedics and Pulmonology.

To find a physician for your child, call **1.800.833.3100** or visit **ChildrensOmaha.org.**

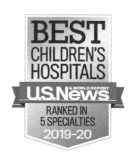

Education • Research • Advocacy • Care

Children's Miracle Network Hospitals® congratulates the 10 Honor Rollees that are all members of our network.

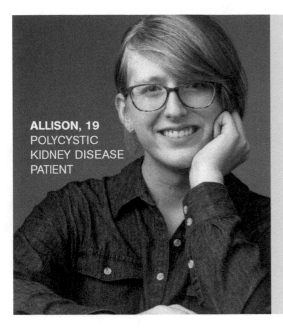

ALLISON, 19
POLYCYSTIC
KIDNEY DISEASE
PATIENT

1. Boston Children's Hospital, Boston, MA
2. Children's Hospital of Philadelphia, Philadelphia, PA
3. (tie) Cincinnati Children's Hospital Medical Center, Cincinnati, OH
3. (tie) Texas Children's Hospital, Houston, TX
5. Children's Hospital Los Angeles, Los Angeles, CA
6. Children's National Medical Center, Washington, DC
7. Nationwide Children's Hospital, Columbus, OH
8. UPMC Children's Hospital of Pittsburgh, Pittsburgh, PA
9. Johns Hopkins Children's Center, Baltimore, MD
10. Seattle Children's Hospital, Seattle, WA

Coincidence? We think not.
Thanks to local donations, Children's Miracle Network Hospitals are able to provide the best care for kids. Congratulations to the following member hospitals on being recognized among the best children's hospitals in the country.

Akron Children's Hospital, Akron, OH

Ann and Robert H. Lurie Children's Hospital of Chicago, Chicago, IL

Arkansas Children's Hospital, Little Rock, AR

Arnold Palmer Hospital for Children, Orlando, FL

Boston Children's Hospital, Boston, MA

Children's Healthcare of Atlanta, Atlanta, GA

Children's Hospital and Medical Center, Omaha, NE

Children's Hospital Colorado, Aurora, CO

Children's Hospital Los Angeles, Los Angeles, CA

Children's Hospital of Alabama at UAB, Birmingham, AL

Children's Hospital of Philadelphia, Philadelphia, PA

Children's Hospital of Wisconsin, Milwaukee, WI

Children's Medical Center, Dallas, TX

Children's National Medical Center, Washington, DC

CHOC Children's Hospital, Orange, CA

Cincinnati Children's Hospital Medical Center, Cincinnati, OH

Cohen Children's Medical Center, New Hyde Park, NY

Connecticut Children's Medical Center, Hartford, CT

Cook Children's Medical Center, Fort Worth, TX

Dayton Children's Hospital, Dayton, OH

Doernbecher Children's Hospital at Oregon Health and Science University, Portland, OR

Duke Children's Hospital and Health Center, Durham, NC

Johns Hopkins All Children's Hospital, St. Petersburg, FL

Johns Hopkins Children's Center, Baltimore, MD

Le Bonheur Children's Hospital, Memphis, TN

Levine Children's Hospital, Charlotte, NC

Monroe Carell Jr. Children's Hospital at Vanderbilt, Nashville, TN

MUSC Health-Children's Hospital, Charleston, SC

Nationwide Children's Hospital, Columbus, OH

Nicklaus Children's Hospital, Miami, FL

Norton Children's Hospital, Louisville, KY

Penn State Children's Hospital, Hershey, PA

Phoenix Children's Hospital, Phoenix, AZ

Primary Children's Hospital, Salt Lake City, UT

Rady Children's Hospital-San Diego, San Diego, CA

Rainbow Babies and Children's Hospital, Cleveland, OH

Riley Hospital for Children at UI Health, Indianapolis, IN

Seattle Children's Hospital, Seattle, WA

Spectrum Health Helen DeVos Children's Hospital, Grand Rapids, MI

SSM Health Cardinal Glennon Children's Hospital, St. Louis, MO

St. Louis Children's Hospital, St. Louis, MO

Texas Children's Hospital, Houston, TX

UCSF Benioff Children's Hospitals, San Francisco and Oakland, CA

UF Health Shands Children's Hospital, Gainesville, FL

University of California Davis Children's Hospital, Sacramento, CA

University of Iowa Stead Family Children's Hospital, Iowa City, IA

University of Rochester-Golisano Children's Hospital, Rochester, NY

University of Virginia Children's Hospital, Charlottesville, VA

UPMC Children's Hospital of Pittsburgh, Pittsburgh, PA

Valley Children's Healthcare and Hospital, Madera, CA

Wolfson Children's Hospital, Jacksonville, FL

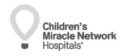

Children's Miracle Network Hospitals®

CHANGE KIDS' HEALTH
CHANGE THE FUTURE

CMNHospitals.org

▼

Cancer

Rank	Hospital	U.S. News score	Five-year survival score (15=best)	Bone marrow transplant survival score (6=best)	Infection prevention score, overall (36=best)	Infection prevention score, ICU (15=best)	Patient volume score (30=best)	Nurse-patient ratio (higher is better)	A Nurse Magnet hospital	Palliative care score (8=best)	% of specialists recommending hospital
1	Dana-Farber/Boston Children's Cancer and Blood Disorders Center	100.0	15	5	36	8	29	4.2	Yes	8	55.8%
2	St. Jude Children's Research Hospital, Memphis, Tenn.	96.1	14	5	35	10	30	4.6	Yes	8	36.9%
3	Texas Children's Hospital, Houston	95.5	12	5	35	12	30	4.1	Yes	8	38.0%
4	Nationwide Children's Hospital, Columbus, Ohio	95.1	15	6	35	12	30	3.3	Yes	8	13.1%
5	Johns Hopkins Children's Center, Baltimore	95.0	14	6	36	12	30	3.2	Yes	8	16.5%
6	Cincinnati Children's Hospital Medical Center	94.9	14	4	36	10	30	4.3	Yes	8	44.1%
7	Children's Hospital of Philadelphia	94.7	13	4	36	8	29	4.1	Yes	8	57.3%
8	Children's Healthcare of Atlanta	92.9	13	5	35	12	30	4.4	Yes	8	20.7%
9	Children's National Medical Center, Washington, D.C.	92.7	14	5	35	15	30	3.8	Yes	8	14.8%
10	Children's Hospital Los Angeles	92.0	15	4	34	12	28	3.8	Yes	8	26.9%
11	Seattle Children's Hospital	87.9	13	5	35	8	18	3.2	Yes	8	33.2%
12	UCSF Benioff Children's Hospitals, San Francisco and Oakland	85.8	13	5	34	10	25	3.9	Yes	7	11.8%
13	Memorial Sloan Kettering Children's Cancer Center, New York	85.1	12	5	34	4	28	4.6	Yes	8	17.1%
14*	Children's Hospital Colorado, Aurora	85.0	12	4	35	10	30	3.1	Yes	8	17.9%
14	Monroe Carell Jr. Children's Hospital at Vanderbilt, Nashville, Tenn.	84.2	15	5	35	10	29	3.4	Yes	8	1.8%
15	Riley Hospital for Children at IU Health, Indianapolis	83.4	12	6	33	11	23	3.7	Yes	8	1.5%
17	Ann and Robert H. Lurie Children's Hospital of Chicago	81.8	9	5	31	10	30	3.7	Yes	8	13.2%
18	Lucile Packard Children's Hospital Stanford, Palo Alto, Calif.	81.6	13	6	35	9	22	3.7	No	7	7.0%
19	CHOC Children's Hospital, Orange, Calif.	81.5	12	6	35	13	17	3.8	Yes	8	2.1%
20	Cleveland Clinic Children's Hospital	81.2	11	6	35	8	24	3.7	Yes	8	1.0%
21	Children's Medical Center Dallas	80.9	11	5	34	10	30	3.2	Yes	8	4.1%
22	C.S. Mott Children's Hospital-Michigan Medicine, Ann Arbor	80.4	13	4	36	13	30	3.6	Yes	8	4.0%
23	Rady Children's Hospital, San Diego	79.8	11	6	33	10	18	2.3	Yes	8	2.5%
24	St. Louis Children's Hospital-Washington University	79.2	10	5	36	11	13	3.7	Yes	8	4.5%
25	UF Health Shands Children's Hospital, Gainesville, Fla.	79.1	14	6	31	12	12	2.6	Yes	8	1.2%
26	Duke Children's Hospital and Health Center, Durham, N.C.	78.9	13	5	36	10	16	3.3	Yes	7	4.2%
27	Cohen Children's Medical Center, New Hyde Park, N.Y.	78.1	12	5	35	12	10	3.5	Yes	8	1.7%
28	Levine Children's Hospital, Charlotte, N.C.	77.1	13	6	33	11	9	3.0	Yes	8	0.7%
28	UCLA Mattel Children's Hospital, Los Angeles	77.1	14	4	31	12	17	4.9	Yes	8	2.3%
30	Children's Mercy Kansas City, Mo.	76.8	9	6	36	6	21	4.2	Yes	7	2.2%
30	Nemours Alfred I. duPont Hosp. for Children, Wilmington, Del.	76.8	13	5	32	10	21	3.4	Yes	8	1.1%
30	Primary Children's Hospital, Salt Lake City	76.8	13	5	33	10	25	2.9	No	8	2.1%
33	UPMC Children's Hospital of Pittsburgh	76.1	11	4	35	9	16	3.5	Yes	8	4.8%
34	Children's Hospital of Wisconsin, Milwaukee	75.7	13	4	30	10	15	4.5	Yes	8	2.6%
35	Phoenix Children's Hospital	75.6	13	4	33	12	28	3.0	No	8	2.6%
36	North Carolina Children's Hospital at UNC, Chapel Hill	75.1	8	6	36	12	25	5.0	Yes	7	0.5%
37	NY-Presby. Morgan Stanley-Komansky Children's Hospital, N.Y.	74.5	12	5	35	8	27	3.0	No	8	4.8%
37	Rainbow Babies and Children's Hospital, Cleveland	74.5	11	4	36	10	15	2.8	Yes	8	3.2%
39	University of Minnesota Masonic Children's Hospital, Minneapolis	74.4	12	5	29	10	25	3.0	No	7	3.3%
40	MUSC Health-Children's Hospital, Charleston, S.C.	74.3	12	5	34	13	16	3.0	Yes	8	0.6%
41	Children's Hospital of Alabama at UAB, Birmingham	74.1	12	5	30	13	26	3.4	No	8	2.3%
42	Spectrum Hlth. Helen DeVos Children's Hosp., Grand Rapids, Mich.	73.4	11	6	30	11	13	2.4	Magnet	6	1.2%
42	Yale New Haven Children's Hospital, New Haven, Conn.	73.4	13	4	34	8	23	4.4	Yes	8	1.4%
44	Hackensack Meridian Hlth. Sanzari & Hovnanian Children's Hosp., N.J.	73.3	10	6	31	15	10	2.5	Yes	8	0.6%
44	Johns Hopkins All Children's Hospital, St. Petersburg, Fla.	73.3	14	5	35	9	20	3.6	No	8	1.6%
46	University of Iowa Stead Family Children's Hospital, Iowa City	73.0	10	6	31	9	23	3.6	Yes	8	0.5%
47	Doernbecher Children's Hosp. at Oregon Hlth. & Science U., Portland	72.8	12	4	27	12	13	4.0	Yes	8	2.0%
48	Penn State Children's Hospital, Hershey, Pa.	72.7	11	6	27	8	10	3.8	Yes	8	0.9%
49	Children's Cancer Hosp.-U. of Texas M.D. Anderson Cancer Ctr., Houston	71.2	7	5	31	10	24	3.0	Yes	8	6.1%
50	Wolfson Children's Hospital, Jacksonville, Fla.	70.4	13	4	29	14	14	2.3	Yes	7	0.6%

*The scores of the hospitals tied at No. 14 are different because Children's Hospital Colorado was initially misranked due to a data error. The hospital's rank was corrected, and no other hospitals' ranks were affected.

Terms are explained on Page 178.

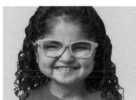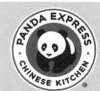

Cardiology & Heart Surgery

Rank	Hospital	U.S. News score	Risk-adjusted surgical survival score (5=best)	Norwood/ hybrid surgery survival score (24=best)	Infection prevention score, overall (41=best)	Infection prevention score, ICU (5=best)	Surgery volume score (15=best)	Catheter procedure volume score (57=best)	Nurse-patient ratio (higher is better)	A Nurse Magnet hospital	% of specialists recommending hospital
1	Texas Children's Hospital, Houston	100.0	5	22	39	4	13	57	4.1	Yes	49.0%
2	Ann and Robert H. Lurie Children's Hospital of Chicago	89.8	5	19	35	4	8	35	3.7	Yes	16.4%
3	UPMC Children's Hospital of Pittsburgh	86.2	5	24	39	3	8	37	3.5	Yes	11.0%
4	Children's Hospital Los Angeles	86.1	4	24	38	4	14	45	3.8	Yes	16.7%
5	Boston Children's Hospital	84.0	3	19	39	2	15	53	4.2	Yes	68.9%
6	Cincinnati Children's Hospital Medical Center	80.8	3	21	40	2	12	46	4.3	Yes	30.2%
7	Children's Hospital of Philadelphia	80.0	3	22	40	2	15	55	4.1	Yes	60.4%
7	MUSC Children's Heart Network of South Carolina, Charleston	80.0	5	22	38	5	8	39	3.0	Yes	7.4%
9	Riley Hospital for Children at IU Health, Indianapolis	79.8	5	17	37	3	10	34	3.7	Yes	2.6%
10	Le Bonheur Children's Hospital, Memphis, Tenn.	79.3	5	20	39	4	6	34	2.7	Yes	2.9%
11	UF Health Shands Children's Hospital, Gainesville, Fla.	78.5	5	24	35	4	6	20	2.6	Yes	0.9%
12	Children's Hospital Colorado, Aurora	77.3	3	20	39	2	12	48	3.1	Yes	12.8%
13	Advocate Children's Heart Institute, Oak Lawn and Park Ridge, Ill.	77.2	5	23	36	3	10	34	4.6	Yes	2.4%
14	Phoenix Children's Hospital	75.8	5	17	39	4	11	39	3.0	No	2.6%
15	C.S. Mott Children's Hospital-Michigan Medicine, Ann Arbor	75.5	3	20	40	3	14	48	3.6	Yes	36.1%
16	Seattle Children's Hospital	74.2	3	21	40	2	12	49	3.2	Yes	13.8%
17	Children's Medical Center Dallas	73.8	3	24	38	4	9	44	3.2	Yes	4.2%
18	UCSF Benioff Children's Hospitals, San Francisco and Oakland	73.0	4	14	39	4	9	43	3.9	Yes	7.6%
19	Levine Children's Hospital, Charlotte, N.C.	72.8	4	23	37	3	9	40	3.0	Yes	2.4%
20	Children's Mercy Kansas City, Mo.	72.7	3	20	40	2	10	44	4.2	Yes	3.6%
21	NY-Presby. Morgan Stanley-Komansky Children's Hospital, N.Y.	72.5	3	24	39	2	13	44	3.0	No	18.8%
22	St. Louis Children's Hospital-Washington University	72.1	3	16	40	3	9	52	3.7	Yes	3.5%
23	Cook Children's Medical Center, Fort Worth	70.7	5	24	32	4	11	33	3.4	Yes	1.1%
24	Nemours Alfred I. duPont Hosp. for Children, Wilmington, Del.	69.9	4	22	36	4	6	20	3.4	Yes	0.4%
25	Johns Hopkins Children's Center, Baltimore	69.8	3	22	40	4	7	32	3.2	Yes	2.4%
26	Children's Memorial Hermann Hospital, Houston	69.7	5	19	35	3	8	36	3.1	Yes	0.9%
27	Penn State Children's Hospital, Hershey, Pa.	69.0	5	24	30	2	5	22	3.8	Yes	1.0%
28	Lucile Packard Children's Hospital Stanford, Palo Alto, Calif.	68.3	1	18	39	3	14	46	3.7	Yes	39.6%
29	Children's Hospital of Wisconsin, Milwaukee	68.0	4	21	34	2	9	30	4.5	Yes	8.3%
30	Mayo Clinic Children's Center, Rochester, Minn.	66.8	3	20	38	2	9	30	3.8	Yes	5.3%
31	Rady Children's Hospital, San Diego	66.6	3	22	37	4	9	46	2.3	Yes	3.9%
32	University of Maryland Children's Hospital, Baltimore	66.1	4	18	37	4	5	22	2.9	Yes	0.6%
33	Spectrum Hlth. Helen DeVos Children's Hosp., Grand Rapids, Mich.	63.1	5	22	34	3	5	27	2.4	Yes	0.7%
34	Children's Healthcare of Atlanta	62.9	1	16	39	4	15	52	4.4	Yes	22.4%
35	Children's Hospital and Medical Center, Omaha	62.7	3	20	38	1	8	36	4.0	Yes	1.1%
36	Monroe Carell Jr. Children's Hospital at Vanderbilt, Nashville, Tenn.	62.1	2	19	39	4	12	54	3.4	Yes	6.0%
37	University of Virginia Children's Hospital, Charlottesville	61.8	3	21	37	1	7	31	2.8	Yes	1.3%
38	Arnold Palmer Hospital for Children, Orlando	61.6	4	22	35	5	6	32	3.2	Yes	0.7%
39	American Family Children's Hospital, Madison, Wis.	61.2	4	24	32	3	5	24	3.3	Yes	0.9%
40	Ochsner Hospital for Children, New Orleans	60.9	3	10	33	5	5	36	2.9	Yes	1.6%
41	Primary Children's Hospital, Salt Lake City	60.1	2	20	38	2	12	48	2.9	No	5.4%
42	Children's National Medical Center, Washington, D.C.	59.9	1	16	39	5	8	46	3.8	Yes	11.3%
43	Nationwide Children's Hospital, Columbus, Ohio	59.4	1	16	39	2	10	49	3.3	Yes	13.4%
44	Children's Hospital of Alabama at UAB, Birmingham	59.3	3	20	33	3	8	44	3.4	No	1.3%
45	Cleveland Clinic Children's Hospital	58.8	2	22	39	2	7	37	3.7	Yes	1.6%
46	UCLA Mattel Children's Hospital, Los Angeles	58.0	2	16	35	4	7	45	4.9	Yes	4.7%
46	Yale-New Haven/Connecticut Children's Medical Ctrs., New Haven	58.0	3	10	38	4	5	33	4.4	Yes	1.4%
48	SSM Hlth. Cardinal Glennon Children's Hosp.-St. Louis U., St. Louis	57.2	4	19	36	1	6	21	3.0	No	0.8%
49	Arkansas Children's Hospital, Little Rock	57.1	3	19	34	4	8	34	3.3	Yes	1.0%
50	Nicklaus Children's Hospital, Miami	54.1	2	18	36	4	9	29	2.9	Yes	2.1%

Terms are explained on Page 178.

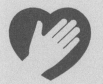

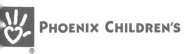
PHOENIX CHILDREN'S

10 out of 10,
three times over

For the third time, Phoenix Children's is ranked in 10 out of 10 specialties as one of U.S. News & World Report's Best Children's Hospitals.

Patients and families are at the center of everything we do. From research and state-of-the-art facilities to renowned clinical expertise, our multidisciplinary approach to care makes Phoenix Children's the only children's hospital in Arizona recognized by U.S. News & World Report. Phoenix Children's is the Southwest's premier destination for compassionate, family-centric pediatric care.

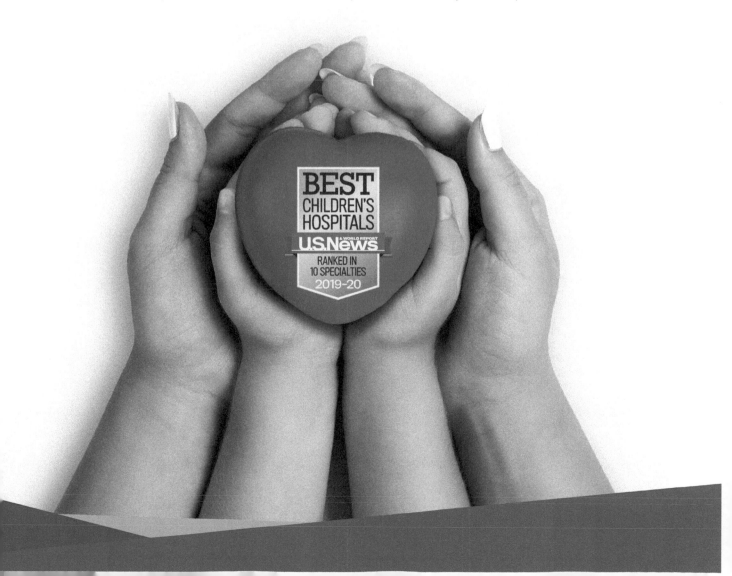

Diabetes & Endocrinology

Rank	Hospital	U.S. News score	Diabetes management score (48=best)	Hypothyroid management score (3=best)	Infection prevention score, overall (36=best)	Patient volume score (36=best)	Procedure volume score (24=best)	Nurse-patient ratio (higher is better)	A Nurse Magnet hospital	No. of best practices (109=best)	% of specialists recommending hospital
1	Children's Hospital of Philadelphia	100.0	41	3	36	36	24	4.1	Yes	108	56.5%
2	Boston Children's Hospital	94.7	36	3	35	34	24	4.2	Yes	104	50.6%
3	Yale New Haven Children's Hospital, New Haven, Conn.	91.0	45	3	34	32	24	4.4	Yes	105	15.7%
4	Children's Hospital Los Angeles	90.3	42	3	33	36	18	3.8	Yes	105	23.0%
5	Cincinnati Children's Hospital Medical Center	86.5	30	3	35	34	19	4.3	Yes	108	28.9%
6	UPMC Children's Hospital of Pittsburgh	86.0	37	3	33	35	20	3.5	Yes	107	21.4%
7	Children's Hospital Colorado, Aurora	85.6	33	3	33	33	22	3.1	Yes	99	28.3%
8	Texas Children's Hospital, Houston	84.1	30	3	34	36	24	4.1	Yes	104	20.5%
9	Lucile Packard Children's Hospital Stanford, Palo Alto, Calif.	79.6	39	3	33	31	14	3.7	No	91	14.3%
10	Seattle Children's Hospital	78.9	29	3	35	36	24	3.2	Yes	103	13.4%
11	UCSF Benioff Children's Hospitals, San Francisco and Oakland	77.0	28	3	33	34	20	3.9	Yes	94	14.6%
12	Nationwide Children's Hospital, Columbus, Ohio	76.1	28	3	34	35	24	3.3	Yes	102	8.2%
13	Riley Hospital for Children at IU Health, Indianapolis	76.0	29	3	32	35	18	3.7	Yes	95	10.6%
14	Children's National Medical Center, Washington, D.C.	75.0	28	3	35	35	20	3.8	Yes	106	5.7%
15	Mayo Clinic Children's Center, Rochester, Minn.	74.6	36	3	32	29	20	3.8	Yes	100	3.8%
16	Mount Sinai Kravis Children's Hospital, New York	73.9	36	3	33	32	20	3.5	Yes	107	2.8%
16	North Carolina Children's Hospital at UNC, Chapel Hill	73.9	34	3	34	33	20	5.0	Yes	104	2.3%
18	Children's Medical Center Dallas	73.4	31	3	32	34	24	3.2	Yes	93	6.9%
19	UF Health Shands Children's Hospital, Gainesville, Fla.	73.1	30	3	30	28	14	2.6	Yes	100	8.1%
20	Holtz Children's Hospital at UM-Jackson Memorial Med. Ctr., Miami	72.9	47	3	27	29	23	2.7	No	107	1.6%
21	University of Iowa Stead Family Children's Hospital, Iowa City	72.6	38	3	29	33	17	3.6	Yes	93	1.0%
22	St. Louis Children's Hospital-Washington University	72.5	27	3	34	33	22	3.7	Yes	96	4.1%
23	Monroe Carell Jr. Children's Hospital at Vanderbilt, Nashville, Tenn.	71.9	27	3	33	34	23	3.4	Yes	95	6.3%
24	CHOC Children's Hospital, Orange, Calif.	71.6	35	3	34	33	22	3.8	Yes	103	1.5%
25	Ann and Robert H. Lurie Children's Hospital of Chicago	70.9	31	3	29	32	21	3.7	Yes	91	7.4%
25	NY-Presby. Morgan Stanley-Komansky Children's Hospital, N.Y.	70.9	33	3	33	31	22	3.0	No	98	8.0%
27	University of Virginia Children's Hospital, Charlottesville	70.6	35	3	31	23	11	2.8	Yes	100	1.3%
28	Cohen Children's Medical Center, New Hyde Park, N.Y.	69.9	28	3	35	33	23	3.5	Yes	105	2.8%
29	Children's Mercy Kansas City, Mo.	69.8	24	3	34	33	17	4.2	Yes	101	4.7%
29	Rady Children's Hospital, San Diego	69.8	31	3	31	34	24	2.3	Yes	96	2.4%
31	Rainbow Babies and Children's Hospital, Cleveland	69.4	23	3	36	31	19	2.8	Yes	104	6.0%
32	Valley Children's Healthcare and Hospital, Madera, Calif.	69.0	39	3	35	31	13	3.1	Yes	98	1.1%
33	Johns Hopkins Children's Center, Baltimore	68.7	23	3	35	27	9	3.2	Yes	102	10.6%
34	UCLA Mattel Children's Hospital, Los Angeles	68.4	32	3	29	22	20	4.9	Yes	92	5.1%
35	Nemours Alfred I. duPont Hosp. for Children, Wilmington, Del.	67.5	32	3	31	32	18	3.4	Yes	92	0.4%
36	Children's Healthcare of Atlanta	67.2	21	3	33	35	23	4.4	Yes	100	2.6%
37	Children's Hospital and Medical Center, Omaha	66.1	31	3	35	33	13	4.0	Yes	93	0.1%
38	Duke Children's Hospital and Health Center, Durham, N.C.	66.0	24	3	34	32	20	3.3	Yes	99	1.7%
39	C.S. Mott Children's Hospital-Michigan Medicine, Ann Arbor	65.5	24	3	34	31	19	3.6	Yes	96	2.5%
39	Cleveland Clinic Children's Hospital	65.5	24	3	35	35	18	3.7	Yes	99	1.9%
41	NYU Winthrop Hospital Children's Medical Center, Mineola, N.Y.	65.2	28	3	34	28	10	4.5	Yes	103	1.3%
42	Children's Minnesota, Minneapolis	64.2	32	3	29	32	19	3.3	Yes	91	1.3%
43	Connecticut Children's Medical Center, Hartford	63.5	32	3	33	30	16	2.8	No	93	1.5%
43	MassGeneral Hospital for Children, Boston	63.5	20	3	29	30	24	2.8	Yes	102	4.3%
45	Children's Hospital of Wisconsin, Milwaukee	62.9	23	3	30	28	21	4.5	Yes	93	2.1%
46	University of Minnesota Masonic Children's Hospital, Minneapolis	62.4	28	3	29	32	17	3.0	No	101	2.0%
47	UC Davis Children's Hospital, Sacramento	62.0	25	3	34	23	14	6.9	Yes	100	0.8%
48	Nicklaus Children's Hospital, Miami	61.8	31	3	30	33	17	2.9	Yes	81	1.0%
49	Norton Children's Hospital, Louisville, Ky.	61.4	22	3	35	36	24	3.2	No	94	1.3%
50	Phoenix Children's Hospital	60.9	23	3	34	34	24	3.0	No	95	0.9%

Terms are explained on Page 178.

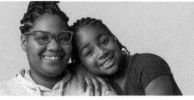

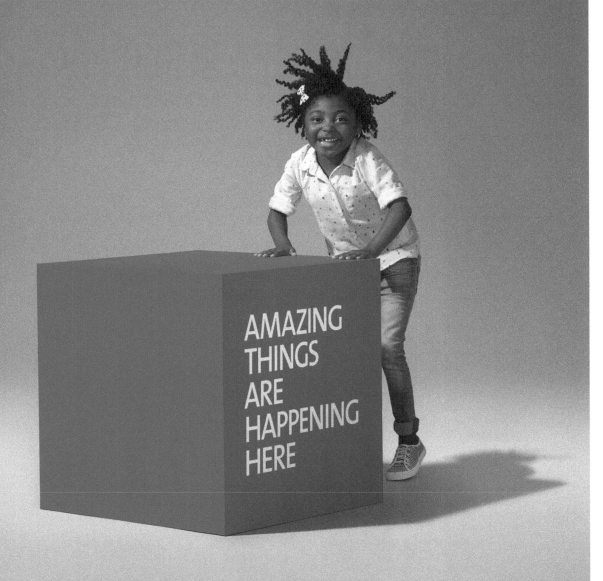

Proud to be New York's #1 Children's Hospital.

With two sites — NewYork-Presbyterian Morgan Stanley Children's Hospital at Columbia and NewYork-Presbyterian Komansky Children's Hospital at Weill Cornell Medicine — children are never far from amazing care.

Learn more at nyp.org/pediatrics

⊣ **NewYork-Presbyterian**

⚕ **Weill Cornell Medicine** | ⊣NewYork-Presbyterian | ♕ COLUMBIA

Gastroenterology & GI Surgery

Rank	Hospital	U.S. News score	Selected treatments success score (9=best)	Liver transplant survival score (6=best)	Infection prevention score, overall (42=best)	Infection prevention score, ICU (5=best)	Patient volume score (27=best)	Surgery volume score (12=best)	Nonsurgical procedure volume score (18=best)	Nurse-patient ratio (higher is better)	A Nurse Magnet hospital	% of specialists recom-mending hospital
1	Children's Hospital of Philadelphia	100.0	8	6	42	2	27	12	18	4.1	Yes	53.5%
2	Texas Children's Hospital, Houston	99.3	9	5	40	4	27	12	18	4.1	Yes	32.8%
3	Cincinnati Children's Hospital Medical Center	97.1	8	5	42	2	27	11	17	4.3	Yes	55.1%
4	Boston Children's Hospital	94.6	7	5	42	2	27	10	18	4.2	Yes	57.0%
5	Children's Healthcare of Atlanta	93.3	9	6	40	4	27	12	18	4.4	Yes	8.9%
6	Children's Hospital Colorado, Aurora	88.7	8	4	41	2	27	12	17	3.1	Yes	32.4%
7	UPMC Children's Hospital of Pittsburgh	88.6	8	6	39	3	24	10	11	3.5	Yes	19.6%
8	Ann and Robert H. Lurie Children's Hospital of Chicago	88.0	7	6	37	4	26	11	17	3.7	Yes	19.8%
9	Children's Hospital Los Angeles	87.2	7	6	40	4	24	9	18	3.8	Yes	14.2%
10	Children's Medical Center Dallas	86.6	8	6	39	4	27	10	18	3.2	Yes	7.6%
11	Johns Hopkins Children's Center, Baltimore	84.5	9	3	42	2	27	11	14	3.2	Yes	8.6%
12	Children's Hospital at Montefiore, New York	83.7	9	6	42	5	18	8	14	5.4	No	2.9%
13	Children's National Medical Center, Washington, D.C.	83.4	7	6	41	5	26	12	17	3.8	Yes	3.6%
14	UCSF Benioff Children's Hospitals, San Francisco and Oakland	82.8	7	6	40	4	25	9	13	3.9	Yes	7.6%
15	Nationwide Children's Hospital, Columbus, Ohio	82.2	9	NR	41	2	26	11	16	3.3	Yes	37.7%
16	Riley Hospital for Children at IU Health, Indianapolis	81.9	8	6	39	3	24	8	16	3.7	Yes	3.7%
17	Monroe Carell Jr. Children's Hosp. at Vanderbilt, Nashville, Tenn.	81.5	8	5	41	4	26	9	17	3.4	Yes	4.1%
18	Seattle Children's Hospital	81.3	7	5	42	2	24	8	17	3.2	Yes	19.8%
19	UCLA Mattel Children's Hospital, Los Angeles	80.0	9	4	37	4	18	8	12	4.9	Yes	5.6%
20	St. Louis Children's Hospital-Washington University	78.7	7	6	42	3	21	8	13	3.7	Yes	5.4%
21	Rady Children's Hospital, San Diego	78.3	8	6	38	4	24	6	14	2.3	Yes	2.9%
22	Children's Mercy Kansas City, Mo.	76.6	8	4	41	2	24	9	14	4.2	Yes	4.8%
23	MassGeneral Hospital for Children, Boston	75.8	6	6	36	5	19	8	14	2.8	Yes	4.6%
24	Le Bonheur Children's Hospital, Memphis, Tenn.	74.8	9	4	41	4	15	8	10	2.7	Yes	1.4%
25	Duke Children's Hospital and Health Center, Durham, N.C.	74.3	7	6	42	4	21	8	11	3.3	Yes	1.7%
26	NY-Presby. Morgan Stanley-Komansky Children's Hospital, N.Y.	73.0	8	4	39	2	23	10	18	3.0	No	7.0%
27	Cleveland Clinic Children's Hospital	72.2	6	5	39	2	24	9	18	3.7	Yes	3.5%
28	Mount Sinai Kravis Children's Hospital, New York	71.6	7	5	39	3	16	9	13	3.5	Yes	2.0%
29	C.S. Mott Children's Hospital-Michigan Medicine, Ann Arbor	71.5	7	4	40	3	27	9	17	3.6	Yes	3.2%
30	Children's Hospital of Wisconsin, Milwaukee	70.8	6	5	35	2	24	9	17	4.5	Yes	5.3%
30	Nemours Alfred I. duPont Hosp. for Children, Wilmington, Del.	70.8	7	5	37	4	17	8	9	3.4	Yes	1.1%
32	Phoenix Children's Hospital	70.1	7	5	39	4	23	10	12	3.0	No	2.1%
33	Primary Children's Hospital, Salt Lake City	69.8	7	6	38	2	25	9	16	2.9	No	2.2%
34	Lucile Packard Children's Hospital Stanford, Palo Alto, Calif.	69.5	5	5	41	3	23	10	14	3.7	No	10.4%
35	Children's Hospital of Michigan, Detroit	69.0	8	6	37	2	23	4	12	3.4	No	0.3%
36	North Carolina Children's Hospital at UNC, Chapel Hill	68.7	8	3	42	2	19	6	11	5.0	Yes	1.7%
37	Yale New Haven Children's Hospital, New Haven, Conn.	68.1	6	5	38	4	17	7	6	4.4	Yes	2.1%
38	MUSC Health-Children's Hospital, Charleston, S.C.	65.6	6	4	36	5	23	9	17	3.0	Yes	0.5%
39	Cohen Children's Medical Center, New Hyde Park, N.Y.	65.3	8	NA	41	4	16	8	16	3.5	Yes	1.3%
40	Rainbow Babies and Children's Hospital, Cleveland	65.1	9	NA	42	4	16	6	14	2.8	Yes	1.7%
41	University of Minnesota Masonic Children's Hosp., Minneapolis	64.1	7	5	36	2	23	6	13	3.0	No	0.9%
42	Levine Children's Hospital, Charlotte, N.C.	63.7	6	4	39	3	19	6	15	3.0	Yes	1.3%
43	Valley Children's Healthcare and Hospital, Madera, Calif.	63.4	9	NA	41	4	21	8	18	3.1	Yes	0.6%
44	Mayo Clinic Children's Center, Rochester, Minn.	61.7	4	5	39	2	19	5	16	3.8	Yes	2.7%
45	Akron Children's Hospital, Ohio	61.2	9	NA	40	4	16	4	7	3.5	Yes	0.6%
46	Children's Hospital and Medical Center, Omaha	60.5	9	NA	37	1	13	9	11	4.0	Yes	1.0%
47	University of Virginia Children's Hospital, Charlottesville	60.4	6	6	36	1	14	7	9	2.8	Yes	1.0%
48	Ochsner Hospital for Children, New Orleans	59.8	6	5	33	5	10	4	10	2.9	Yes	0.6%
49	Holtz Children's Hosp. at UM-Jackson Memorial Med. Ctr., Miami	59.2	6	5	33	5	19	8	12	2.7	No	1.2%
50	American Family Children's Hospital, Madison, Wis.	58.7	6	5	35	3	8	4	6	3.3	Yes	0.3%

NA=not applicable. NR=not reported. Terms are explained on Page 178.

Best in Northern California in 5 Specialties

CANCER | CARDIOLOGY & HEART SURGERY
GASTROENTEROLOGY & GI SURGERY | NEONATOLOGY
NEUROLOGY & NEUROSURGERY

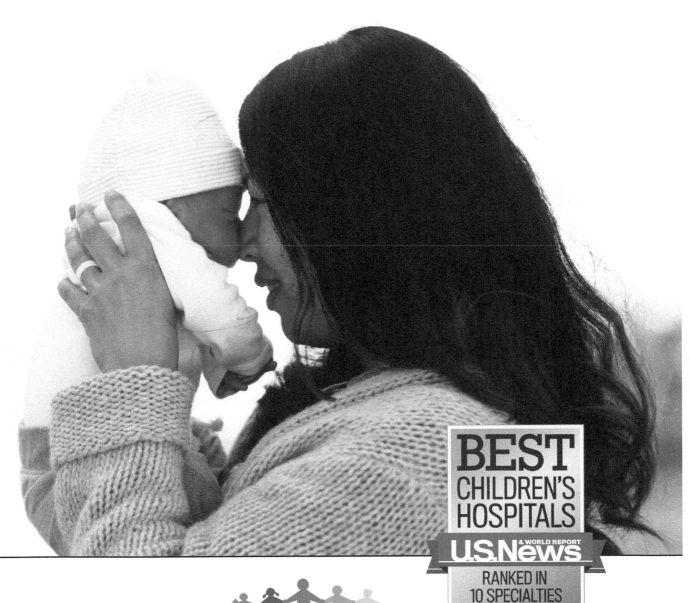

BEST
CHILDREN'S
HOSPITALS
U.S.News & WORLD REPORT
RANKED IN
10 SPECIALTIES
2019-20

UCSF Benioff Children's Hospitals

Neonatology

Rank	Hospital	U.S. News score	Leaves NICU on breast milk score (3=best)	Keeping breathing tube in place score (5=best)	Infection prevention score, overall (42=best)	Infection prevention score, NICU (5=best)	Patient volume score (33=best)	Nurse-patient ratio (higher is better)	A Nurse Magnet hospital	No. of best practices (101=best)	% of specialists recommending hospital
1	Children's National Medical Center, Washington, D.C.	100.0	3	5	41	5	29	3.4	Yes	100	17.5%
2	Boston Children's Hospital	92.6	3	4	42	3	22	3.8	Yes	101	35.4%
3	Children's Hospital of Philadelphia	91.7	3	5	42	2	33	3.8	Yes	95	43.7%
4	Cincinnati Children's Hospital Medical Center	91.6	2	4	41	4	29	4.0	Yes	99	28.4%
5	UCSF Benioff Children's Hospitals, San Francisco and Oakland	88.5	3	4	41	4	29	3.4	Yes	99	13.3%
6	Lucile Packard Children's Hospital Stanford, Palo Alto, Calif.	86.7	3	3	40	5	20	4.6	No	98	15.9%
7	Rainbow Babies and Children's Hospital, Cleveland	82.2	2	4	42	4	13	4.6	Yes	98	17.0%
7	Texas Children's Hospital, Houston	82.2	3	3	41	3	30	2.9	Yes	101	17.9%
9	Children's Hospital Los Angeles	82.0	3	5	40	4	30	3.6	Yes	101	9.8%
10	St. Louis Children's Hospital-Washington University	81.4	2	4	42	4	28	4.0	Yes	97	9.1%
11	Rady Children's Hospital, San Diego	80.9	3	4	40	4	25	3.0	Yes	95	6.3%
12	Johns Hopkins Children's Center, Baltimore	80.0	2	5	42	4	24	3.0	Yes	84	11.9%
13	Children's Mercy Kansas City, Mo.	79.9	2	3	42	5	27	4.0	Yes	99	5.3%
14	Seattle Children's Hospital	79.3	3	5	35	3	28	3.6	Yes	93	15.6%
15	Nationwide Children's Hospital, Columbus, Ohio	78.9	2	3	41	4	32	2.8	Yes	95	15.9%
16	University of Iowa Stead Family Children's Hospital, Iowa City	78.2	3	5	32	5	17	3.1	Yes	89	4.4%
17	Children's Medical Center Dallas-Parkland Memorial Hospital	77.2	2	4	40	5	27	2.5	Yes	95	3.7%
18	Children's Hospital Colorado, Aurora	76.1	3	4	41	2	27	3.2	Yes	99	12.7%
19	Doernbecher Children's Hosp. at Oregon Hlth. & Science U., Portland	75.9	3	5	33	5	19	2.7	Yes	94	0.9%
20	Duke Children's Hospital and Health Center, Durham, N.C.	75.6	2	4	42	5	21	2.5	Yes	90	4.9%
21	C.S. Mott Children's Hospital-Michigan Medicine, Ann Arbor	75.2	2	3	42	5	25	2.6	Yes	87	4.4%
21	NY-Presby. Morgan Stanley-Komansky Children's Hospital, N.Y.	75.2	3	4	41	3	31	2.9	No	97	11.9%
23	Ann & Robert H. Lurie Children's Hosp.-Prentice Women's Hosp., Chicago	74.3	2	4	36	4	25	2.8	Yes	91	10.3%
24	Cohen Children's Medical Center, New Hyde Park, N.Y.	74.0	3	3	38	5	25	2.0	Yes	96	1.9%
25	Yale New Haven Children's Hospital, New Haven, Conn.	73.8	2	4	39	5	21	2.6	Yes	94	2.7%
26	Children's Hospital at Montefiore, New York	72.5	3	4	42	4	13	3.8	No	100	2.0%
27	Phoenix Children's Hospital	72.2	3	5	40	4	28	3.2	No	94	0.7%
28	Monroe Carell Jr. Children's Hospital at Vanderbilt, Nashville, Tenn.	71.6	2	4	34	4	27	2.8	Yes	93	6.4%
29	UCLA Mattel Children's Hospital, Los Angeles	71.5	3	5	27	4	12	4.5	Yes	91	4.4%
30	UC Davis Children's Hospital, Sacramento	70.6	2	5	42	4	20	3.7	Yes	95	1.0%
31	AdventHealth for Children, Orlando	69.4	2	5	35	5	15	2.4	Yes	94	1.0%
32	Cleveland Clinic Children's Hospital	68.3	2	3	41	4	17	2.9	Yes	99	1.8%
32	Primary Children's Hospital, Salt Lake City	68.3	3	5	40	3	27	3.4	No	92	2.8%
34	Children's Healthcare of Atlanta	67.6	2	4	41	4	30	3.4	Yes	96	4.7%
34	Children's Hosp. at St. Peter's University Hosp., New Brunswick, N.J.	67.6	2	5	40	5	4	3.2	Yes	100	0.0%
34	Connecticut Children's Medical Center, Hartford	67.6	3	5	39	5	11	2.3	No	96	1.2%
37	Children's Hospital of Alabama at UAB, Birmingham	66.6	3	4	36	3	31	3.1	No	98	5.5%
38	University of Rochester-Golisano Children's Hospital, N.Y.	66.5	2	4	37	4	16	2.9	Yes	99	1.9%
39	Akron Children's Hospital, Ohio	66.4	2	4	39	5	15	3.3	Yes	95	1.2%
40	University of Virginia Children's Hospital, Charlottesville	65.6	2	5	34	4	16	2.5	Yes	93	1.4%
41	CHOC Children's Hospital, Orange, Calif.	65.5	2	4	41	3	28	3.4	Yes	98	2.9%
42	Norton Children's Hospital, Louisville, Ky.	65.4	2	3	42	5	22	2.1	No	95	1.8%
43	Children's Minnesota, Minneapolis	65.0	3	3	32	5	26	3.2	Yes	76	0.4%
44	Valley Children's Healthcare and Hospital, Madera, Calif.	64.8	2	3	41	5	22	3.1	Yes	90	0.9%
45	Levine Children's Hospital, Charlotte, N.C.	64.6	2	3	38	5	22	2.4	Yes	84	2.4%
46	MassGeneral Hospital for Children, Boston	64.5	3	3	34	5	16	1.9	Yes	93	0.9%
47	Le Bonheur Children's Hospital, Memphis, Tenn.	64.3	2	2	42	4	20	2.7	Yes	96	1.2%
48	UPMC Children's Hospital of Pittsburgh	63.6	2	3	41	2	25	3.1	Yes	100	6.7%
49	American Family Children's Hospital, Madison, Wis.	63.1	3	3	34	4	14	4.3	Yes	92	0.1%
49	Nicklaus Children's Hospital, Miami	63.1	3	5	34	3	20	3.3	Yes	85	1.2%

Terms are explained on Page 178.

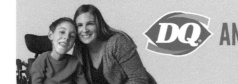

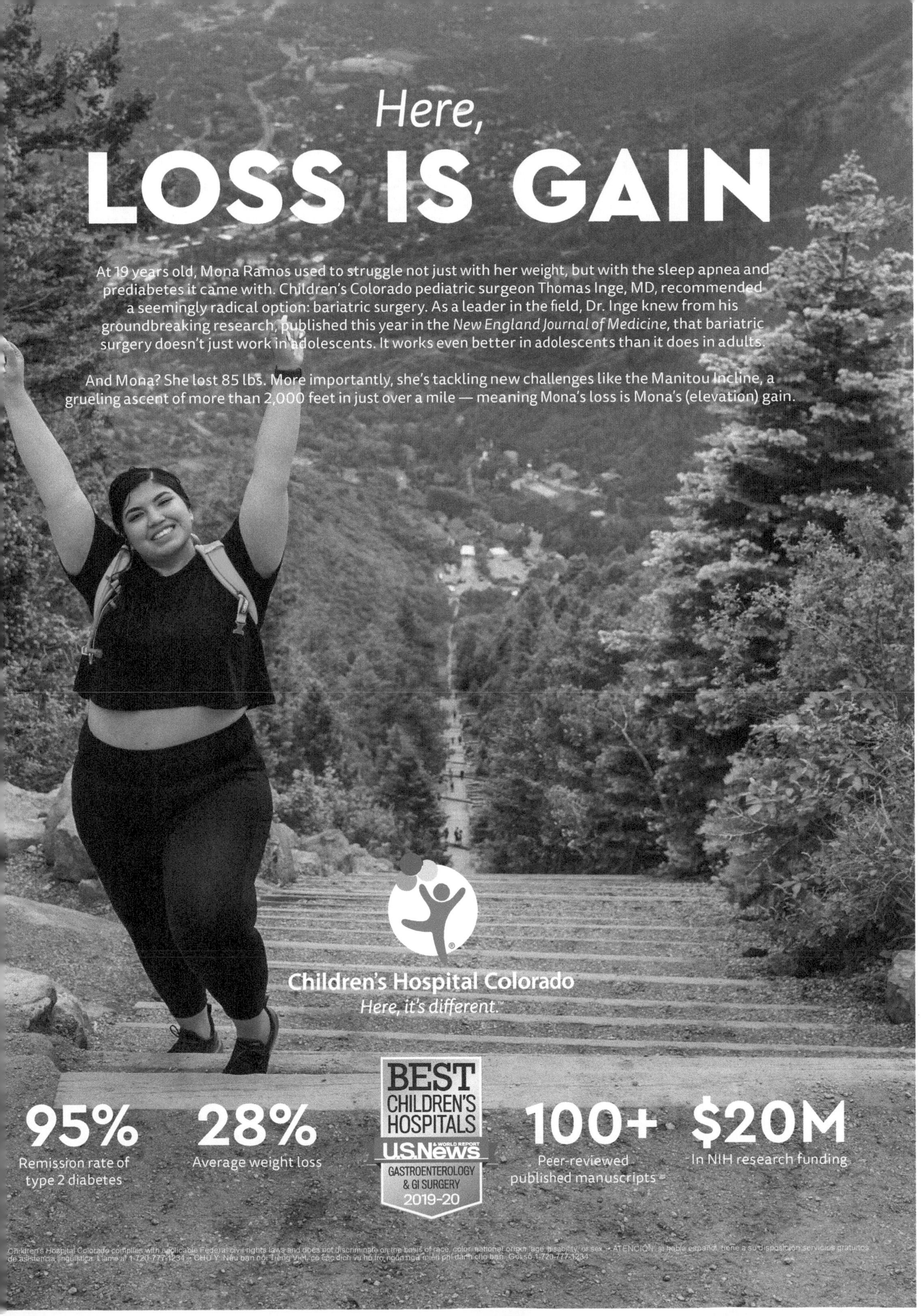

Here,
LOSS IS GAIN
At 19 years old, Mona Ramos used to struggle not just with her weight, but with the sleep apnea and prediabetes it came with. Children's Colorado pediatric surgeon Thomas Inge, MD, recommended a seemingly radical option: bariatric surgery. As a leader in the field, Dr. Inge knew from his groundbreaking research, published this year in the New England Journal of Medicine, that bariatric surgery doesn't just work in adolescents. It works even better in adolescents than it does in adults.
And Mona? She lost 85 lbs. More importantly, she's tackling new challenges like the Manitou Incline, a grueling ascent of more than 2,000 feet in just over a mile — meaning Mona's loss is Mona's (elevation) gain.
Children's Hospital Colorado
Here, it's different.™
95%
Remission rate of type 2 diabetes
28%
Average weight loss
BEST CHILDREN'S HOSPITALS
U.S.News & WORLD REPORT
GASTROENTEROLOGY & GI SURGERY
2019-20
100+
Peer-reviewed published manuscripts
$20M
In NIH research funding
Children's Hospital Colorado complies with applicable Federal civil rights laws and does not discriminate on the basis of race, color, national origin, age, disability, or sex. • ATENCIÓN: si habla español, tiene a su disposición servicios gratuitos de asistencia lingüística. Llame al 1-720-777-1234. • CHÚ Ý: Nếu bạn nói Tiếng Việt, có các dịch vụ hỗ trợ ngôn ngữ miễn phí dành cho bạn. Gọi số 1-720-777-1234.

Nephrology

Rank	Hospital	U.S. News score	Kidney transplant survival score (24=best)	Biopsy complications prevention score (6=best)	Dialysis management score (12=best)	Infection prevention score, overall (59=best)	Infection prevention score, ICU (5=best)	Infection prevention score, dialysis (9=best)	Patient volume score (14=best)	Nurse-patient ratio (higher is better)	A Nurse Magnet hospital	% of specialists recommending hospital
1	Boston Children's Hospital	100.0	23	6	12	59	2	8	13	4.2	Yes	51.9%
2	Texas Children's Hospital, Houston	98.5	23	6	12	58	4	9	14	4.1	Yes	30.2%
3	Cincinnati Children's Hospital Medical Center	98.0	23	6	11	59	2	9	14	4.3	Yes	49.3%
4	Children's Hospital of Philadelphia	96.2	23	6	12	59	2	7	13	4.1	Yes	45.3%
5	Children's Healthcare of Atlanta	95.6	23	6	12	58	4	8	14	4.4	Yes	23.9%
6	Children's National Medical Center, Washington, D.C.	94.7	23	6	12	58	5	9	14	3.8	Yes	10.1%
7	Children's Mercy Kansas City, Mo.	94.6	24	6	12	59	2	9	13	4.2	Yes	20.9%
8	Seattle Children's Hospital	93.2	24	6	12	59	2	6	14	3.2	Yes	45.6%
9	Johns Hopkins Children's Center, Baltimore	92.5	23	6	12	59	4	7	9	3.2	Yes	18.7%
10	Ann and Robert H. Lurie Children's Hospital of Chicago	91.2	23	6	12	54	4	9	14	3.7	Yes	12.5%
11	Lucile Packard Children's Hospital Stanford, Palo Alto, Calif.	90.9	24	6	12	56	3	8	14	3.7	No	26.7%
12	Nationwide Children's Hospital, Columbus, Ohio	87.6	21	6	12	58	2	8	13	3.3	Yes	19.8%
13	UPMC Children's Hospital of Pittsburgh	87.5	24	6	12	58	3	8	11	3.5	Yes	8.7%
14	UCSF Benioff Children's Hospitals, San Francisco and Oakland	85.9	24	6	11	55	4	8	11	3.9	Yes	7.8%
15	Riley Hospital for Children at IU Health, Indianapolis	84.0	23	6	12	55	3	9	13	3.7	Yes	5.5%
16	Children's Hospital Los Angeles	83.9	23	6	12	57	4	9	13	3.8	Yes	3.6%
17	UCLA Mattel Children's Hospital, Los Angeles	82.1	23	3	10	52	4	8	12	4.9	Yes	16.5%
18	Children's Medical Center Dallas	81.6	22	6	10	53	4	8	12	3.2	Yes	7.6%
19	C.S. Mott Children's Hospital-Michigan Medicine, Ann Arbor	81.5	24	6	12	58	3	6	12	3.6	Yes	10.9%
20	Children's Hospital Colorado, Aurora	80.2	24	6	8	58	2	9	14	3.1	Yes	6.5%
21	Duke Children's Hospital and Health Center, Durham, N.C.	80.1	24	6	12	59	4	8	11	3.3	Yes	5.5%
22	Children's Hospital at Montefiore, New York	79.6	22	6	12	59	5	5	12	5.4	No	5.9%
23	St. Louis Children's Hospital-Washington University	78.0	22	5	12	58	3	7	12	3.7	Yes	3.9%
24	Monroe Carell Jr. Children's Hosp. at Vanderbilt, Nashville, Tenn.	77.4	22	6	8	58	4	9	11	3.4	Yes	2.9%
25	MUSC Health-Children's Hospital, Charleston, S.C.	77.1	23	6	11	57	5	8	13	3.0	Yes	1.1%
26	Mount Sinai Kravis Children's Hospital, New York	77.0	23	6	12	56	3	9	7	3.5	Yes	2.9%
27	Levine Children's Hospital, Charlotte, N.C.	76.9	24	6	9	56	3	9	12	3.0	Yes	3.0%
28	U. Minn. Masonic Children's Hosp.-Children's Minn., Minneapolis	76.0	22	6	11	52	2	6	13	3.0	Yes	5.9%
29	Doernbecher Children's Hospital, Portland, Ore.	75.9	24	6	12	50	4	7	11	4.0	Yes	1.2%
30	North Carolina Children's Hospital at UNC, Chapel Hill	75.7	24	6	12	58	2	8	12	5.0	Yes	2.0%
31	Rady Children's Hospital, San Diego	75.6	24	5	10	56	4	9	12	2.3	Yes	2.9%
32	Phoenix Children's Hospital	73.5	22	6	11	56	4	8	14	3.0	No	1.7%
33	UC Davis Children's Hospital, Sacramento	72.9	21	6	12	59	1	6	9	6.9	Yes	1.8%
34	Children's Hospital of Michigan, Detroit	72.1	23	6	12	56	2	8	11	3.4	No	1.5%
35	Cleveland Clinic Children's Hospital	72.0	17	6	10	58	2	9	10	3.7	Yes	2.6%
36	Cohen Children's Medical Center, New Hyde Park, N.Y.	71.6	12	4	12	58	4	8	11	3.5	Yes	0.8%
37	Le Bonheur Children's Hospital, Memphis, Tenn.	71.4	20	5	8	56	4	8	12	2.7	Yes	3.3%
37	NY-Presby. Morgan Stanley-Komansky Children's Hospital, N.Y.	71.4	23	6	11	58	2	7	14	3.0	No	4.6%
39	Spectrum Hlth. Helen DeVos Children's Hosp., Grand Rapids, Mich.	71.1	22	6	12	52	3	8	9	2.4	Yes	1.1%
39	University of Iowa Stead Family Children's Hospital, Iowa City	71.1	24	6	7	54	3	5	10	3.6	Yes	5.2%
41	University of Rochester-Golisano Children's Hospital, N.Y.	70.8	24	6	12	52	4	8	6	3.3	Yes	0.9%
42	Nemours Alfred I. duPont Hosp. for Children, Wilmington, Del.	70.7	24	6	8	54	4	7	13	3.4	Yes	2.1%
42	Yale New Haven Children's Hospital, New Haven, Conn.	70.7	18	6	12	57	4	5	11	4.4	Yes	1.8%
44	Primary Children's Hospital, Salt Lake City	70.2	24	6	11	56	2	7	12	2.9	No	1.4%
45	American Family Children's Hospital, Madison, Wis.	68.7	22	6	12	51	3	8	6	3.3	Yes	0.9%
46	Arkansas Children's Hospital, Little Rock	68.2	20	6	11	52	4	7	9	3.3	Yes	0.4%
47	University of Virginia Children's Hospital, Charlottesville	67.9	23	6	11	56	1	9	8	2.8	Yes	2.2%
48	Children's Hospital of Wisconsin, Milwaukee	67.6	23	4	6	54	2	7	11	4.5	Yes	2.4%
49	Holtz Children's Hosp. at UM-Jackson Memorial Med. Ctr., Miami	67.5	24	5	10	50	5	8	13	2.7	No	3.0%
50	Children's Hospital of Alabama at UAB, Birmingham	67.3	22	6	7	53	3	5	11	3.4	No	4.7%

Terms are explained on Page 178.

DONATE TO CMN HOSPITALS FOR LIFE-SAVING MEDICAL EQUIPMENT

Children's Miracle Network Hospitals

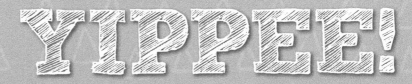

Neurology & Neurosurgery

Rank	Hospital	U.S. News score	Surgical survival score (12=best)	Surgical complications prevention score (22=best)	Epilepsy management score (6=best)	Infection prevention score, overall (40=best)	Surgery volume score (39=best)	Nurse-patient ratio (higher is better)	A Nurse Magnet hospital	% of specialists recommending hospital
1	Boston Children's Hospital	100.0	12	21	6	40	39	4.2	Yes	55.0%
2	Children's Hospital of Philadelphia	98.6	12	21	6	40	34	4.1	Yes	47.5%
3	Texas Children's Hospital, Houston	94.5	12	19	6	39	39	4.1	Yes	31.5%
4	Cincinnati Children's Hospital Medical Center	94.3	12	20	6	40	32	4.3	Yes	27.5%
5	Children's National Medical Center, Washington, D.C.	93.3	12	22	6	39	34	3.8	Yes	19.6%
6	St. Louis Children's Hospital-Washington University	91.9	12	21	6	40	34	3.7	Yes	20.8%
7	Nationwide Children's Hospital, Columbus, Ohio	91.7	12	22	6	39	34	3.3	Yes	16.9%
8	Johns Hopkins Children's Center, Baltimore	89.4	12	19	6	40	31	3.2	Yes	22.7%
9	Children's Hospital Los Angeles	88.4	11	22	6	38	38	3.8	Yes	10.7%
10	Seattle Children's Hospital	87.3	11	20	6	40	29	3.2	Yes	20.7%
11	Ann and Robert H. Lurie Children's Hospital of Chicago	87.0	12	20	6	34	37	3.7	Yes	14.6%
12	Children's Medical Center Dallas	84.9	12	21	6	38	36	3.2	Yes	4.4%
13	Children's Hospital Colorado, Aurora	84.1	11	13	6	39	34	3.1	Yes	19.7%
13	UCSF Benioff Children's Hospitals, San Francisco and Oakland	84.1	12	15	5	39	35	3.9	Yes	14.6%
15	UPMC Children's Hospital of Pittsburgh	83.8	11	18	6	38	27	3.5	Yes	10.3%
16	Nicklaus Children's Hospital, Miami	81.5	12	19	6	36	25	2.9	Yes	8.0%
17	Cohen Children's Medical Center, New Hyde Park, N.Y.	81.1	12	22	6	39	32	3.5	Yes	1.3%
17	Le Bonheur Children's Hospital, Memphis, Tenn.	81.1	12	17	6	40	25	2.7	Yes	5.9%
19	Children's Healthcare of Atlanta	81.0	12	19	5	39	31	4.4	Yes	3.6%
20	Rady Children's Hospital, San Diego	80.9	12	21	6	36	39	2.3	Yes	1.7%
21	NY-Presby. Morgan Stanley-Komansky Children's Hospital, N.Y.	80.7	12	20	6	39	29	3.0	No	7.1%
22	Cleveland Clinic Children's Hospital	80.4	12	22	3	39	24	3.7	Yes	10.2%
23	Children's Mercy Kansas City, Mo.	80.3	12	16	6	40	27	4.2	Yes	2.9%
24	Riley Hospital for Children at IU Health, Indianapolis	79.6	11	17	6	37	35	3.7	Yes	3.1%
25	Lucile Packard Children's Hospital Stanford, Palo Alto, Calif.	79.5	12	21	4	39	31	3.7	No	11.3%
26	C.S. Mott Children's Hospital-Michigan Medicine, Ann Arbor	78.8	12	19	5	40	26	3.6	Yes	6.2%
27	Primary Children's Hospital, Salt Lake City	77.5	12	18	5	37	35	2.9	No	8.3%
28	CHOC Children's Hospital, Orange, Calif.	77.3	12	16	6	39	28	3.8	Yes	2.2%
29	Doernbecher Children's Hospital, Portland, Ore.	77.2	11	20	6	31	24	4.0	Yes	2.1%
30	Children's Hospital of Alabama at UAB, Birmingham	77.0	12	18	6	34	36	3.4	No	6.4%
31	UCLA Mattel Children's Hospital, Los Angeles	76.8	12	16	6	35	14	4.9	Yes	5.9%
32	Mayo Clinic Children's Center, Rochester, Minn.	76.5	12	16	4	37	26	3.8	Yes	7.1%
33	University of Virginia Children's Hospital, Charlottesville	76.1	12	20	6	37	15	2.8	Yes	1.7%
34	Monroe Carell Jr. Children's Hospital at Vanderbilt, Nashville, Tenn.	75.7	11	15	5	39	34	3.4	Yes	4.6%
35	Yale New Haven Children's Hospital, New Haven, Conn.	75.0	12	21	4	38	16	4.4	Yes	1.3%
36	Children's Hospital at Montefiore, New York	74.1	12	21	3	40	25	5.4	No	3.1%
36	Levine Children's Hospital, Charlotte, N.C.	74.1	12	21	5	37	25	3.0	Yes	1.1%
38	Arkansas Children's Hospital, Little Rock	73.9	12	18	6	33	21	3.3	Yes	0.2%
38	Phoenix Children's Hospital	73.9	12	12	6	39	34	3.0	No	3.5%
40	Children's Hospital of Michigan, Detroit	73.4	11	19	6	36	28	3.4	No	0.5%
41	Children's Memorial Hermann Hospital, Houston	73.2	12	18	6	35	26	3.1	Yes	1.1%
42	Akron Children's Hospital, Ohio	73.0	12	15	6	38	23	3.5	Yes	1.6%
42	UF Health Shands Children's Hospital, Gainesville, Fla.	73.0	12	17	6	36	15	2.6	Yes	1.0%
44	Mount Sinai Kravis Children's Hospital, New York	72.2	12	22	4	37	19	3.5	Yes	0.2%
45	Nemours Alfred I. duPont Hosp. for Children, Wilmington, Del.	71.2	12	18	6	35	15	3.4	Yes	0.4%
46	Duke Children's Hospital and Health Center, Durham, N.C.	71.1	12	11	5	40	29	3.3	Yes	4.1%
47	Children's Hospital of Wisconsin, Milwaukee	70.8	12	10	5	35	21	4.5	Yes	3.3%
48	Wolfson Children's Hospital, Jacksonville, Fla.	70.5	12	14	6	34	18	2.3	Yes	0.5%
49	Cook Children's Medical Center, Fort Worth	69.2	10	19	5	32	25	3.4	Yes	2.5%
49	Joseph M. Sanzari Children's Hosp. at Hackensack U. Med. Ctr., N.J.	69.2	12	20	6	36	15	2.5	Yes	0.6%

Terms are explained on Page 178.

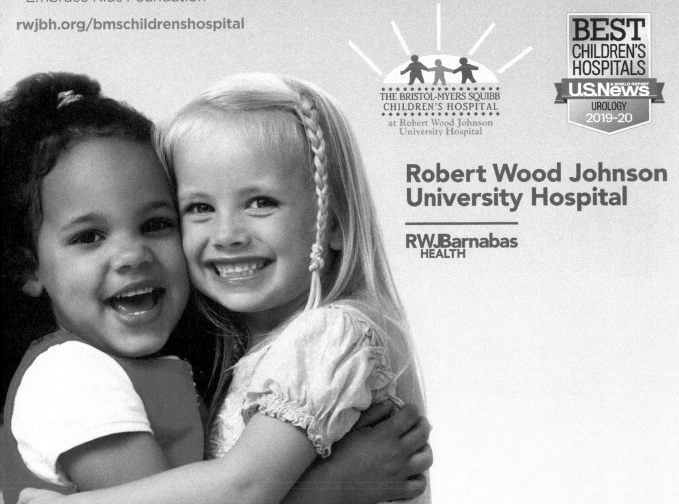

CHANGE KIDS' HEALTH
CHANGE THE FUTURE

More than 10 million kids enter a Children's Miracle Network Hospital every year. To provide the best care for kids, children's hospitals rely on donations and community support, as government and insurance programs do not fully cover the cost of care.

These organizations address the funding gap by providing financial donations through partnerships with Children's Miracle Network Hospitals.® Together, CMN Hospitals and its partners work to save and improve the lives of children at 170 local children's hospitals. Donations remain local to fund charitable care, education, life-saving medical equipment, patient and advancement services.

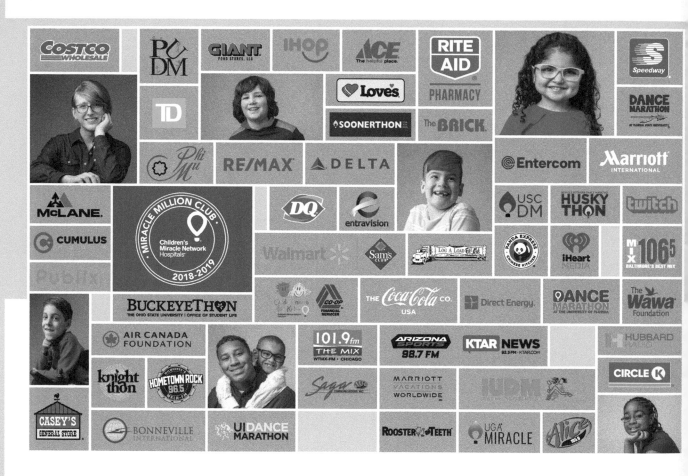

Our Miracle Million Club partners raised more than **$296 million** last year for children's hospitals.

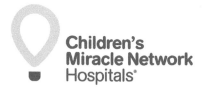

CMNHospitals.org

Panda Express

Thank you *Panda Cares* for 20 years of sharing good fortune with those less fortunate. As the philanthropic arm of Panda Express, *Panda Cares* was created to serve the health and education needs of underserved youth and foster the spirit of giving. Since 2007, Panda has donated more than $59 million to support the physical, spiritual, emotional and mental wellbeing of kids at 134 Children's Miracle Network Hospitals.

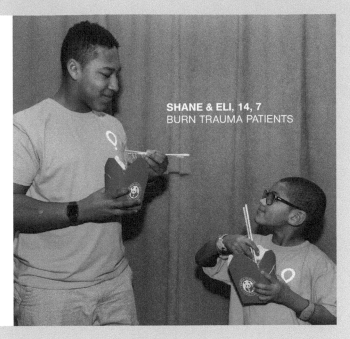

SHANE & ELI, 14, 7
BURN TRAUMA PATIENTS

Changing Kids Health for:

35 YEARS	30 YEARS	25 YEARS	20 YEARS
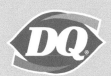	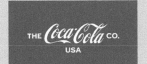	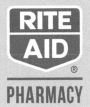	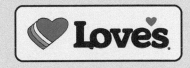

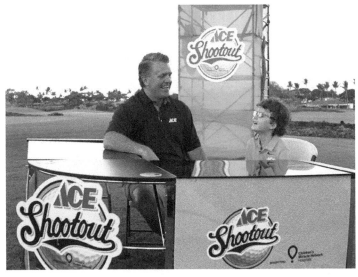

Explore how these companies save and improve the lives of children in local communities.
cmnhospitals.org/toughquestions

Tough Questions

Does your company solve social problems? Kids ask executives Tough Questions.

Orthopedics

Rank	Hospital	U.S. News score	Fracture repair score (7=best)	Surgical complications prevention score (12=best)	Infection prevention score, overall (37=best)	Patient volume score (21=best)	Procedure volume score (23=best)	Nurse-patient ratio (higher is better)	A Nurse Magnet hospital	No. of best practices (69=best)	% of specialists recommending hospital
1	Boston Children's Hospital	100.0	7	12	37	21	23	4.2	Yes	69	55.4%
2	Children's Medical Ctr. Dallas-Texas Scottish Rite Hosp. for Children	96.2	7	12	35	21	23	3.2	Yes	69	46.9%
3	Children's Hospital of Philadelphia	95.4	6	12	37	21	22	4.1	Yes	69	49.4%
4	Cincinnati Children's Hospital Medical Center	93.1	7	12	37	19	21	4.3	Yes	69	23.8%
5	Children's Hospital Los Angeles	90.9	7	12	35	21	20	3.8	Yes	69	19.6%
6	Children's Healthcare of Atlanta	86.0	7	11	36	21	22	4.4	Yes	66	11.5%
7	Rady Children's Hospital, San Diego	85.9	7	9	34	20	18	2.3	Yes	68	40.2%
8	UC Davis Children's Hospital/Shriners Hospitals N. Calif., Sacramento	84.5	7	12	37	21	21	6.9	Yes	65	7.7%
9	Nationwide Children's Hospital, Columbus, Ohio	83.8	7	12	36	20	21	3.3	Yes	65	7.2%
10	Texas Children's Hospital, Houston	82.7	7	10	36	21	22	4.1	Yes	69	7.6%
11	Rainbow Babies and Children's Hospital, Cleveland	82.6	7	12	37	20	22	2.8	Yes	67	7.5%
12	St. Louis Children's Hospital-Washington University/Shriners Hospital	82.3	7	10	37	17	23	3.7	Yes	67	9.8%
13	Children's Mercy Kansas City, Mo.	81.9	7	11	37	21	21	4.2	Yes	69	4.8%
14	Nemours Alfred I. duPont Hosp. for Children, Wilmington, Del.	81.0	7	9	33	21	20	3.4	Yes	68	19.0%
15	Le Bonheur Children's Hospital, Memphis, Tenn.	80.8	7	12	37	17	17	2.7	Yes	68	4.8%
16	Children's National Medical Center, Washington, D.C.	80.5	6	12	36	20	19	3.8	Yes	69	6.1%
17	Seattle Children's Hospital	80.0	7	10	37	18	20	3.2	Yes	65	10.8%
18	UCLA Mattel Children's Hospital, Los Angeles	79.8	7	12	32	18	17	4.9	Yes	68	3.2%
19	Johns Hopkins Children's Center, Baltimore	78.9	7	10	37	13	19	3.2	Yes	69	6.6%
20	Children's Hospital Colorado, Aurora	78.1	6	10	36	19	20	3.1	Yes	59	14.4%
21	C.S. Mott Children's Hospital-Michigan Medicine, Ann Arbor	78.0	7	11	37	14	13	3.6	Yes	65	3.4%
22	Lerner Children's Pavilion-Hospital for Special Surgery, New York	76.9	6	12	37	14	20	4.1	Yes	69	4.2%
23	North Carolina Children's Hospital at UNC, Chapel Hill	76.8	7	12	37	10	15	5.0	Yes	65	0.8%
24	Mayo Clinic Children's Center, Rochester, Minn.	76.7	7	12	35	7	14	3.8	Yes	67	3.5%
25	UCSF Benioff Children's Hospitals, San Francisco and Oakland	76.6	7	11	36	16	11	3.9	Yes	63	3.0%
26	Monroe Carell Jr. Children's Hospital at Vanderbilt, Nashville, Tenn.	75.8	7	9	36	16	19	3.4	Yes	67	6.1%
27	Ann and Robert H. Lurie Children's Hospital of Chicago	75.6	7	12	32	13	20	3.7	Yes	58	4.9%
28	NY-Presby. Morgan Stanley-Komansky Children's Hospital, N.Y.	74.4	7	12	36	11	13	3.0	No	57	6.1%
29	University of Iowa Stead Family Children's Hospital, Iowa City	74.2	7	12	32	19	13	3.6	Yes	60	2.2%
30	Children's Hospital at Montefiore, New York	74.0	7	12	37	13	11	5.4	No	67	0.9%
31	Lucile Packard Children's Hospital Stanford, Palo Alto, Calif.	73.6	7	11	36	10	16	3.7	No	65	3.4%
32	Cohen Children's Medical Center, New Hyde Park, N.Y.	73.0	6	12	36	16	16	3.5	Yes	69	0.6%
33	Joe DiMaggio Children's Hospital at Memorial, Hollywood, Fla.	71.7	7	12	35	18	22	3.2	No	68	1.6%
33	Valley Children's Healthcare and Hospital, Madera, Calif.	71.7	7	12	36	17	16	3.1	Yes	65	0.5%
35	Levine Children's Hospital, Charlotte, N.C.	71.1	7	11	34	13	13	3.0	Yes	61	1.7%
36	Nicklaus Children's Hospital, Miami	70.9	7	11	33	12	11	2.9	Yes	62	2.6%
37	Primary Children's Hosp.-Shriners Hosps. for Children, Salt Lake City	70.8	7	9	35	20	20	2.9	No	55	8.7%
38	Cook Children's Medical Center, Fort Worth	68.4	7	12	29	16	12	3.4	Yes	61	0.4%
39	Phoenix Children's Hospital	68.2	7	9	36	15	22	3.0	No	66	1.3%
40	Arnold Palmer Hospital for Children, Orlando	68.0	6	12	32	15	9	3.2	Yes	62	3.5%
40	MUSC Health-Children's Hospital, Charleston, S.C.	68.0	7	12	35	9	7	3.0	A	57	0.6%
40	Riley Hospital for Children at IU Health, Indianapolis	68.0	6	10	34	13	16	3.7	Yes	64	1.7%
43	Duke Children's Hospital and Health Center, Durham, N.C.	65.0	6	10	37	9	15	3.3	Yes	67	1.1%
44	Children's Hospital of Wisconsin, Milwaukee	64.5	5	10	32	14	14	4.5	Yes	66	1.0%
45	UPMC Children's Hospital of Pittsburgh	64.4	7	6	36	18	16	3.5	Yes	58	1.0%
46	Children's Hospital of Michigan, Detroit	64.2	6	10	34	19	14	3.4	No	69	0.4%
47	Akron Children's Hospital, Ohio	63.0	6	8	35	15	12	3.5	Yes	62	3.1%
48	Arkansas Children's Hospital, Little Rock	62.9	7	10	31	11	8	3.3	Yes	57	0.5%
48	Children's Hospital and Medical Center, Omaha	62.9	7	8	36	12	10	4.0	Yes	61	1.2%
50	Doernbecher Children's Hosp. at Oregon Hlth. & Science U., Portland	62.2	6	12	28	7	9	4.0	Yes	51	0.1%

Terms are explained on Page 178.

Pulmonology & Lung Surgery

Rank	Hospital	U.S. News score	Asthma inpatient care score (5=best)	Lung transplant survival score (5=best)	Cystic fibrosis management score (16=best)	Infection prevention score, overall (49=best)	Infection prevention score, ICU (5=best)	Patient volume score (17=best)	Nurse-patient ratio (higher is better)	A Nurse Magnet hospital	% of specialists recommending hospital
1	Texas Children's Hospital, Houston	100.0	5	5	13	47	4	17	4.1	Yes	39.9%
2	Children's Hospital of Philadelphia	98.2	5	5	14	49	2	17	4.1	Yes	56.3%
3	Boston Children's Hospital	92.4	5	2	12	49	2	16	4.2	Yes	49.0%
4	Cincinnati Children's Hospital Medical Center	89.2	4	2	13	47	2	16	4.3	Yes	51.4%
5	St. Louis Children's Hospital-Washington University	83.7	4	4	13	46	3	11	3.7	Yes	17.2%
6	UPMC Children's Hospital of Pittsburgh	82.9	3	5	13	45	3	15	3.5	Yes	21.1%
7	Children's Hospital Colorado, Aurora	82.8	4	NA	12	47	2	14	3.1	Yes	46.9%
8	Lucile Packard Children's Hospital Stanford, Palo Alto, Calif.	82.7	5	5	12	47	3	17	3.7	No	14.0%
9	Children's National Medical Center, Washington, D.C.	80.3	5	NA	13	48	5	14	3.8	Yes	6.7%
10	Nationwide Children's Hospital, Columbus, Ohio	80.1	5	0	14	48	2	16	3.3	Yes	20.3%
11	Johns Hopkins Children's Center, Baltimore	79.4	4	NR	13	49	4	15	3.2	Yes	18.4%
12	Seattle Children's Hospital	78.4	5	NA	13	48	2	12	3.2	Yes	31.9%
13	Children's Hospital Los Angeles	76.2	5	NA	10	47	4	14	3.8	Yes	13.7%
14	Rainbow Babies and Children's Hospital, Cleveland	75.9	5	NR	13	48	4	11	2.8	Yes	11.7%
15	Monroe Carell Jr. Children's Hospital at Vanderbilt, Nashville, Tenn.	75.7	5	NR	13	46	4	12	3.4	Yes	10.3%
16	North Carolina Children's Hospital at UNC, Chapel Hill	74.9	4	3	11	47	2	12	5.0	Yes	18.4%
17	Riley Hospital for Children at IU Health, Indianapolis	74.1	4	1	12	45	3	13	3.7	Yes	18.0%
18	Ann and Robert H. Lurie Children's Hospital of Chicago	71.8	4	NA	14	42	4	11	3.7	Yes	9.2%
19	Children's Healthcare of Atlanta	71.7	5	0	12	44	4	15	4.4	Yes	2.2%
20	NY-Presby. Morgan Stanley-Komansky Children's Hospital, N.Y.	68.9	4	5	12	42	2	15	3.0	No	5.3%
21	Rady Children's Hospital, San Diego	68.7	5	NA	14	45	4	10	2.3	Yes	3.4%
22	UF Health Shands Children's Hospital, Gainesville, Fla.	67.8	5	3	10	45	4	12	2.6	Yes	0.3%
23	Le Bonheur Children's Hospital, Memphis, Tenn.	67.3	5	NA	11	47	4	10	2.7	Yes	3.9%
24	MassGeneral Hospital for Children, Boston	67.1	5	NA	11	43	5	7	2.8	Yes	2.9%
25	C.S. Mott Children's Hospital-Michigan Medicine, Ann Arbor	66.0	4	NA	13	48	3	11	3.6	Yes	3.2%
26	Yale New Haven Children's Hospital, New Haven, Conn.	65.9	5	NA	14	47	4	9	4.4	Yes	2.2%
27	CHOC Children's Hospital, Orange, Calif.	65.8	5	NA	11	48	5	12	3.8	Yes	1.3%
27	Children's Mercy Kansas City, Mo.	65.8	5	NA	10	48	2	11	4.2	Yes	2.7%
29	UCSF Benioff Children's Hospitals, San Francisco and Oakland	65.5	4	NA	10	46	4	8	3.9	Yes	3.9%
30	Cohen Children's Medical Center, New Hyde Park, N.Y.	65.2	5	NA	12	47	4	9	3.5	Yes	0.7%
31	University of Minnesota Masonic Children's Hospital, Minneapolis	65.1	5	5	13	41	2	8	3.0	No	0.3%
32	Children's Medical Center Dallas	65.0	5	NA	13	45	4	14	3.2	Yes	2.0%
33	NYU Winthrop Hospital Children's Medical Center, Mineola, N.Y.	64.3	4	NA	14	47	5	7	4.5	Yes	0.6%
34	Children's Hospital of Wisconsin, Milwaukee	64.0	4	NA	15	38	2	13	4.5	Yes	1.9%
35	Children's Hospital of Alabama at UAB, Birmingham	63.4	5	NA	14	37	3	14	3.4	No	7.3%
36	Duke Children's Hospital and Health Center, Durham, N.C.	63.1	4	0	12	49	4	8	3.3	Yes	1.9%
37	Akron Children's Hospital, Ohio	62.9	5	NA	14	40	4	7	3.5	Yes	1.3%
38	Children's Minnesota, Minneapolis	62.1	4	NA	13	41	4	13	3.3	Yes	1.7%
39	Dayton Children's Hospital, Ohio	62.0	5	NA	11	46	5	10	3.5	Yes	1.2%
40	Phoenix Children's Hospital	61.7	5	NA	13	44	4	13	3.0	No	1.0%
41	Doernbecher Children's Hosp. at Oregon Hlth. & Science U., Portland	61.6	5	NA	13	39	4	8	4.0	Yes	1.3%
42	Nicklaus Children's Hospital, Miami	61.4	4	NA	14	44	4	9	2.9	Yes	0.8%
43	Cleveland Clinic Children's Hospital	60.5	3	NA	15	43	2	11	3.7	Yes	2.0%
44	Johns Hopkins All Children's Hospital, St. Petersburg, Fla.	59.7	5	NA	14	48	3	9	3.6	No	0.7%
45	Arkansas Children's Hospital, Little Rock	58.8	5	NA	12	39	4	8	3.3	Yes	1.2%
45	UCLA Mattel Children's Hospital, Los Angeles	58.8	4	NA	10	44	4	6	4.9	Yes	2.9%
47	Arnold Palmer Hospital for Children, Orlando	58.7	5	NA	13	44	5	7	3.2	Yes	0.9%
47	Mount Sinai Kravis Children's Hospital, New York	58.7	5	NA	12	46	3	5	3.5	Yes	0.7%
49	University of Virginia Children's Hospital, Charlottesville	58.1	5	3	14	43	1	6	2.8	Yes	0.6%
50	Children's Hospital and Medical Center, Omaha	57.8	4	NA	11	48	1	10	4.0	Yes	0.4%

NA=not applicable. NR=not reported. Terms are explained on Page 178.

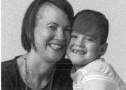
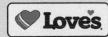

Urology

Rank	Hospital	U.S. News score	Surgical complications prevention score (15=best)	Testicular torsion care score (2=best)	Infection prevention score, overall (31=best)	Patient volume score (30=best)	Surgery volume score (20=best)	Minimally invasive volume score (9=best)	Nurse-patient ratio (higher is better)	A Nurse Magnet hospital	% of specialists recommending hospital
1	Boston Children's Hospital	100.0	14	2	31	30	20	9	4.2	Yes	67.2%
2	Children's Hospital of Philadelphia	96.5	12	2	31	30	20	9	4.1	Yes	70.0%
3	Riley Hospital for Children at IU Health, Indianapolis	92.4	13	2	28	27	18	9	3.7	Yes	45.7%
4	Cincinnati Children's Hospital Medical Center	92.1	12	2	31	27	17	8	4.3	Yes	45.3%
5	Ann and Robert H. Lurie Children's Hospital of Chicago	90.8	13	2	26	28	16	9	3.7	Yes	43.7%
6	Texas Children's Hospital, Houston	90.7	12	2	30	30	19	9	4.1	Yes	35.7%
7	Monroe Carell Jr. Children's Hospital at Vanderbilt, Nashville, Tenn.	90.1	13	2	30	28	18	8	3.4	Yes	34.8%
8	Johns Hopkins Children's Center, Baltimore	89.5	15	2	31	21	15	8	3.2	Yes	17.8%
9	Nationwide Children's Hospital, Columbus, Ohio	84.0	11	2	30	27	19	9	3.3	Yes	23.3%
10	Children's Healthcare of Atlanta	83.9	13	2	30	29	20	9	4.4	Yes	9.3%
10	UPMC Children's Hospital of Pittsburgh	83.9	13	2	30	24	16	9	3.5	Yes	11.5%
12	Children's Medical Center Dallas	83.4	13	2	29	26	15	9	3.2	Yes	15.4%
13	Children's Hospital Los Angeles	83.3	13	2	29	27	19	9	3.8	Yes	14.3%
14	Children's Hospital Colorado, Aurora	81.6	12	2	30	27	17	8	3.1	Yes	11.6%
15	Seattle Children's Hospital	80.1	9	2	31	22	18	8	3.2	Yes	35.3%
16	Yale-New Haven/Connecticut Children's Medical Ctrs., New Haven	79.0	14	2	29	20	15	8	4.4	Yes	3.9%
17	Children's Mercy Kansas City, Mo.	78.5	13	2	31	24	20	8	4.2	Yes	1.7%
18	C.S. Mott Children's Hospital-Michigan Medicine, Ann Arbor	77.8	13	2	31	20	14	7	3.6	Yes	4.3%
19	Children's National Medical Center, Washington, D.C.	77.7	9	2	30	26	18	8	3.8	Yes	14.9%
20	UC Davis Children's Hospital/Shriners Hospitals N. Calif., Sacramento	77.2	15	2	31	20	12	7	6.9	Yes	1.4%
21	Rady Children's Hospital, San Diego	76.8	13	2	28	23	12	8	2.3	Yes	7.9%
22	St. Louis Children's Hospital-Washington University	75.6	12	2	31	22	14	7	3.7	Yes	3.1%
23	UCSF Benioff Children's Hospitals, San Francisco and Oakland	74.0	9	2	30	26	16	8	3.9	Yes	8.0%
24	Cleveland Clinic Children's Hospital	73.3	13	2	30	14	10	7	3.7	Yes	0.8%
24	Le Bonheur Children's Hospital, Memphis, Tenn.	73.3	13	2	31	15	16	7	2.7	Yes	4.2%
26	CHOC Children's Hospital, Orange, Calif.	70.6	10	2	30	22	15	7	3.8	Yes	5.0%
26	Duke Children's Hospital and Health Center, Durham, N.C.	70.6	11	2	31	24	13	5	3.3	Yes	5.9%
26	University of Iowa Stead Family Children's Hospital, Iowa City	70.6	12	2	26	22	14	7	3.6	Yes	2.9%
29	UCLA Mattel Children's Hospital, Los Angeles	70.1	12	2	26	13	8	3	4.9	Yes	3.8%
30	West Virginia U. Children's Hospital, Morgantown	69.9	14	2	28	13	11	6	3.4	Yes	0.5%
31	Akron Children's Hospital, Ohio	69.8	13	2	29	20	12	7	3.5	Yes	2.3%
32	Children's Hospital of Wisconsin, Milwaukee	69.5	10	2	26	23	18	9	4.5	Yes	2.2%
32	Rainbow Babies and Children's Hospital, Cleveland	69.5	13	2	31	10	8	3	2.8	Yes	2.1%
34	Children's Hospital of Michigan, Detroit	69.1	13	2	28	15	13	5	3.4	No	2.0%
35	Norton Children's Hospital, Louisville, Ky.	68.6	13	2	31	23	11	5	3.2	No	0.2%
36	Mayo Clinic Children's Center, Rochester, Minn.	68.3	9	2	29	26	11	5	3.8	Yes	8.6%
37	North Carolina Children's Hospital at UNC, Chapel Hill	67.8	10	2	31	15	13	5	5.0	Yes	1.4%
38	Bristol-Myers Squibb Children's Hosp., New Brunswick, N.J.	67.3	15	2	26	11	8	3	2.6	Yes	0.2%
39	Cohen Children's Medical Center, New Hyde Park, N.Y.	66.7	12	1	30	23	12	8	3.5	Yes	4.8%
39	Spectrum Hlth. Helen DeVos Children's Hosp., Grand Rapids, Mich.	66.7	13	2	25	17	12	7	2.4	Yes	0.6%
41	Phoenix Children's Hospital	66.0	10	2	30	29	17	9	3.0	No	1.9%
42	Primary Children's Hospital, Salt Lake City	65.9	9	2	29	29	18	8	2.9	No	5.9%
43	Valley Children's Healthcare and Hospital, Madera, Calif.	65.4	12	2	30	16	15	7	3.1	Yes	1.4%
44	MassGeneral Hospital for Children, Boston	65.3	12	2	25	13	8	3	2.8	Yes	1.3%
45	Nicklaus Children's Hospital, Miami	65.2	10	2	27	15	13	8	2.9	Yes	3.6%
46	NYU Winthrop Hospital Children's Medical Center, Mineola, N.Y.	65.1	15	2	29	8	6	2	4.5	Yes	0.9%
47	University of Virginia Children's Hospital, Charlottesville	64.9	11	2	28	10	9	4	2.8	Yes	2.7%
48	Children's Hospital at Montefiore, New York	64.7	12	2	31	15	7	3	5.4	No	0.0%
49	Lucile Packard Children's Hospital Stanford, Palo Alto, Calif.	63.3	7	2	30	24	12	6	3.7	No	5.0%
50	NY-Presby. Morgan Stanley-Komansky Children's Hospital, N.Y.	63.2	10	2	30	15	17	5	3.0	No	2.6%

Terms are explained on Page 178.

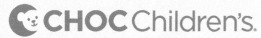
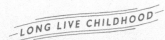

CHOC Children's.

LONG LIVE CHILDHOOD

WORLD-CLASS CARE DEDICATED TO PRESERVING THE MAGIC OF CHILDHOOD

- Leading destination for 2nd opinions

- Phase 1 clinical trials as a member of the Children's Oncology Group

- Trained 57 urology fellows from 12 different countries

- Level 4 Epilepsy Center

- Pioneered third ventriculostomy for hydrocephalus

- A robust urology research program that includes a dedicated clinical epidemiologist

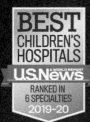

BEST CHILDREN'S HOSPITALS
U.S.News & WORLD REPORT
RANKED IN 6 SPECIALTIES 2019-20

CHOC.ORG

Thanks to our patients, physicians, nurses & staff for making us

#16 IN THE NATION

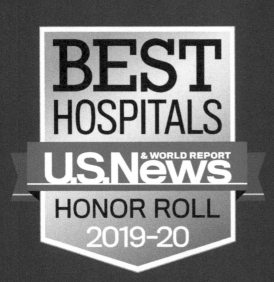

CHAPTER 6

Best Regional Hospitals

BEST REGIONAL HOSPITALS
U.S.News & WORLD REPORT
2019-20

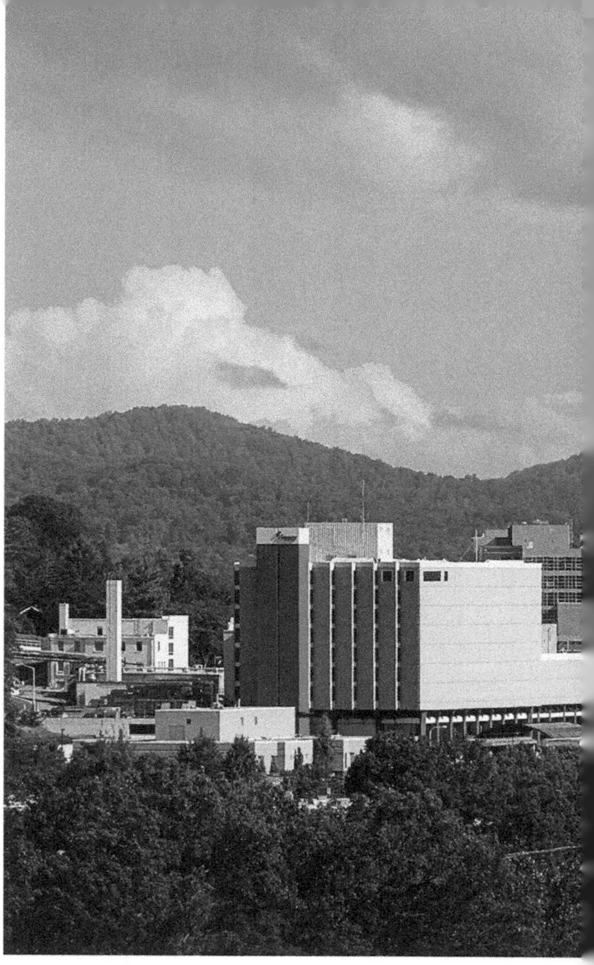

Great Care Near Home

How we identified and ranked the top hospitals state by state

by **Ben Harder**

IF YOU'RE LIKE MOST PEOPLE facing hospitalization, you would much prefer to stay close to home. You'll feel more comfortable, and lower stress can lead to faster recovery. Your family can visit without racking up hotel bills. And a battle with your health insurer over coverage at an out-of-network facility might be avoidable.

Since 2011, our Best Regional Hospitals listings have showcased hundreds of facilities around the U.S. that offer high-quality care across a range of clinical services. These services include both complex, highly specialized care for the sickest patients – the focus of the Best Hospitals specialty rankings (Page 117) – and safe, effective treatment for those whose medical needs are more commonplace, such as patients seeking hip or knee replacement surgery for age-related arthritis. Found in their entirety at usnews.com/bestregionalhospitals, the Best Regional Hospitals rankings offer readers in most parts of the country a number of high-quality choices near home.

These evaluations include ratings of how well hospitals handle nine relatively common procedures and conditions in addition to their assessments in 12 specialties.* The nine areas of care are heart bypass surgery, aortic valve surgery, abdominal aortic aneurysm repair, heart failure, hip replacement, knee replacement, colon cancer surgery, lung cancer surgery and chronic obstructive pulmonary disease. Hospitals are assigned a rating of "high performing," "average" or "below average" in each area in which they treated enough patients to be evaluated.

Recognition as a 2019-20 Best Regional Hospital means a hospital was nationally ranked in at least one of the 12 Best Hospitals specialties that use objective data, or that it earned at least three "high

---

*Cancer; cardiology & heart surgery; diabetes & endocrinology; ear, nose & throat; gastroenterology & GI surgery; geriatrics; gynecology; nephrology; neurology & neurosurgery; orthopedics; pulmonology & lung surgery; and urology.

performing" ratings across the nine procedures and conditions. (An FAQ at usnews.com/best-hospitals offers more details.)

This year, 569 hospitals merited Best Regional Hospitals status. They appear ranked by state on the following pages. Hospitals are numerically ordered according to the following rules:

1. The higher rank went to the hospital with the better status in the Best Hospitals Honor Roll ranking (Page 112), if any.

2. Next, the higher rank went to the hospital that earned more points according to the following three rules: (a) A hospital received two points for each of the 12 specialties in which it was ranked among the top 50. (b) A hospital received one point for each specialty, procedure or condition in which it was rated high performing. (c) A hospital lost one point for each procedure or condition in which it was rated below average.

Based on the same rules, hospitals in major met-

USNEWS.COM/BESTHOSPITALS

Visit usnews.com regularly while researching your health care choices, as U.S. News often adds content aimed at helping patients and families make decisions about their medical care. We also update the Best Hospitals, Best Children's Hospitals and Best Regional Hospitals data on the website when new data become available.

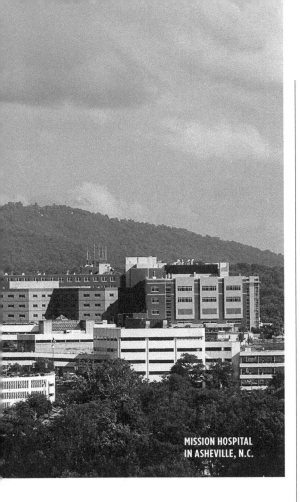

MISSION HOSPITAL
IN ASHEVILLE, N.C.

Tops at Routine Care

U.S. NEWS EVALUATED more than 4,500 hospitals for their handling of two chronic conditions – chronic obstructive pulmonary disease and heart failure – and seven surgical procedures: colon cancer surgery, lung cancer surgery, heart bypass surgery, aortic valve surgery, abdominal aortic aneurysm repair, knee replacement and hip replacement. Nearly a third of those hospitals earned at least one top rating of "high performing." But only these 57 standouts, barely 1 percent of the hospitals evaluated, got the top rating in all nine procedures and conditions:

- **Abbott Northwestern Hospital,** Minneapolis
- **AdventHealth Orlando,** Fla.
- **Aurora St. Luke's Medical Center,** Milwaukee
- **Banner Boswell Medical Center,** Sun City, Ariz.
- **Barnes-Jewish Hospital,** St. Louis
- **Bronson Methodist Hospital,** Kalamazoo, Mich.
- **Cedars-Sinai Medical Center,** Los Angeles
- **Christ Hospital,** Cincinnati
- **Christiana Care Hospitals,** Newark, Del.
- **Cleveland Clinic**
- **Cleveland Clinic Florida,** Weston
- **Duke University Hospital,** Durham, N.C.
- **Emory St. Joseph's Hospital,** Atlanta
- **Emory University Hospital,** Atlanta
- **Fairview Southdale Hospital,** Edina, Minn.
- **Hackensack University Medical Center,** N.J.
- **Hoag Memorial Hospital Presbyterian,** Newport Beach, Calif.
- **Houston Methodist Hospital**
- **John Muir Health-Concord Medical Center,** Concord, Calif.
- **Maine Medical Center,** Portland
- **Massachusetts General Hospital,** Boston
- **Mayo Clinic,** Rochester, Minn.
- **Mayo Clinic-Jacksonville,** Fla.
- **Mayo Clinic-Phoenix**
- **Mission Hospital,** Asheville, N.C.
- **Morristown Medical Center,** N.J.
- **Morton Plant Hospital,** Clearwater, Fla.
- **Munson Medical Center,** Traverse City, Mich.
- **New York-Presbyterian Hospital-Columbia and Cornell,** New York
- **North Shore University Hospital,** Manhasset, N.Y.
- **NorthShore University HealthSystem-Metro Chicago,** Evanston, Ill.
- **Northwestern Medicine Central DuPage Hospital,** Winfield, Ill.
- **Northwestern Memorial Hospital,** Chicago
- **NYU Langone Hospitals,** New York
- **Piedmont Atlanta Hospital**
- **Providence St. Vincent Medical Center,** Portland, Ore.
- **Regions Hospital,** St. Paul, Minn.
- **Sanford USD Medical Center,** Sioux Falls, S.D.
- **Sarasota Memorial Hospital,** Fla.
- **Scripps La Jolla Hospitals,** La Jolla, Calif.
- **Spectrum Health-Butterworth and Blodgett Campuses,** Grand Rapids, Mich.
- **St. Cloud Hospital,** St. Cloud, Minn.
- **St. Luke's Regional Medical Center,** Boise, Idaho
- **St. Luke's University Hospital-Bethlehem Campus,** Pa.
- **Stanford Health Care-Stanford Hospital,** Palo Alto, Calif.
- **Sutter Medical Center,** Sacramento, Calif.
- **Torrance Memorial Medical Center,** Torrance, Calif.
- **UC San Diego Health-Jacobs Medical Center**
- **UNC Rex,** Raleigh, N.C.
- **United Hospital,** St. Paul, Minn.
- **University of Maryland St. Joseph Medical Center,** Towson
- **University of Michigan Hospitals-Michigan Medicine,** Ann Arbor
- **University of Virginia Medical Center,** Charlottesville
- **University of Wisconsin Hospitals,** Madison
- **UPMC Presbyterian Shadyside,** Pittsburgh
- **Vanderbilt University Medical Center,** Nashville
- **Yale New Haven Hospital,** Conn.

ropolitan areas also received rankings that compare them to other top hospitals in the same metropolis. Our website displays these rankings for 89 metro areas with at least 500,000 residents. The website also lists top hospitals in more than 100 U.S. News-defined regions, such as Southern Indiana and Texas' Hill Country, to help consumers outside the biggest urban centers searching for high-quality care.

Our goal with the state and metro area rankings is to identify general medical-surgical hospitals that offer both high-quality care and breadth of care, so only hospitals that deliver a wide range of clinical services for adult patients were considered for Best Regional Hospitals status. Consequently, specialty hospitals such as dedicated cancer centers, surgical hospitals and children's hospitals were not considered in the regional rankings. Also, how a hospital performed in pediatric care and in four adult specialties – ophthalmology, psychiatry, rehabilitation and rheumatology – did not factor into the regional rankings.

That these specialties are important is undeniable. But pediatric hospital care is such a distinct domain of medicine, and so few hospitals specialize in it, that we've chosen to rank Best Children's Hospitals separately. And in the four adult specialties, objective data on which to compare performance are either not available or do not meet our analytical standards.

When choosing a hospital, you'll want to consult with your physician or other health professional and combine your research with ours to find the best possible care. ●

COMPLEX SPECIALTY CARE
- ● Nationally ranked
- ● High performing

COMMON PROCEDURES & CONDITIONS
- ● High performing
- ● Average
- ● Below average

COMPLEX SPECIALTY CARE   **COMMON PROCEDURES & CONDITIONS**

Columns (Complex Specialty Care): CANCER · CARDIOLOGY & HEART SURGERY · DIABETES & ENDOCRINOLOGY · EAR, NOSE & THROAT · GASTROENTEROLOGY & GI SURGERY · GERIATRICS · GYNECOLOGY · NEPHROLOGY · NEUROLOGY & NEUROSURGERY · ORTHOPEDICS · PULMONOLOGY · UROLOGY

Columns (Common Procedures & Conditions): COLON CANCER SURGERY · LUNG CANCER SURGERY · HEART BYPASS SURGERY · HEART FAILURE · HEART VALVE SURGERY · ABDOMINAL AORTIC ANEURYSM · HIP REPLACEMENT · KNEE REPLACEMENT · COPD

State Rank — Hospital

ALABAMA
Rank	Hospital
1	University of Alabama at Birmingham Hospital, Birmingham
2	Huntsville Hospital
3	Princeton Baptist Medical Center, Birmingham
3	St. Vincent's Birmingham Hospital
5	Mobile Infirmary Medical Center, Mobile

ARIZONA
Rank	Hospital
1	Mayo Clinic-Phoenix
2	Banner Boswell Medical Center, Sun City
2	Banner University Medical Center Phoenix
2	Flagstaff Medical Center
5	Chandler Regional Medical Center, Chandler
5	St. Joseph's Hospital and Medical Center, Phoenix
7	TMC Healthcare-Tucson
8	Banner Del E. Webb Medical Center, Sun City West
8	Mercy Gilbert Medical Center, Gilbert
10	Banner Baywood Medical Center, Mesa
10	Banner Desert Medical Center, Mesa
10	HonorHealth Scottsdale Shea Medical Center, Scottsdale
10	Oro Valley Hospital, Oro Valley
14	Northwest Medical Center, Tucson
15	Yuma Regional Medical Center

ARKANSAS
Rank	Hospital
1	UAMS Medical Center, Little Rock
2	CHI St. Vincent Infirmary, Little Rock
2	Washington Regional Medical Center, Fayetteville
4	Mercy Hospital Fort Smith, Fort Smith
5	Mercy Hospital Rogers, Rogers

CALIFORNIA
Rank	Hospital
1	UCLA Medical Center, Los Angeles[1]
2	UCSF Medical Center, San Francisco
3	Cedars-Sinai Medical Center, Los Angeles
4	Stanford Health Care-Stanford Hospital, Palo Alto
5	Keck Hospital of USC, Los Angeles[2]
6	UC Davis Medical Center, Sacramento
7	Scripps La Jolla Hospitals, La Jolla
8	Hoag Memorial Hospital Presbyterian, Newport Beach[3]
8	UC San Diego Health-Jacobs Medical Center[4]
10	Huntington Memorial Hospital, Pasadena
10	UC Irvine Medical Center, Orange
12	Torrance Memorial Medical Center, Torrance
13	John Muir Health-Walnut Creek Medical Center, Walnut Creek
13	Mission Hospital, Mission Viejo
15	John Muir Health-Concord Medical Center, Concord
15	MemorialCare Long Beach Memorial Medical Center, Long Beach

In complex care specialties, (-) indicates hospital is not nationally ranked or high performing.
In procedures and conditions, (-) indicates care not offered or hospital has too few Medicare patients to be rated.

A footnote indicates that another hospital's results are included, that the hospital has a different name in one or more areas of care, or both.
[1] Santa Monica-UCLA Medical Center and Orthopedic Hospital. [2] USC Norris Cancer Hospital-Keck Medical Center of USC. [3] Hoag Orthopedic Institute.
[4] UC San Diego Health-Moores Cancer Center; UC San Diego Health-Sulpizio Cardiovascular Center.

More @ usnews.com/bestregionalhospitals

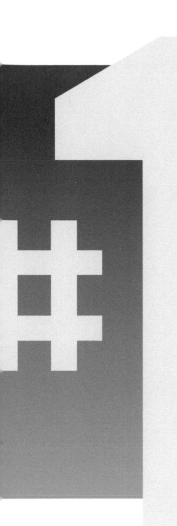

UCLA Health ranked #1 in California

#6 in the Nation

U.S. News & World Report

Putting U first keeps us first

At UCLA Health, we're proud to be ranked #1. According to *U.S. News & World Report's* annual best hospital rankings, UCLA Health is #1 in Los Angeles and #1 in California. We also happen to be #6 in the nation — we know this comes from putting patients first, with a culture that always strives to make healthcare the best it can be. With four hospitals and over 180 neighborhood locations, everything we do...begins with U.

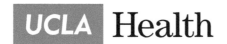 it begins with U

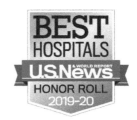

1-800-UCLA-MD1 or visit uclahealth.org

LAW/USN

COMPLEX SPECIALTY CARE
- ● Nationally ranked
- ● High performing

COMMON PROCEDURES & CONDITIONS
- ● High performing
- ● Average
- ● Below average

State Rank / Hospital	Cancer	Cardiology & Heart Surgery	Diabetes & Endocrinology	Ear, Nose & Throat	Gastroenterology & GI Surgery	Geriatrics	Gynecology	Nephrology	Neurology & Neurosurgery	Orthopedics	Pulmonology	Urology	Colon Cancer Surgery	Lung Cancer Surgery	Heart Bypass Surgery	Heart Failure	Heart Valve Surgery	Abdominal Aortic Aneurysm	Hip Replacement	Knee Replacement	COPD
CALIFORNIA (CONTINUED)																					
17 **Adventist Health-Glendale**, Los Angeles	–	–	●	–	●	●	–	●	●	●	–	●	●	●	●	●	●	●	●	●	●
18 **California Pacific Medical Center**, San Francisco	●	–	–	–	●	●	●	●	–	●	–	●	●	●	●	●	●	●	●	●	●
18 **Providence Tarzana Medical Center**, Tarzana	–	–	●	–	●	●	–	●	●	●	–	●	●	●	●	●	●	●	●	●	●
18 **Sutter Medical Center**, Sacramento	–	–	–	–	–	●	●	●	–	●	–	●	●	●	●	●	●	●	●	●	●
21 **Eisenhower Medical Center**, Rancho Mirage	–	–	–	–	●	●	–	●	●	●	–	●	●	●	●	●	●	●	●	●	●
22 **Loma Linda University Medical Center**	–	–	–	–	●	●	●	–	●	–	–	●	●	●	●	●	●	●	●	●	●
22 **MemorialCare Saddleback Memorial Medical Center**, Laguna Hills	–	–	–	–	●	●	–	●	–	●	–	●	●	●	●	●	●	●	●	●	●
22 **St. Jude Medical Center**, Fullerton	–	–	–	–	–	●	–	●	●	●	–	●	●	●	●	●	●	●	●	●	●
25 **El Camino Hospital**, Mountain View	–	–	–	–	–	–	–	●	–	●	–	●	●	●	●	●	●	●	●	●	●
25 **PIH Health Hospital-Whittier**	–	–	–	–	●	●	–	●	–	●	–	●	●	●	●	●	●	●	●	●	●
25 **Sharp Memorial Hospital**, San Diego	–	–	–	–	–	–	–	●	–	●	–	●	●	●	●	●	●	●	●	●	●
28 **Kaiser Permanente Los Angeles Medical Center**	–	–	–	–	–	–	–	●	–	●	–	–	–	–	●	●	●	–	●	●	●
28 **Providence Holy Cross Medical Center**, Mission Hills	–	–	–	–	–	–	–	–	●	●	–	●	●	●	●	●	●	●	●	●	●
28 **Sequoia Hospital**, Redwood City	–	–	–	–	–	–	–	–	–	●	–	●	●	●	●	●	●	●	●	●	●
28 **St. Joseph Hospital**, Orange	–	–	–	–	–	–	–	–	–	●	–	●	●	●	●	●	●	●	●	●	●
28 **Sutter Roseville Medical Center**, Roseville	–	–	–	–	–	–	–	–	–	●	–	●	●	●	–	●	–	●	●	●	●
33 **Community Hospital of the Monterey Peninsula**, Monterey	–	–	–	–	–	–	–	–	–	●	–	●	●	●	●	●	●	–	●	●	●
33 **Kaiser Permanente Santa Clara Medical Center**, Santa Clara	–	–	–	–	–	–	–	–	–	–	–	●	●	●	●	●	–	●	●	●	●
33 **Mercy General Hospital**, Sacramento	–	–	–	–	–	–	–	–	–	–	–	●	●	●	●	●	●	●	●	●	●
33 **Providence St. John's Health Center**, Santa Monica	–	–	–	–	–	–	●	●	–	●	–	●	●	●	●	●	●	●	●	●	●
37 **Enloe Medical Center**, Chico	–	–	–	–	–	–	–	–	–	–	–	●	●	●	●	●	●	●	●	●	●
37 **Kaiser Permanente Anaheim and Irvine Medical Centers**, Anaheim	–	–	–	–	●	–	–	–	–	●	–	–	–	–	●	●	●	–	●	●	●
37 **Kaiser Permanente Fontana and Ontario Medical Centers**, Fontana	–	–	–	–	–	–	–	–	–	–	–	●	●	●	●	●	●	–	●	●	●
37 **Kaiser Permanente Sacramento Medical Center**	–	–	–	–	–	–	–	–	–	–	–	●	●	●	●	●	●	–	●	●	●
37 **Mills-Peninsula Health Services-Burlingame**, Burlingame	–	–	–	–	–	–	–	–	●	–	–	●	●	●	●	●	●	●	●	●	●
37 **Oroville Hospital**	–	–	–	–	●	●	–	●	–	–	●	●	●	–	●	●	–	–	●	●	●
37 **Santa Barbara Cottage Hospital**	–	–	–	–	–	–	–	–	–	–	–	●	●	●	●	●	●	●	●	●	●
37 **Sharp Grossmont Hospital**, La Mesa	–	–	–	–	–	–	–	–	–	–	–	●	●	●	●	●	●	●	●	●	●
45 **Alta Bates Summit Medical Center**, Berkeley	–	–	–	–	–	–	–	–	–	●	–	●	●	●	●	●	●	●	●	●	●
45 **Kaiser Permanente Riverside Medical Center**, Riverside	–	–	–	–	–	–	–	–	–	–	–	–	●	●	●	●	●	●	●	●	●
45 **Kaiser Permanente South Bay Medical Center**, Harbor City	–	–	–	–	–	–	–	–	–	–	–	●	●	●	●	●	●	●	●	●	●
45 **Kaiser Permanente South Sacramento Medical Center**	–	–	–	–	–	–	–	–	–	–	–	●	●	●	●	●	●	●	●	●	●
45 **Palomar Medical Center Escondido**, Escondido	–	–	–	–	–	–	–	–	–	–	–	●	●	●	●	●	●	●	●	●	●
45 **Providence Little Company of Mary Medical Center Torrance**	–	–	–	–	–	–	–	–	●	–	–	●	●	●	●	●	–	●	●	●	●
45 **Providence St. Joseph Medical Center**, Burbank	–	–	–	–	–	–	–	–	–	–	–	●	●	●	●	●	●	●	●	●	●
52 **Adventist Health St. Helena**, St. Helena	–	–	–	–	–	–	–	–	–	–	–	●	●	●	●	●	●	●	●	●	●
52 **Alta Bates Summit Medical Center**, Oakland	–	–	–	–	–	–	–	–	–	–	–	●	●	●	●	●	●	–	●	●	●
52 **Desert Regional Medical Center**, Palm Springs	–	–	–	–	–	–	–	–	–	–	–	●	●	●	●	●	●	●	●	●	●
52 **Kaiser Permanente Baldwin Park Medical Center**, Baldwin Park	–	–	–	–	–	–	–	–	–	–	–	–	–	–	●	●	–	–	●	●	●
52 **Kaiser Permanente Downey Medical Center**, Downey	–	–	–	–	–	–	–	–	–	–	–	●	●	●	●	●	●	●	●	●	●
52 **Kaweah Delta Medical Center**, Visalia	–	–	–	–	–	–	–	–	–	–	–	●	●	●	●	●	●	●	●	●	●
52 **Mercy San Juan Medical Center**, Carmichael	–	–	–	–	–	–	–	–	–	–	–	●	●	●	●	●	●	●	●	●	●
52 **Scripps Memorial Hospital-Encinitas**	–	–	–	–	–	–	–	–	–	–	–	●	●	●	●	●	–	●	●	●	●
52 **Scripps Mercy Hospital**, San Diego	–	–	–	–	–	–	–	–	–	–	–	●	●	●	●	●	●	●	●	●	●
52 **Sharp Chula Vista Medical Center**, Chula Vista	–	–	–	–	–	–	–	–	–	–	–	●	●	●	●	●	●	●	●	●	●

In complex care specialties, (-) indicates hospital is not nationally ranked or high performing.
In procedures and conditions, (-) indicates care not offered or hospital has too few Medicare patients to be rated.

▶ **More** @ usnews.com/bestregionalhospitals

COMPLEX SPECIALTY CARE
- ● Nationally ranked
- ◉ High performing

COMMON PROCEDURES & CONDITIONS
- ◉ High performing
- ◉ Average
- ● Below average

COMPLEX SPECIALTY CARE — **COMMON PROCEDURES & CONDITIONS**

State Rank / Hospital	Cancer	Cardiology & Heart Surgery	Diabetes & Endocrinology	Ear, Nose & Throat	Gastroenterology & GI Surgery	Geriatrics	Gynecology	Nephrology	Neurology & Neurosurgery	Orthopedics	Pulmonology	Urology	Colon Cancer Surgery	Lung Cancer Surgery	Heart Bypass Surgery	Heart Failure	Heart Valve Surgery	Abdominal Aortic Aneurysm	Hip Replacement	Knee Replacement	COPD
CALIFORNIA (CONTINUED)																					
52 St. Agnes Medical Center, Fresno	–	–	–	–	–	–	–	–	–	–	–	–	●	●	●	●	●	●	●	●	●
52 Stanford Health Care-ValleyCare, Pleasanton	–	–	–	–	–	–	–	–	–	–	–	–	●	●	●	●	●	●	●	●	●
64 Washington Hospital, Fremont	–	–	–	–	–	–	–	–	–	–	–	–	●	●	●	●	●	●	●	●	●
COLORADO																					
1 University of Colorado Hospital, Aurora[5]	●	●	●	–	●	●	●	–	●	●	●	●	●	●	●	●	●	●	●	●	●
2 Porter Adventist Hospital, Denver	–	–	–	–	–	–	–	–	–	–	–	–	●	●	●	●	●	●	●	●	●
3 Penrose-St. Francis Health Services-Colorado Springs	–	–	–	–	–	–	–	–	–	–	–	–	●	●	●	●	●	●	●	●	●
3 Sky Ridge Medical Center, Lone Tree	–	–	–	–	–	●	–	–	–	●	–	–	●	●	●	●	●	–	●	●	●
5 SCL Health St. Joseph Hospital, Denver	–	–	–	–	–	–	–	–	–	–	–	–	●	●	●	●	●	●	●	●	●
6 St. Mary's Hospital and Medical Center, Grand Junction	–	–	–	–	–	–	–	–	–	–	–	–	●	●	●	●	●	●	●	●	●
7 Parker Adventist Hospital, Parker	–	–	–	–	–	–	–	–	●	–	–	–	●	–	●	●	●	●	●	●	●
7 Parkview Medical Center, Pueblo	–	–	–	–	–	–	–	–	–	–	–	–	●	●	●	●	●	●	●	●	●
7 UCHealth Medical Center of the Rockies, Loveland	–	–	–	–	–	–	–	–	–	–	–	–	●	●	●	●	●	●	●	●	●
7 UCHealth Memorial Hospital, Colorado Springs	–	–	–	–	–	–	–	–	–	–	–	–	●	●	●	●	●	●	●	●	●
11 St. Anthony Hospital, Lakewood	–	–	–	–	–	–	–	–	–	–	–	–	●	●	●	●	●	●	●	●	●
11 UCHealth Poudre Valley Hospital, Fort Collins	–	–	–	–	–	–	–	–	–	–	–	–	●	–	–	●	–	–	–	●	●
CONNECTICUT																					
1 Yale New Haven Hospital[6]	●	●	●	●	●	●	●	●	●	●	●	●	●	●	●	●	●	●	●	●	●
2 Hartford Hospital, Hartford	–	–	–	–	–	–	●	–	–	–	–	–	●	●	●	●	●	●	●	●	●
3 St. Francis Hospital and Medical Center, Hartford	–	–	–	–	–	–	–	–	–	–	–	–	●	●	●	●	●	●	●	●	●
DELAWARE																					
1 Christiana Care Hospitals, Newark	–	–	–	–	●	●	●	●	–	–	–	–	●	●	●	●	●	●	●	●	●
2 Beebe Healthcare-Lewes, Lewes	–	–	–	–	–	–	–	–	–	–	–	–	●	●	●	●	●	●	●	●	●
FLORIDA																					
1 AdventHealth Orlando	●	●	●	–	●	●	●	●	●	●	●	●	●	●	●	●	●	●	●	●	●
2 UF Health Shands Hospital, Gainesville	●	–	●	–	●	–	●	●	●	●	●	●	●	●	●	●	●	●	●	●	●
3 Mayo Clinic-Jacksonville	●	–	–	●	●	●	–	●	●	●	●	●	●	●	●	●	●	●	●	●	●
4 Tampa General Hospital	–	–	●	–	●	●	–	●	●	●	●	●	●	●	●	●	●	●	●	●	●
5 Baptist Medical Center Jacksonville	–	–	●	–	●	●	●	●	●	●	●	●	●	●	●	●	●	●	●	●	●
5 Cleveland Clinic Florida, Weston	–	–	–	–	●	–	●	–	●	●	●	●	●	●	●	●	●	●	●	●	●
7 Baptist Hospital of Miami[7]	–	–	–	–	–	–	●	–	●	●	–	–	●	●	●	●	●	●	●	●	●
8 Sarasota Memorial Hospital	–	–	–	–	–	●	–	–	–	●	–	–	●	●	●	●	●	●	●	●	●
9 Morton Plant Hospital, Clearwater	–	–	–	–	–	–	–	–	–	●	–	–	●	●	●	●	●	●	●	●	●
9 University of Miami Hospital and Clinics-UHealth Tower	–	–	–	●	–	–	–	–	–	–	–	–	●	●	●	●	●	●	●	●	●
11 Mount Sinai Medical Center, Miami Beach	–	–	–	–	–	–	–	–	–	–	–	–	●	●	●	●	●	●	●	●	●
11 Orlando Regional Medical Center	–	–	–	–	–	–	–	–	–	–	●	–	●	●	●	●	●	●	●	●	●
13 St. Joseph's Hospital, Tampa	–	–	–	–	●	–	–	–	–	–	–	–	●	●	●	●	●	●	●	●	●
14 Lee Memorial Hospital, Fort Myers	–	–	–	–	–	–	–	–	–	–	–	–	●	●	●	●	●	●	●	●	●
14 NCH Baker Hospital, Naples	–	–	–	–	–	–	–	–	–	–	–	–	●	●	●	●	●	●	●	●	●
16 Flagler Hospital, St. Augustine	–	–	●	–	–	–	–	–	–	–	–	–	●	●	●	●	●	●	●	●	●
16 Holy Cross Hospital, Fort Lauderdale	–	–	–	–	–	–	–	–	●	–	–	–	●	●	●	●	●	●	●	●	●
16 Memorial Regional Hospital, Hollywood	–	–	–	–	–	–	–	–	–	–	–	–	●	●	●	●	●	●	●	●	●
16 South Miami Hospital[8]	–	–	–	–	●	–	–	–	–	–	–	–	●	●	●	●	●	●	●	●	●

In complex care specialties, (-) indicates hospital is not nationally ranked or high performing.
In procedures and conditions, (-) indicates care not offered or hospital has too few Medicare patients to be rated.

A footnote indicates that another hospital's results are included, that the hospital has a different name in one or more areas of care, or both. [5]National Jewish Health, Denver-University of Colorado Hospital, Aurora. [6]Smilow Cancer Hospital at Yale New Haven. [7]Miami Cancer Institute at Baptist Hospital of Miami; Miami Cardiac & Vascular Institute at Baptist Hospital of Miami; Baptist Health Neuroscience Center at Baptist Hospital of Miami; Miami Orthopedics & Sports Medicine Institute at Baptist Hospital of Miami. [8]Miami Cancer Institute at South Miami Hospital; Miami Cardiac & Vascular Institute at South Miami Hospital; Miami Neuroscience Center at South Miami Hospital; Miami Orthopedic & Sports Medicine Institute at South Miami Hospital.

		COMPLEX SPECIALTY CARE											COMMON PROCEDURES & CONDITIONS									
State Rank Hospital	CANCER	CARDIOLOGY & HEART SURGERY	DIABETES & ENDOCRINOLOGY	EAR, NOSE & THROAT	GASTROENTEROLOGY & GI SURGERY	GERIATRICS	GYNECOLOGY	NEPHROLOGY	NEUROLOGY & NEUROSURGERY	ORTHOPEDICS	PULMONOLOGY	UROLOGY	COLON CANCER SURGERY	LUNG CANCER SURGERY	HEART BYPASS SURGERY	HEART FAILURE	HEART VALVE SURGERY	ABDOMINAL AORTIC ANEURYSM	HIP REPLACEMENT	KNEE REPLACEMENT	COPD
FLORIDA (CONTINUED)																					
16 UF Health-Jacksonville	–	–	–	●	–	–	–	●	–	–	–	–	●	●	●	●	●	●	●	●	●
21 Boca Raton Regional Hospital	–	–	–	–	–	–	–	–	–	–	–	–	●	●	●	●	●	●	●	●	●
21 Gulf Coast Medical Center, Fort Myers	–	–	–	–	–	–	–	–	–	–	–	–	●	–	–	●	–	●	●	●	●
21 Health First Holmes Regional Medical Center, Melbourne	–	–	–	–	–	–	–	–	–	–	–	–	●	●	●	●	●	●	●	●	●
21 Heart of Florida Regional Medical Center, Davenport	–	–	–	–	–	–	–	–	–	–	–	–	●	–	●	●	–	–	●	●	●
21 Jackson Health System-Miami	–	–	–	–	–	–	●	–	–	–	–	–	●	–	●	●	●	–	●	●	●
21 Lakeland Regional Health Medical Center, Lakeland	–	–	–	–	–	–	–	–	–	–	–	–	●	●	●	●	●	●	●	●	●
27 AdventHealth Daytona Beach	–	–	–	–	–	–	–	–	–	–	–	–	●	●	●	●	●	●	●	●	●
27 Baptist Hospital, Pensacola	–	–	–	–	–	–	–	–	–	–	–	–	●	●	●	●	●	●	●	●	●
27 Broward Health Medical Center, Fort Lauderdale	–	–	–	–	–	–	–	–	–	–	–	–	●	●	●	●	●	●	●	●	●
27 Indian River Medical Center, Vero Beach	–	–	–	–	–	–	–	–	–	–	–	–	●	●	●	●	●	●	●	●	●
27 Leesburg Regional Medical Center	–	–	–	–	–	–	–	–	–	–	–	–	●	●	●	●	●	●	●	●	●
27 Mease Countryside Hospital, Safety Harbor	–	–	–	–	–	–	–	–	–	–	–	–	●	–	●	●	●	–	●	●	●
27 Memorial Hospital West, Pembroke Pines	–	–	–	–	–	–	–	–	–	–	–	–	●	●	●	●	–	–	●	●	●
27 St. Vincent's Medical Center Riverside, Jacksonville	–	–	–	–	–	–	–	–	–	–	–	–	●	●	●	●	●	●	●	●	●
27 Winter Haven Hospital	–	–	–	–	–	–	–	–	–	–	–	–	●	●	●	●	●	●	●	●	●
36 AdventHealth Tampa	–	–	–	–	–	–	–	–	–	–	–	–	●	●	●	●	●	●	●	●	●
36 Bethesda Hospital East, Boynton Beach	–	–	–	–	–	–	–	–	–	–	–	–	●	●	●	●	●	●	●	●	●
36 Munroe Regional Medical Center, Ocala	–	–	–	–	–	–	–	–	–	–	–	–	●	●	●	●	●	●	●	●	●
39 Ocala Regional Medical Center	–	–	–	–	–	–	–	–	–	–	–	–	●	●	●	●	●	●	●	●	●
40 Blake Medical Center, Bradenton	–	–	–	–	–	–	–	–	–	–	–	–	●	●	●	●	●	●	●	●	●
GEORGIA																					
1 Emory University Hospital, Atlanta[9]	●	●	●	–	●	●	●	●	●	●	–	●	●	●	●	●	●	●	●	●	●
2 Emory St. Joseph's Hospital, Atlanta	–	●	–	–	●	●	–	●	●	●	●	–	●	●	●	●	●	●	●	●	●
3 Piedmont Atlanta Hospital[10]	–	–	–	–	●	–	–	●	–	●	–	–	●	●	●	●	●	●	●	●	●
4 Northeast Georgia Medical Center, Gainesville	–	–	–	–	–	–	–	–	–	–	–	–	●	●	●	●	●	●	●	●	●
5 Emory University Hospital Midtown, Atlanta	–	–	–	●	–	–	–	–	–	–	–	–	●	●	●	●	●	●	●	●	●
5 Northside Hospital, Atlanta	●	–	–	–	–	–	–	–	–	–	–	–	●	●	●	–	●	–	●	●	●
5 WellStar Kennestone Hospital, Marietta	–	–	–	–	–	–	–	–	–	–	–	–	●	●	●	●	●	●	●	●	●
8 Gwinnett Medical Center, Lawrenceville	–	–	–	–	–	–	–	–	–	–	–	–	●	●	●	●	●	●	●	●	●
9 Memorial Health University Medical Center, Savannah	–	–	–	–	–	–	–	–	–	–	–	–	●	●	●	●	●	●	●	●	●
9 Northside Hospital-Forsyth, Cumming	–	–	–	–	–	–	–	–	–	–	–	–	●	●	●	●	●	●	●	●	●
9 University Hospital, Augusta	–	–	–	–	–	–	–	–	–	–	–	–	●	●	●	●	●	●	●	●	●
12 Piedmont Athens Regional Medical Center, Athens	–	–	–	–	–	–	–	–	–	–	–	–	●	●	●	●	●	●	●	●	●
12 St. Joseph's Hospital, Savannah	–	–	–	–	–	–	–	●	–	–	–	–	●	●	●	●	●	●	●	●	●
14 WellStar Cobb Hospital, Austell	–	–	–	–	–	–	–	–	–	–	–	–	●	–	●	–	●	–	●	●	●
15 Navicent Health Medical Center, Macon	–	–	–	–	–	–	–	–	–	–	–	–	●	●	●	●	●	●	●	●	●
15 St. Francis Hospital, Columbus	–	–	–	–	–	–	–	–	–	–	–	–	●	●	●	●	●	●	●	●	●
HAWAII																					
1 Queen's Medical Center, Honolulu	●	–	●	–	–	●	–	●	●	●	●	●	●	●	●	●	●	●	●	●	●
2 Straub Medical Center, Honolulu	–	–	–	–	–	–	–	–	–	–	–	–	●	●	●	●	●	●	●	●	●
IDAHO																					
1 St. Luke's Regional Medical Center, Boise	–	–	●	–	●	●	–	–	–	●	–	●	●	●	●	●	●	●	●	●	●
2 St. Alphonsus Regional Medical Center, Boise	–	–	–	–	–	–	–	–	–	–	–	–	●	●	●	●	●	●	●	●	●

COMPLEX SPECIALTY CARE
● Nationally ranked
● High performing

COMMON PROCEDURES & CONDITIONS
● High performing
● Average
● Below average

In complex care specialties, (-) indicates hospital is not nationally ranked or high performing.
In procedures and conditions, (-) indicates care not offered or hospital has too few Medicare patients to be rated.

A footnote indicates that another hospital's results are included, that the hospital has a different name in one or more areas of care, or both.
[9]Emory University Hospital at Wesley Woods. [10]Piedmont Heart Institute at Piedmont Atlanta Hospital.

COMPLEX SPECIALTY CARE
● Nationally ranked
● High performing

COMMON PROCEDURES & CONDITIONS
● High performing
● Average
● Below average

State Rank / Hospital	Cancer	Cardiology & Heart Surgery	Diabetes & Endocrinology	Ear, Nose & Throat	Gastroenterology & GI Surgery	Geriatrics	Gynecology	Nephrology	Neurology & Neurosurgery	Orthopedics	Pulmonology	Urology	Colon Cancer Surgery	Lung Cancer Surgery	Heart Bypass Surgery	Heart Failure	Heart Valve Surgery	Abdominal Aortic Aneurysm	Hip Replacement	Knee Replacement	COPD
IDAHO (CONTINUED)																					
3 Kootenai Health-Coeur D'Alene	−	−	−	−	−	−	−	−	−	−	−	−	●	●	●	●	●	●	●	●	●
3 Portneuf Medical Center, Pocatello	−	−	−	−	−	−	−	−	−	−	−	−	●	●	●	●	●	●	●	●	●
ILLINOIS																					
1 Northwestern Memorial Hospital, Chicago	●	●	●	●	●	●	−	●	●	●	●	●	●	●	●	●	●	●	●	●	●
2 University of Chicago Medical Center	●	−	−	●	●	●	●	●	●	●	−	●	●	●	●	●	●	●	●	●	●
3 NorthShore University Health System-Metro Chicago, Evanston	−	−	−	−	●	●	●	−	●	●	−	−	●	●	●	●	●	●	●	●	●
3 Rush University Medical Center, Chicago	●	●	−	−	●	●	●	●	●	●	−	−	●	●	●	●	●	●	●	●	●
5 Loyola University Medical Center, Maywood	●	●	−	−	●	−	−	●	●	−	●	−	●	●	●	●	●	●	●	●	●
6 Northwestern Medicine Central DuPage Hospital, Winfield	−	−	−	−	−	−	−	−	−	●	●	−	●	●	●	●	●	●	●	●	●
6 OSF Healthcare St. Francis Medical Center, Peoria	−	−	−	−	−	−	−	●	−	−	−	−	●	●	●	●	●	●	●	●	●
8 Advocate Christ Medical Center, Oak Lawn	−	●	−	−	−	−	−	−	−	−	−	−	●	●	●	●	●	●	●	●	●
8 Advocate Lutheran General Hospital, Park Ridge	−	−	−	−	●	−	−	●	−	−	−	−	●	●	●	●	●	●	●	●	●
10 Advocate Good Samaritan Hospital, Downers Grove	−	−	−	−	−	−	−	−	−	−	−	−	●	●	●	●	●	●	●	●	●
10 Edward Hospital, Naperville[11]	−	−	−	−	−	−	−	−	−	−	−	−	●	●	●	●	●	●	●	●	●
10 Memorial Medical Center, Springfield	−	−	−	−	−	−	−	−	−	−	−	−	●	●	●	●	●	●	●	●	●
13 AMITA Health Adventist Medical Center-Hinsdale	−	−	−	−	●	−	−	−	−	●	−	−	●	●	●	●	●	−	●	●	●
14 Advocate Condell Medical Center, Libertyville	−	−	−	−	−	−	●	−	−	−	−	−	●	●	●	●	●	●	●	●	●
14 Advocate Sherman Hospital, Elgin	−	−	−	−	●	−	−	−	−	−	−	−	●	●	●	●	●	●	●	●	●
14 HSHS St. John's Hospital, Springfield	−	−	−	−	●	−	−	−	−	−	−	−	●	●	●	●	●	●	●	●	●
14 Northwest Community Hospital, Arlington Heights	−	−	−	−	●	−	−	−	−	−	−	−	●	●	●	●	●	●	●	●	●
18 Advocate Good Shepherd Hospital, Barrington	−	−	−	−	●	−	−	−	−	−	−	−	●	●	●	●	●	●	●	●	●
18 Northwestern Medicine Delnor, Geneva	−	−	−	−	−	−	−	−	−	●	−	−	●	●	●	●	−	−	●	●	●
18 UnityPoint Health-Peoria	−	−	−	−	−	−	−	−	−	−	−	−	●	●	●	●	●	●	●	●	●
21 AMITA Health Elk Grove Village	−	−	−	−	−	−	−	−	−	−	−	−	●	●	●	●	●	●	●	●	●
21 AMITA Saints Mary and Elizabeth Medical Center Chicago	−	−	−	−	●	−	●	−	−	−	−	−	●	−	●	●	−	−	●	●	●
21 OSF St. Anthony Medical Center, Rockford	−	−	−	−	−	−	−	−	−	−	−	−	●	●	●	●	●	●	●	●	●
21 Palos Community Hospital, Palos Heights	−	−	−	−	−	−	−	−	−	−	−	−	●	●	●	●	●	●	●	●	●
25 Centegra Hospital-McHenry	−	−	−	−	−	−	−	−	−	−	−	−	●	●	●	●	●	●	●	●	●
25 Rush-Copley Medical Center, Aurora	−	−	−	−	−	−	−	−	−	−	−	−	●	●	●	●	●	●	●	●	●
INDIANA																					
1 Indiana University Health Medical Center, Indianapolis	●	−	−	−	●	●	−	●	●	−	●	−	●	●	●	●	●	●	●	●	●
2 Deaconess Hospital, Evansville	−	−	−	−	−	−	−	−	−	−	−	−	●	●	●	●	−	●	●	●	●
2 Elkhart General Hospital, Elkhart	−	−	−	−	−	−	−	−	−	−	−	−	●	●	●	●	●	●	●	●	●
4 Memorial Hospital of South Bend	−	−	−	−	−	−	−	−	−	−	−	−	●	●	●	●	●	●	●	●	●
5 Community Hospital East, Indianapolis	−	−	−	−	−	−	−	−	−	−	−	−	●	●	●	●	●	●	●	●	●
5 Indiana University Health Ball Memorial Hospital, Muncie	−	−	−	−	−	−	−	−	−	−	−	−	●	●	●	●	●	●	●	●	●
5 St. Vincent Indianapolis Hospital	−	−	−	−	−	−	−	−	−	−	−	−	●	●	●	●	●	●	●	●	●
8 Goshen Hospital, Goshen[12]	−	−	−	−	−	−	−	−	−	−	−	−	●	●	−	●	−	●	●	●	●
8 Indiana University Health Arnett Hospital, Lafayette	−	−	−	−	−	−	−	−	−	−	−	−	●	●	●	●	●	●	●	●	●
8 Indiana University Health Bloomington Hospital, Bloomington	−	−	−	−	−	−	−	−	−	−	−	−	●	●	●	●	●	●	●	●	●
8 St. Joseph Health System-Mishawaka	−	−	−	−	−	−	−	−	−	−	−	−	●	●	●	●	●	●	●	●	●
12 Lutheran Hospital of Indiana, Fort Wayne	−	−	−	−	−	−	−	−	−	−	−	−	●	●	●	●	●	●	●	●	●
12 Parkview Regional Medical Center, Fort Wayne	−	−	−	−	−	−	−	−	−	−	−	−	●	●	●	●	●	●	●	●	●

In complex care specialties, (-) indicates hospital is not nationally ranked or high performing.
In procedures and conditions, (-) indicates care not offered or hospital has too few Medicare patients to be rated.

A footnote indicates that another hospital's results are included, that the hospital has a different name in one or more areas of care, or both.
[11] Edward Cancer Center; Edward Heart Hospital. [12] Goshen Center for Cancer Care; Goshen Heart & Vascular Center.

BEST REGIONAL HOSPITALS

COMPLEX SPECIALTY CARE
- ● Nationally ranked
- ● High performing

COMMON PROCEDURES & CONDITIONS
- ● High performing
- ● Average
- ● Below average

State Rank / Hospital	CANCER	CARDIOLOGY & HEART SURGERY	DIABETES & ENDOCRINOLOGY	EAR, NOSE & THROAT	GASTROENTEROLOGY & GI SURGERY	GERIATRICS	GYNECOLOGY	NEPHROLOGY	NEUROLOGY & NEUROSURGERY	ORTHOPEDICS	PULMONOLOGY	UROLOGY	COLON CANCER SURGERY	LUNG CANCER SURGERY	HEART BYPASS SURGERY	HEART FAILURE	HEART VALVE SURGERY	ABDOMINAL AORTIC ANEURYSM	HIP REPLACEMENT	KNEE REPLACEMENT	COPD
IOWA																					
1 University of Iowa Hospitals and Clinics, Iowa City	●	–	–	●	–	●	●	–	–	●	●	●	●	●	●	●	●	●	●	●	●
2 MercyOne Des Moines Medical Center	–	–	–	–	–	–	–	–	–	–	–	–	●	●	●	●	●	●	●	●	●
3 UnityPoint Health-St. Luke's Hospital, Cedar Rapids	–	–	–	–	–	–	–	–	–	–	–	●	●	●	●	●	●	●	●	●	●
4 UnityPoint Health-Iowa Methodist Medical Center, Des Moines	–	–	–	–	–	–	–	–	–	–	–	–	●	●	●	●	●	●	●	●	●
KANSAS																					
1 University of Kansas Hospital, Kansas City	●	●	●	●	●	●	–	●	●	●	●	●	●	●	●	●	●	●	●	●	●
2 Stormont Vail Hospital, Topeka	–	–	–	–	–	–	–	–	–	–	●	–	●	●	●	●	●	●	●	●	●
3 Shawnee Mission Medical Center, Shawnee Mission	–	–	–	–	–	–	–	–	–	–	–	–	●	●	●	●	●	●	●	●	●
KENTUCKY																					
1 University of Kentucky Albert B. Chandler Hospital, Lexington	●	–	–	–	–	–	–	–	–	–	–	●	●	●	●	●	●	●	●	●	●
2 St. Elizabeth Healthcare Edgewood-Covington Hospitals, Edgewood	–	–	–	–	–	–	–	–	–	–	–	–	●	●	●	●	●	●	●	●	●
3 Baptist Health Lexington	–	–	–	–	–	–	–	–	–	–	–	–	●	●	●	●	●	●	●	●	●
3 Baptist Health Louisville	–	–	–	–	–	–	–	–	–	–	–	–	●	●	●	●	●	●	●	●	●
5 Norton Hospital, Louisville	–	–	–	–	–	–	–	–	–	–	–	–	●	●	●	●	●	●	●	●	●
6 Baptist Health Paducah	–	–	–	–	–	–	–	–	–	–	–	–	●	●	●	●	●	●	●	●	●
LOUISIANA																					
1 Ochsner Medical Center, New Orleans	●	–	–	–	●	–	–	–	●	–	–	–	●	●	●	●	●	●	●	●	●
2 Willis-Knighton Medical Center, Shreveport	–	–	–	–	–	–	–	–	–	–	–	–	●	●	●	●	●	●	●	●	●
3 Our Lady of the Lake Regional Medical Center, Baton Rouge	–	–	–	–	–	–	–	–	–	–	–	–	●	●	●	●	●	●	●	●	●
4 Lafayette General Medical Center, Lafayette	–	–	–	–	–	–	–	–	–	–	–	–	●	●	●	●	●	●	●	●	●
MAINE																					
1 Maine Medical Center, Portland	–	–	–	–	●	–	●	–	–	–	–	●	●	●	●	●	●	●	●	●	●
2 Eastern Maine Medical Center, Bangor	–	–	–	–	–	–	–	–	–	–	–	–	●	●	●	●	●	●	●	●	●
2 Mercy Hospital of Portland	–	–	–	–	–	–	–	–	–	–	–	–	●	●	–	●	–	●	–	–	●
MARYLAND																					
1 Johns Hopkins Hospital, Baltimore	●	●	●	●	●	●	●	●	●	●	●	●	●	●	●	●	●	●	–	–	●
2 University of Maryland Medical Center, Baltimore	●	–	–	●	●	–	–	●	–	–	–	●	●	●	●	●	●	●	●	●	●
3 University of Maryland St. Joseph Medical Center, Towson	–	–	–	–	–	–	–	–	–	–	–	–	●	●	●	●	●	●	●	●	●
4 Anne Arundel Medical Center, Annapolis	–	–	–	–	–	–	–	–	–	–	–	–	●	●	●	●	●	●	●	●	●
4 MedStar Union Memorial Hospital, Baltimore	–	–	–	–	–	–	–	–	–	–	–	–	●	●	●	●	●	●	●	●	●
6 Greater Baltimore Medical Center	–	–	–	–	–	–	–	–	–	–	–	–	●	●	●	●	●	●	●	●	●
7 Carroll Hospital Center, Westminster	–	–	–	–	–	–	–	–	–	–	–	–	●	●	●	●	●	–	●	●	●
7 Peninsula Regional Medical Center, Salisbury	–	–	–	–	–	–	–	–	–	–	–	–	●	●	●	●	●	●	●	●	●
7 U. of Maryland Baltimore Washington Medical Ctr., Glen Burnie	–	–	–	–	–	–	–	–	–	–	–	–	●	●	●	●	●	●	●	●	●
10 Holy Cross Hospital, Silver Spring	–	–	–	–	–	–	–	–	–	–	–	–	●	●	●	●	●	●	●	●	●
10 MedStar Franklin Square Medical Center, Baltimore	–	–	–	–	–	–	–	–	–	–	–	–	●	●	●	●	–	●	●	●	●
10 Suburban Hospital, Bethesda	–	–	–	–	–	–	–	–	–	–	–	–	●	●	●	●	●	●	●	●	●
MASSACHUSETTS																					
1 Massachusetts General Hospital, Boston[13]	●	●	●	●	●	●	●	●	●	●	●	●	●	●	●	●	●	●	●	●	●
2 Brigham and Women's Hospital, Boston[14]	●	●	●	–	●	●	●	●	●	●	●	●	●	●	●	●	●	●	●	●	●
3 Beth Israel Deaconess Medical Center, Boston	●	–	●	–	●	●	●	●	●	–	●	●	●	●	●	●	●	●	●	●	●
4 Lahey Hospital and Medical Center, Burlington	–	–	●	–	●	–	–	●	–	–	●	●	●	●	●	●	●	●	●	●	●
5 Baystate Medical Center, Springfield	–	–	–	–	–	–	–	●	–	–	●	–	●	●	●	●	●	●	●	●	●
6 Newton-Wellesley Hospital, Newton Lower Falls	–	–	–	–	–	–	–	–	–	–	–	–	●	●	●	●	–	●	●	●	●

In complex care specialties, (-) indicates hospital is not nationally ranked or high performing.
In procedures and conditions, (-) indicates care not offered or hospital has too few Medicare patients to be rated.

A footnote indicates that another hospital's results are included, that the hospital has a different name in one or more areas of care, or both.
[13]Massachusetts Eye and Ear Infirmary, Massachusetts General Hospital. [14]Dana-Farber/Brigham and Women's Cancer Center.

More @ usnews.com/bestregionalhospitals

	COMPLEX SPECIALTY CARE												COMMON PROCEDURES & CONDITIONS								
State Rank / Hospital	CANCER	CARDIOLOGY & HEART SURGERY	DIABETES & ENDOCRINOLOGY	EAR, NOSE & THROAT	GASTROENTEROLOGY & GI SURGERY	GERIATRICS	GYNECOLOGY	NEPHROLOGY	NEUROLOGY & NEUROSURGERY	ORTHOPEDICS	PULMONOLOGY	UROLOGY	COLON CANCER SURGERY	LUNG CANCER SURGERY	HEART BYPASS SURGERY	HEART FAILURE	HEART VALVE SURGERY	ABDOMINAL AORTIC ANEURYSM	HIP REPLACEMENT	KNEE REPLACEMENT	COPD
MASSACHUSETTS (CONTINUED)																					
6 UMass Memorial Medical Center, Worcester	–	–	–	–	–	–	–	–	–	–	–	–	●	●	●	●	●	●	●	●	●
8 Southcoast Charlton Memorial Hospital, Fall River	–	–	–	–	–	–	–	–	–	–	●	–	●	●	●	●	●	●	●	●	●
9 Tufts Medical Center, Boston	–	–	–	–	–	–	–	–	–	–	–	–	●	●	●	●	●	●	●	●	●
MICHIGAN																					
1 University of Michigan Hospitals-Michigan Medicine, Ann Arbor	●	●	●	●	●	●	●	●	●	●	●	●	●	●	●	●	●	●	●	●	●
2 Beaumont Hospital-Royal Oak	–	●	●	●	●	●	●	●	●	●	●	●	●	●	●	●	●	●	●	●	●
3 Beaumont Hospital-Troy	–	●	●	●	●	●	–	●	●	●	●	●	●	●	●	●	●	●	●	●	●
4 Beaumont Hospital-Grosse Pointe	–	–	●	–	●	●	–	●	●	●	●	●	●	●	–	●	–	●	●	●	●
5 Spectrum Health-Butterworth and Blodgett Campuses, Grand Rapids	–	–	–	–	–	–	–	●	●	●	–	●	●	●	●	●	●	●	●	●	●
6 DMC Harper University Hospital, Detroit	–	–	●	–	●	●	–	●	●	–	●	●	●	●	●	●	●	●	●	●	●
7 Munson Medical Center, Traverse City	–	–	–	–	–	–	–	–	–	–	–	–	●	●	●	●	●	●	●	●	●
8 Bronson Methodist Hospital, Kalamazoo	–	–	–	–	–	–	–	–	–	–	–	–	●	●	●	●	●	●	●	●	●
8 Henry Ford Hospital, Detroit	–	–	●	–	●	●	–	●	●	–	●	●	●	●	●	●	●	●	●	●	●
8 St. Joseph Mercy Ann Arbor Hospital, Ypsilanti	–	–	–	–	–	●	–	–	–	–	●	–	●	●	●	●	●	●	●	●	●
11 Ascension Providence Hospital-Southfield	–	–	–	–	–	–	–	–	–	–	–	–	●	●	●	●	●	●	●	●	●
12 McLaren Northern Michigan Hospital, Petoskey	–	–	–	–	–	–	–	–	–	–	–	–	●	●	●	●	●	●	●	●	●
13 Henry Ford Macomb Hospitals, Clinton Township	–	–	–	–	–	–	–	–	–	–	–	–	●	●	●	●	●	●	●	●	●
13 Lakeland Medical Center, St. Joseph	–	–	–	–	–	–	–	–	–	–	–	–	●	●	●	●	●	●	●	●	●
13 McLaren Flint Hospital, Flint	–	–	●	–	–	–	–	–	–	–	–	–	●	●	●	●	●	●	●	●	●
13 Mercy Health St. Mary's Campus, Grand Rapids	–	–	–	–	–	●	–	–	●	–	–	–	●	●	–	●	–	●	●	●	●
17 Ascension St. John Hospital, Detroit	–	–	–	–	–	–	–	–	–	–	–	–	●	●	●	●	●	●	●	●	●
17 Borgess Medical Center, Kalamazoo	–	–	–	–	–	–	–	–	–	–	–	–	●	●	●	●	●	●	●	●	●
17 Genesys Regional Medical Center, Grand Blanc	–	–	–	–	–	●	–	–	–	–	–	–	●	●	●	●	●	●	●	●	●
17 St. Joseph Mercy Oakland Hospital, Pontiac	–	–	–	–	–	–	–	–	–	–	–	–	●	●	●	●	●	●	●	●	●
21 Ascension Crittenton Hospital Medical Center, Rochester	–	–	–	–	–	–	–	–	–	–	–	–	●	●	●	●	●	–	●	●	●
21 Beaumont Hospital-Dearborn	–	–	–	–	–	–	–	–	–	–	–	–	●	●	●	●	●	●	●	●	●
21 Beaumont Hospital-Trenton	–	–	–	–	–	–	–	–	–	–	–	–	●	–	–	●	●	●	●	●	●
21 MidMichigan Medical Center-Midland	–	–	–	–	–	–	–	–	–	–	–	–	●	●	●	●	●	●	●	●	●
21 Sparrow Hospital, Lansing	–	–	–	–	–	–	–	–	–	–	–	–	●	●	●	●	●	●	●	●	●
26 McLaren Greater Lansing Hospital	–	–	–	–	–	–	–	–	–	–	–	–	●	●	●	●	●	●	●	●	●
MINNESOTA																					
1 Mayo Clinic, Rochester	●	●	●	●	●	●	●	●	●	●	●	●	●	●	●	●	●	●	●	●	●
2 Abbott Northwestern Hospital, Minneapolis[15]	–	●	●	–	●	●	–	●	●	●	●	●	●	●	●	●	●	●	●	●	●
3 St. Cloud Hospital, St. Cloud	–	●	–	–	●	●	–	–	●	●	–	–	●	●	●	●	●	●	●	●	●
4 Mercy Hospital, Coon Rapids	–	–	–	–	●	●	–	–	–	●	●	●	●	●	●	●	●	●	●	●	●
5 Fairview Ridges Hospital, Burnsville	–	–	–	–	●	●	–	●	–	●	●	●	●	–	–	●	–	–	●	●	●
5 Park Nicollet Methodist Hospital, St. Louis Park	–	–	–	–	–	●	–	–	–	●	–	–	●	●	●	●	●	●	●	●	●
5 Regions Hospital, St. Paul	–	–	–	–	–	–	–	–	–	–	–	●	●	●	●	●	●	●	●	●	●
8 Fairview Southdale Hospital, Edina	–	–	–	–	–	–	–	–	–	–	–	–	●	●	●	●	●	●	●	●	●
8 United Hospital, St. Paul	–	–	–	–	–	–	–	–	–	–	–	–	●	●	●	●	●	●	●	●	●
10 Essentia Health-St. Mary's Medical Center, Duluth	–	–	–	–	–	–	–	●	–	–	–	–	●	●	●	●	●	●	●	●	●
11 University of Minnesota Medical Center, Minneapolis	●	–	–	–	–	–	–	–	●	●	–	–	●	●	●	●	●	●	●	●	●
12 St. Joseph's Hospital, St. Paul	–	–	–	–	–	–	–	–	–	–	–	–	●	●	●	●	●	●	●	●	●
13 Woodwinds Health Campus, Woodbury	–	–	–	–	–	–	–	●	–	–	●	–	●	●	–	●	–	–	●	●	●
14 Mayo Clinic Health System-Albert Lea and Austin, Albert Lea	–	–	–	–	–	–	–	–	–	–	–	–	●	●	–	●	●	–	●	●	●

In complex care specialties, (-) indicates hospital is not nationally ranked or high performing.
In procedures and conditions, (-) indicates care not offered or hospital has too few Medicare patients to be rated.
A footnote indicates that another hospital's results are included, that the hospital has a different name in one or more areas of care, or both.
[15]Minneapolis Heart Institute at Abbott Northwestern Hospital.

Legend

COMPLEX SPECIALTY CARE
- ● Nationally ranked
- ○ High performing

COMMON PROCEDURES & CONDITIONS
- ○ High performing
- ○ Average
- ● Below average

State / Rank / Hospital	Cancer	Cardiology & Heart Surgery	Diabetes & Endocrinology	Ear, Nose & Throat	Gastroenterology & GI Surgery	Geriatrics	Gynecology	Nephrology	Neurology & Neurosurgery	Orthopedics	Pulmonology	Urology	Colon Cancer Surgery	Lung Cancer Surgery	Heart Bypass Surgery	Heart Failure	Heart Valve Surgery	Abdominal Aortic Aneurysm	Hip Replacement	Knee Replacement	COPD
MISSISSIPPI																					
1 Mississippi Baptist Medical Center, Jackson	–	–	–	–	●	–	–	–	–	–	–	–	○	○	○	○	○	○	○	○	○
2 North Mississippi Medical Center-Tupelo	–	–	–	–	–	–	–	–	–	–	–	–	○	○	○	○	○	○	○	○	○
3 Memorial Hospital at Gulfport	–	–	–	–	–	–	–	–	–	–	–	–	○	○	○	○	○	○	○	○	○
4 St. Dominic-Jackson Memorial Hospital, Jackson	–	–	–	–	–	–	–	–	–	–	–	–	○	○	○	○	○	○	○	○	○
MISSOURI																					
1 Barnes-Jewish Hospital, St. Louis[16]	●	●	●	●	●	●	●	●	●	○	●	○	○	○	○	○	○	○	○	○	○
2 Saint Luke's Hospital of Kansas City	–	●	–	–	○	○	–	–	●	–	–	○	○	○	○	○	○	○	○	○	○
3 Missouri Baptist Medical Center, St. Louis	–	–	○	–	–	–	–	–	–	–	–	○	○	○	○	○	○	○	○	○	○
4 North Kansas City Hospital	–	–	–	–	–	○	–	–	–	–	–	○	○	○	○	○	○	○	○	○	○
5 Boone Hospital Center, Columbia	–	–	–	–	–	–	–	○	–	–	–	○	○	○	○	○	○	○	○	○	○
5 Mercy Hospital Springfield	–	–	–	–	–	–	–	–	–	–	–	○	○	○	○	○	○	○	○	○	○
5 St. Luke's Hospital, Chesterfield	–	–	–	–	–	–	–	–	–	–	–	○	○	○	○	○	○	○	○	○	○
8 Mercy Hospital St. Louis	–	–	–	–	–	–	–	–	○	–	–	○	○	○	○	○	○	○	○	○	○
9 CoxHealth Springfield	–	–	–	–	–	–	–	–	–	–	–	○	○	○	○	○	○	○	○	○	○
9 SSM Health St. Clare Hospital-Fenton	–	–	–	–	–	–	–	–	–	–	–	○	○	○	○	○	○	○	○	○	○
11 Freeman Health System-Joplin	–	–	–	–	–	–	–	–	–	–	–	○	○	○	○	○	○	○	○	○	○
11 Mercy Hospital South, St. Louis	–	–	–	–	–	–	–	–	–	–	–	○	○	○	○	○	○	○	○	○	○
11 Mercy Hospital Washington	–	–	–	–	–	–	–	–	–	–	–	–	○	–	–	○	–	○	○	○	○
14 SSM Health DePaul Hospital-St. Louis, Bridgeton	–	–	–	–	–	–	–	–	–	–	–	○	○	●	○	●	○	○	○	○	○
MONTANA																					
1 St. Patrick Hospital, Missoula	–	–	–	–	–	–	–	–	–	●	–	○	○	○	○	○	○	○	○	○	○
2 St. Vincent Healthcare-Billings	–	–	–	–	–	–	–	–	–	–	–	○	○	○	○	○	○	○	○	○	○
NEBRASKA																					
1 Nebraska Medicine-Nebraska Medical Center, Omaha	●	–	–	○	–	–	○	–	–	–	○	○	○	○	○	○	○	○	○	○	○
2 Bryan Medical Center, Lincoln	–	–	–	–	–	–	–	–	–	–	–	○	○	○	○	○	○	○	○	○	○
3 Nebraska Methodist Hospital, Omaha	–	–	–	–	–	–	–	–	–	–	–	○	○	○	○	○	○	○	○	○	○
4 Creighton University Medical Center-Bergan Mercy, Omaha	–	–	–	–	–	–	–	–	–	–	–	○	○	○	○	○	○	○	○	○	○
NEVADA																					
1 St. Rose Dominican Hospitals-Siena Campus, Henderson	–	–	–	–	–	–	–	–	–	–	–	○	○	○	○	○	○	○	○	○	○
2 Renown Regional Medical Center, Reno	–	–	–	–	–	–	–	–	–	–	–	○	○	○	○	○	●	○	○	○	○
NEW HAMPSHIRE																					
1 Dartmouth-Hitchcock Medical Center, Lebanon	○	–	–	○	○	–	–	○	–	○	–	○	○	○	○	○	○	○	○	○	○
2 Concord Hospital	–	–	–	–	–	–	–	–	–	–	–	○	○	○	○	○	○	○	○	○	○
3 Catholic Medical Center, Manchester	–	–	–	–	–	–	–	–	–	–	–	○	○	○	○	○	○	○	○	○	○
3 Wentworth-Douglass Hospital, Dover	–	–	–	–	–	–	–	–	–	–	–	○	○	–	○	–	○	○	○	○	○
NEW JERSEY																					
1 Morristown Medical Center	–	●	–	–	○	○	–	○	–	●	○	○	○	○	○	○	○	○	○	○	○
2 Hackensack University Medical Center	○	–	–	–	○	○	–	○	○	–	○	○	○	○	○	○	○	○	○	○	○
3 St. Barnabas Medical Center, Livingston	–	–	●	–	○	○	●	–	○	–	–	○	○	○	○	○	○	○	○	○	○
4 Robert Wood Johnson University Hospital, New Brunswick	○	–	–	–	○	○	–	○	○	–	–	○	○	○	○	○	○	○	○	○	○
5 Jersey Shore University Medical Center, Neptune	–	–	–	–	–	–	–	–	●	–	–	○	○	○	○	○	○	○	○	○	○
6 Valley Hospital, Ridgewood	–	–	–	–	–	–	–	–	○	–	–	○	○	○	○	○	○	○	○	○	○
7 AtlantiCare Regional Medical Center, Atlantic City	–	–	–	–	–	–	–	–	○	–	–	○	○	○	○	○	○	○	○	○	○
7 Virtua Voorhees Hospital, Voorhees	–	–	–	–	–	–	–	–	–	–	–	○	○	○	○	○	–	○	○	○	○

In complex care specialties, (-) indicates hospital is not nationally ranked or high performing.
In procedures and conditions, (-) indicates care not offered or hospital has too few Medicare patients to be rated.

A footnote indicates that another hospital's results are included, that the hospital has a different name in one or more areas of care, or both.
[16]Siteman Cancer Center.

More @ usnews.com/bestregionalhospitals

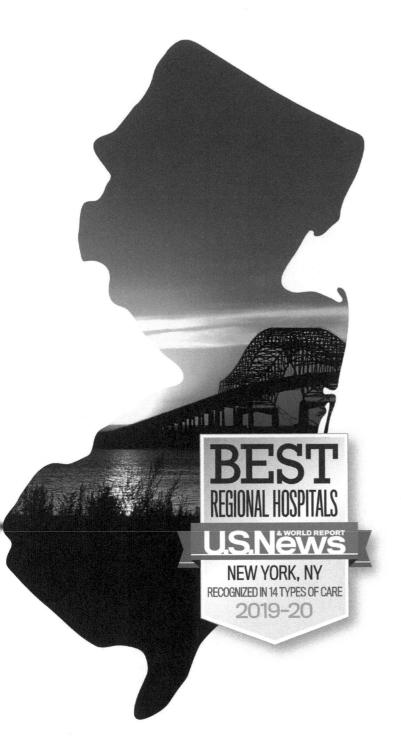

BEST
REGIONAL HOSPITALS
U.S.News & WORLD REPORT
NEW YORK, NY
RECOGNIZED IN 14 TYPES OF CARE
2019-20

Home is where award-winning care is.

Once again, four Hackensack Meridian *Health* hospitals are ranked among the best in New Jersey by *U.S. News & World Report*. Because home is where compassionate, uncompromising care happens every day. Visit hackensackmeridianhealth.org/usnews

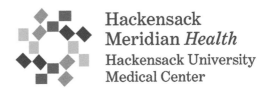

Hackensack
Meridian *Health*
Hackensack University
Medical Center

HACKENSACK UNIVERSITY MEDICAL CENTER / JERSEY SHORE UNIVERSITY MEDICAL CENTER
RIVERVIEW MEDICAL CENTER / OCEAN MEDICAL CENTER

	COMPLEX SPECIALTY CARE	COMMON PROCEDURES & CONDITIONS
COMPLEX SPECIALTY CARE	● Nationally ranked ◐ High performing	
COMMON PROCEDURES & CONDITIONS	◐ High performing ● Average ● Below average	

State Rank / Hospital	CANCER	CARDIOLOGY & HEART SURGERY	DIABETES & ENDOCRINOLOGY	EAR, NOSE & THROAT	GASTROENTEROLOGY & GI SURGERY	GERIATRICS	GYNECOLOGY	NEPHROLOGY	NEUROLOGY & NEUROSURGERY	ORTHOPEDICS	PULMONOLOGY	UROLOGY	COLON CANCER SURGERY	LUNG CANCER SURGERY	HEART BYPASS SURGERY	HEART FAILURE	HEART VALVE SURGERY	ABDOMINAL AORTIC ANEURYSM	HIP REPLACEMENT	KNEE REPLACEMENT	COPD
NEW JERSEY (CONTINUED)																					
9 Hackensack Meridian Health Riverview Medical Center, Red Bank	–	–	–	–	–	–	–	–	–	●	–	–	●	●	–	●	–	●	●	●	●
9 Robert Wood Johnson University Hospital Somerset, Somerville	–	–	–	–	–	–	–	–	●	●	–	–	●	●	–	●	–	●	●	●	●
11 Hackensack Meridian Health Ocean Medical Center, Brick Township	–	–	–	–	–	–	–	–	–	●	–	–	●	●	–	●	–	●	●	●	●
11 Jefferson Health-Stratford, Cherry Hill, and Washington Township	–	–	–	–	–	–	–	–	–	●	–	–	●	●	–	●	–	●	●	●	●
11 Our Lady of Lourdes Medical Center, Camden	–	–	–	–	–	–	–	–	–	●	–	–	●	●	●	●	●	●	●	●	●
11 Overlook Medical Center, Summit	–	–	–	–	–	–	–	–	–	●	–	–	●	●	–	●	–	●	●	●	●
11 Penn Medicine Princeton Medical Center, Plainsboro	–	–	–	–	–	–	–	–	–	●	–	–	●	●	–	●	–	●	●	●	●
NEW MEXICO																					
1 Presbyterian Hospital, Albuquerque	–	–	–	–	–	–	–	–	–	–	–	–	●	●	●	●	●	●	●	●	●
NEW YORK																					
1 New York-Presbyterian Hospital-Columbia and Cornell	●	●	●	●	●	●	●	●	●	●	●	●	●	●	●	●	●	●	●	●	●
2 NYU Langone Hospitals, New York[17]	●	●	●	●	●	●	●	●	●	●	●	●	●	●	●	●	●	●	●	●	●
3 Mount Sinai Hospital, New York	◐	●	●	●	●	●	●	●	●	●	●	●	●	●	●	●	●	●	●	●	●
4 North Shore University Hospital, Manhasset	–	●	●	–	●	●	●	●	●	●	●	●	●	●	●	●	●	●	●	●	●
5 Lenox Hill Hospital, New York[18]	●	●	●	●	●	●	●	●	●	●	●	●	●	●	●	●	●	●	●	●	●
6 Montefiore Medical Center, Bronx	●	●	●	–	●	●	●	●	●	–	●	●	●	●	●	●	●	●	●	●	●
7 NYU Winthrop Hospital, Mineola	–	●	●	–	●	●	●	●	●	●	●	●	●	●	●	●	●	●	●	●	●
8 Long Island Jewish Medical Center, New Hyde Park	◐	–	●	●	◐	●	●	●	–	●	●	●	●	●	●	●	●	●	●	●	●
9 St. Francis Hospital, Roslyn	–	●	–	–	●	●	–	●	●	●	●	●	●	●	●	●	●	●	●	●	●
10 Albany Medical Center	–	–	–	●	–	–	●	●	–	–	●	●	●	●	●	●	●	●	●	●	●
11 Stony Brook University Hospital, Stony Brook	–	–	–	–	●	●	●	●	●	●	●	●	●	●	●	●	●	●	●	●	●
12 Huntington Hospital, Huntington	–	–	–	–	●	●	●	●	●	●	●	●	●	●	–	●	–	●	●	●	●
12 Mount Sinai West and Mount Sinai St. Luke's Hospitals, New York	–	–	●	–	●	●	–	●	●	●	●	●	●	●	●	●	●	●	●	●	●
12 St. Peter's Hospital, Albany	–	–	–	–	–	●	–	●	●	●	●	●	●	●	●	●	●	●	●	●	●
12 Strong Memorial Hospital of the University of Rochester	–	–	–	●	●	●	●	●	●	●	●	●	●	●	●	●	●	–	–	●	●
16 Buffalo General Medical Center[19]	–	–	–	–	●	●	●	●	●	●	●	●	●	●	●	●	●	●	●	●	●
16 Mount Sinai Beth Israel Hospital, New York	●	–	●	–	●	●	–	●	●	●	●	●	●	●	●	●	●	●	●	●	●
16 White Plains Hospital	–	–	–	●	●	–	●	●	●	●	●	●	●	●	–	●	–	●	●	●	●
19 St. Joseph's Health Hospital, Syracuse	–	–	–	–	–	–	–	–	–	●	●	●	●	●	●	●	●	●	●	●	●
20 Rochester General Hospital, Rochester	–	–	–	–	–	–	●	●	–	●	●	●	●	●	●	●	●	●	●	●	●
20 South Nassau Communities Hospital, Oceanside	–	–	–	–	–	●	–	●	●	●	●	●	●	●	–	●	–	●	●	●	●
22 Maimonides Medical Center, Brooklyn	–	●	–	–	●	–	–	●	–	●	●	●	●	●	●	●	●	●	●	●	●
22 Mercy Hospital, Buffalo	–	–	–	–	–	–	–	–	–	●	●	●	●	●	●	●	●	●	●	●	●
22 Staten Island University Hospital	–	–	–	–	–	–	●	–	–	●	●	●	●	●	●	●	●	●	●	●	●
25 Arnot Ogden Medical Center, Elmira	–	–	–	–	–	–	–	–	–	●	●	●	●	●	●	●	●	●	●	●	●
25 Crouse Hospital, Syracuse	–	–	–	–	–	–	–	–	–	●	●	●	●	●	–	●	–	●	●	●	●
25 Highland Hospital, Rochester	–	–	–	–	–	–	–	–	–	●	●	●	●	–	●	–	●	●	●	●	●
25 Kenmore Mercy Hospital, Kenmore	–	–	–	–	–	–	–	–	–	●	●	●	●	–	●	–	●	●	●	●	●
25 Sisters of Charity Hospital of Buffalo	–	–	–	–	–	–	–	–	–	●	●	●	●	–	●	–	●	●	●	●	●
25 St. Elizabeth Medical Center, Utica	–	–	–	–	–	–	–	–	–	●	●	●	●	●	●	●	●	●	●	●	●
25 Vassar Brothers Medical Center, Poughkeepsie	–	–	–	–	–	–	–	–	–	●	●	●	●	●	●	●	●	●	●	●	●
32 Good Samaritan Hospital Medical Center, West Islip	–	–	–	–	–	–	–	–	–	●	●	●	●	●	●	●	●	●	●	●	●
32 New York-Presbyterian Queens Hospital, Flushing	–	–	–	–	–	–	–	–	–	●	●	●	●	●	●	●	●	●	●	●	●
32 NewYork-Presbyterian Brooklyn Methodist Hospital, Brooklyn	–	–	–	–	–	–	–	–	–	●	●	●	●	●	●	●	●	●	●	●	●

In complex care specialties, (-) indicates hospital is not nationally ranked or high performing.
In procedures and conditions, (-) indicates care not offered or hospital has too few Medicare patients to be rated.

A footnote indicates that another hospital's results are included, that the hospital has a different name in one or more areas of care, or both.
[17]NYU Langone Orthopedic Hospital. [18]Lenox Hill Hospital-Manhattan Eye, Ear and Throat Institute. [19]Roswell Park Oishei Children's Cancer and Blood Disorders.

More @ usnews.com/bestregionalhospitals

COMPLEX SPECIALTY CARE

● Nationally ranked
○ High performing

COMMON PROCEDURES & CONDITIONS

○ High performing
○ Average
● Below average

COMPLEX SPECIALTY CARE   **COMMON PROCEDURES & CONDITIONS**

State Rank	Hospital	Cancer	Cardiology & Heart Surgery	Diabetes & Endocrinology	Ear, Nose & Throat	Gastroenterology & GI Surgery	Geriatrics	Gynecology	Nephrology	Neurology & Neurosurgery	Orthopedics	Pulmonology	Urology	Colon Cancer Surgery	Lung Cancer Surgery	Heart Bypass Surgery	Heart Failure	Heart Valve Surgery	Abdominal Aortic Aneurysm	Hip Replacement	Knee Replacement	COPD
NORTH CAROLINA																					
1	Duke University Hospital, Durham	●	●	–	–	●	○	–	●	●	●	●	●	○	○	○	○	○	○	○	○	○
2	University of North Carolina Hospitals, Chapel Hill	●	–	–	●	●	–	●	●	–	–	○	–	○	○	○	○	○	○	○	○	○
3	Vidant Medical Center, Greenville	–	–	–	●	–	–	●	○	–	–	–	–	○	○	○	○	○	○	○	○	○
4	Carolinas Medical Center, Charlotte[20]	○	–	–	○	–	–	–	–	○	–	–	–	○	○	○	○	○	○	○	○	○
5	Wake Forest Baptist Medical Center, Winston-Salem	○	○	–	–	○	–	○	–	–	–	–	–	○	○	○	○	○	○	○	○	○
6	Moses H. Cone Memorial Hospital, Greensboro	–	–	–	–	–	–	–	–	–	●	–	–	○	○	○	○	○	○	○	○	○
7	Mission Hospital, Asheville	–	–	–	–	–	–	–	–	–	–	○	–	○	○	○	○	○	○	○	○	○
7	UNC Rex Hospital, Raleigh	–	–	–	–	–	–	–	–	–	–	○	–	○	○	○	○	○	○	○	○	○
9	FirstHealth Moore Regional Hospital, Pinehurst	–	–	–	–	–	–	–	–	–	–	○	–	○	○	○	○	○	○	○	○	○
10	New Hanover Regional Medical Center, Wilmington	–	–	–	–	–	–	–	–	–	–	○	–	○	○	○	○	○	○	○	○	○
11	CarolinaEast Medical Center, New Bern	–	–	–	–	–	–	–	–	–	–	–	–	○	○	○	○	○	○	○	○	○
11	Duke Regional Hospital, Durham	–	–	–	–	–	–	–	–	–	○	–	–	○	–	○	○	–	–	○	○	○
11	Novant Health Presbyterian Medical Center, Charlotte	–	–	–	–	–	–	–	–	–	–	○	–	○	○	○	○	○	○	○	○	○
11	WakeMed Health and Hospitals-Raleigh Campus, Raleigh	–	–	–	–	–	–	–	–	–	–	○	–	○	○	○	○	○	○	○	○	○
15	CaroMont Regional Medical Center, Gastonia	–	–	–	–	–	–	–	–	–	–	–	–	○	○	○	○	○	○	○	○	○
15	Novant Health Forsyth Medical Center, Winston-Salem	–	–	–	–	–	–	–	–	–	–	○	–	○	○	○	○	○	○	○	○	○
17	Carolinas Healthcare System Pineville, Charlotte	–	–	–	–	–	–	–	–	–	–	○	–	○	–	○	○	○	○	○	○	○
18	Cape Fear Valley Medical Center, Fayetteville	–	–	–	–	–	–	–	–	–	–	○	–	○	●	●	○	●	●	○	○	○
NORTH DAKOTA																					
1	Altru Health System-Grand Forks	–	–	–	–	–	–	–	–	–	○	–	–	○	○	○	○	○	○	○	○	○
2	Sanford Medical Center Bismarck	–	–	–	–	–	–	–	–	–	○	–	–	○	○	○	○	○	○	○	○	○
3	CHI St. Alexius Health-Bismarck	–	–	–	–	–	–	–	–	–	○	–	–	○	○	○	○	○	○	○	○	○
3	Sanford Medical Center Fargo	–	–	–	–	–	–	–	–	–	○	–	–	○	○	○	○	○	○	○	○	○
OHIO																					
1	Cleveland Clinic	●	●	●	●	●	●	●	●	●	●	●	●	○	○	○	○	○	○	○	○	○
2	University Hospitals Cleveland Medical Center[21]	●	●	–	●	●	●	–	●	●	○	–	●	○	○	○	○	○	○	○	○	○
3	Ohio State University Wexner Medical Center, Columbus[22]	●	○	●	●	○	○	–	●	○	–	●	○	○	○	○	○	○	○	○	○	○
4	Cleveland Clinic Fairview Hospital, Cleveland	–	●	○	–	○	○	○	○	○	●	–	○	○	○	○	○	○	○	○	○	○
5	Cleveland Clinic Hillcrest Hospital, Cleveland	–	–	–	●	○	–	○	–	○	●	–	–	○	○	○	○	○	○	○	○	○
6	Miami Valley Hospital, Dayton	–	–	–	–	–	○	–	○	○	●	–	–	○	○	○	○	○	○	○	○	○
7	Christ Hospital, Cincinnati	–	–	–	–	–	○	–	○	–	○	–	–	○	○	○	○	○	○	○	○	○
8	ProMedica Toledo Hospital	–	–	–	–	–	●	–	○	–	–	–	–	○	○	○	○	○	○	○	○	○
9	OhioHealth Riverside Methodist Hospital, Columbus	–	–	–	–	–	–	–	–	–	○	–	–	○	○	○	○	○	○	○	○	○
10	Aultman Hospital, Canton	–	–	–	–	–	–	–	–	–	○	–	–	○	○	○	○	○	○	○	○	○
10	Kettering Medical Center, Kettering	–	–	–	–	–	–	–	–	–	○	–	–	○	○	○	○	○	○	○	○	○
12	Mount Carmel East and West Hospitals, Columbus	–	–	–	–	–	–	–	–	–	○	–	–	○	○	○	○	○	○	○	○	○
12	University Hospitals Ahuja Medical Center, Beachwood	–	–	–	–	–	–	–	–	–	○	–	–	○	–	○	○	–	○	○	○	○
14	Blanchard Valley Hospital, Findlay	–	–	–	–	–	–	–	–	–	○	–	–	○	○	○	○	○	○	○	○	○
14	Cleveland Clinic Akron General, Akron	–	–	–	–	–	–	–	–	–	○	–	–	○	○	○	○	○	○	○	○	○
14	Southwest General Health Center, Middleburg Heights	–	–	–	–	–	–	–	–	–	○	–	–	○	○	○	○	○	○	○	○	○
17	Bethesda North Hospital, Cincinnati	–	–	–	–	–	–	–	–	–	○	–	–	○	○	○	○	○	○	○	○	○
17	Good Samaritan Hospital, Cincinnati	–	–	–	–	–	–	–	–	–	○	–	–	○	○	○	○	○	○	○	○	○
17	Mercy Medical Center, Canton	–	–	–	–	–	–	–	–	–	○	–	–	○	○	○	○	○	○	○	○	○

In complex care specialties, (-) indicates hospital is not nationally ranked or high performing.
In procedures and conditions, (-) indicates care not offered or hospital has too few Medicare patients to be rated.

A footnote indicates that another hospital's results are included, that the hospital has a different name in one or more areas of care, or both.
[20]Levine Cancer Institute; Sanger Heart & Vascular Institute. [21]University Hospitals Seidman Cancer Center. [22]Ohio State University James Cancer Hospital.

COMPLEX SPECIALTY CARE
- ● Nationally ranked
- ○ High performing

COMMON PROCEDURES & CONDITIONS
- ● High performing
- ○ Average
- ● Below average

COMPLEX SPECIALTY CARE   **COMMON PROCEDURES & CONDITIONS**

State Rank / Hospital	CANCER	CARDIOLOGY & HEART SURGERY	DIABETES & ENDOCRINOLOGY	EAR, NOSE & THROAT	GASTROENTEROLOGY & GI SURGERY	GERIATRICS	GYNECOLOGY	NEPHROLOGY	NEUROLOGY & NEUROSURGERY	ORTHOPEDICS	PULMONOLOGY	UROLOGY	COLON CANCER SURGERY	LUNG CANCER SURGERY	HEART BYPASS SURGERY	HEART FAILURE	HEART VALVE SURGERY	ABDOMINAL AORTIC ANEURYSM	HIP REPLACEMENT	KNEE REPLACEMENT	COPD
OHIO (CONTINUED)																					
17 OhioHealth MedCentral Mansfield Hospital, Mansfield	–	–	–	–	–	–	–	–	–	–	–	–	●	–	●	●	●	●	●	●	●
17 St. John Medical Center, Westlake	–	–	–	–	–	–	–	–	–	–	–	–	●	●	●	●	●	●	●	●	●
OKLAHOMA																					
1 St. Francis Hospital, Tulsa	–	–	–	–	–	●	–	–	–	–	–	●	●	●	●	●	●	●	●	●	●
1 OU Medical Center, Oklahoma City	●	–	–	–	–	–	–	–	–	–	–	●	●	●	●	●	●	●	●	●	●
3 Hillcrest Medical Center, Tulsa	–	–	–	–	–	–	–	–	–	–	–	●	●	●	●	●	●	●	●	●	●
3 Integris Baptist Medical Center, Oklahoma City	–	–	–	–	–	–	–	–	–	–	–	●	●	●	●	●	●	●	●	●	●
5 St. John Medical Center, Tulsa	–	–	–	–	–	–	–	–	–	–	–	●	●	●	●	●	●	●	●	●	●
OREGON																					
1 OHSU Hospital, Portland	●	●	–	●	●	●	–	●	●	●	●	●	●	●	●	●	●	●	●	●	●
2 Providence St. Vincent Medical Center, Portland	–	–	–	–	●	–	●	–	–	●	–	●	●	●	●	●	●	●	●	●	●
3 Asante Rogue Regional Medical Center, Medford	–	–	–	–	–	–	–	–	–	–	–	●	●	●	●	●	●	●	●	●	●
3 Providence Portland Medical Center, Portland	–	–	–	●	●	–	●	–	–	–	–	●	●	●	●	●	●	●	●	●	●
5 Salem Hospital, Salem	–	–	–	–	–	–	–	–	–	–	–	●	●	●	●	●	●	●	●	●	●
6 St. Charles Medical Center, Bend	–	–	–	–	–	–	–	–	–	●	–	●	●	●	●	●	●	●	●	●	●
7 Kaiser Permanente Sunnyside Medical Center, Clackamas	–	–	–	–	–	–	–	–	–	–	–	●	–	●	●	●	●	●	●	●	●
7 PeaceHealth Sacred Heart Medical Center at RiverBend, Springfield	–	–	–	–	–	–	–	–	–	–	–	●	●	●	●	●	●	●	●	●	●
9 Good Samaritan Regional Medical Center, Corvallis	–	–	–	–	–	–	–	–	–	–	–	●	●	●	●	●	●	●	●	●	●
9 Kaiser Permanente Westside Medical Center, Hillsboro	–	–	–	–	–	–	–	–	–	–	–	–	–	–	●	●	–	●	●	–	●
9 Legacy Meridian Park Medical Center, Tualatin	–	–	–	–	–	–	–	–	–	–	–	●	●	–	●	●	●	●	●	●	●
9 McKenzie-Willamette Medical Center, Springfield	–	–	–	–	–	–	–	–	–	–	–	●	–	●	●	●	●	●	●	●	●
PENNSYLVANIA																					
1 UPMC Presbyterian, Pittsburgh	●	●	●	●	●	●	–	●	●	●	●	●	●	●	●	●	●	●	●	●	●
2 Hospitals of the U. of Pennsylvania-Penn Presbyterian, Philadelphia	●	●	●	●	●	●	●	●	●	●	●	●	●	●	●	●	●	●	●	●	●
3 Jefferson Health-Thomas Jefferson U. Hospitals, Philadelphia[23]	●	●	–	●	●	●	–	●	●	●	●	●	●	●	●	●	●	●	●	●	●
4 Penn State Health Milton S. Hershey Medical Center, Hershey	●	●	–	–	●	●	●	●	●	●	●	●	●	●	●	●	●	●	●	●	●
5 Lehigh Valley Hospital, Allentown	–	–	–	–	●	–	–	●	–	●	–	●	●	●	●	●	●	●	●	●	●
5 UPMC Pinnacle Harrisburg	–	–	●	–	●	–	–	–	●	–	●	●	●	●	●	●	●	●	●	●	●
7 Penn Medicine Lancaster General Hospital	–	–	–	–	●	–	–	–	●	●	–	●	●	●	●	●	●	●	●	●	●
7 St. Luke's University Hospital-Bethlehem Campus	–	–	–	–	●	–	–	–	●	●	●	●	●	●	●	●	●	●	●	●	●
9 Lankenau Medical Center, Wynnewood	–	–	–	–	●	–	–	–	–	–	–	●	●	●	●	●	●	●	●	●	●
9 Pennsylvania Hospital, Philadelphia	–	–	–	–	●	●	–	●	–	–	–	–	●	●	●	●	–	●	●	●	●
11 Jefferson Health-Abington Hospital, Abington	–	–	–	–	–	–	–	–	–	–	–	●	●	●	●	●	●	●	●	●	●
11 Reading Hospital, West Reading	–	–	–	–	–	–	–	–	–	●	–	●	●	●	●	●	●	●	●	●	●
13 Chester County Hospital, West Chester	–	–	–	–	–	–	●	–	●	–	●	●	●	–	●	●	●	●	●	●	●
13 Doylestown Hospital	–	–	–	–	–	–	–	–	–	–	–	●	●	●	●	●	●	●	●	●	●
15 WellSpan York Hospital, York	–	–	–	–	–	–	–	●	–	●	–	●	●	●	●	●	●	●	●	●	●
16 Bryn Mawr Hospital	–	–	–	–	–	–	●	–	●	–	–	●	●	●	●	●	●	●	●	●	●
16 St. Clair Hospital, Pittsburgh	–	–	–	–	–	–	–	–	–	–	–	●	●	●	●	●	●	●	●	●	●
18 Crozer-Chester Medical Center, Upland	–	–	–	–	–	–	–	–	–	–	–	●	●	●	●	●	●	●	●	●	●
18 St. Mary Medical Center, Langhorne	–	–	–	–	–	–	–	–	–	–	–	●	●	●	●	●	●	●	●	●	●
18 UPMC Passavant, Pittsburgh	–	–	–	–	●	–	–	–	–	–	–	●	●	●	●	●	●	●	●	●	●
21 Allegheny General Hospital, Pittsburgh	–	–	–	–	–	–	–	–	●	–	–	●	●	●	●	●	●	●	●	●	●
21 Chambersburg Hospital, Chambersburg	–	–	–	–	–	–	–	–	●	–	–	●	●	–	●	●	–	●	●	●	●

In complex care specialties, (-) indicates hospital is not nationally ranked or high performing.
In procedures and conditions, (-) indicates care not offered or hospital has too few Medicare patients to be rated.

A footnote indicates that another hospital's results are included, that the hospital has a different name in one or more areas of care, or both.
[23]Rothman Institute at Thomas Jefferson University Hospitals.

You don't **have to**

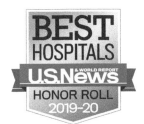

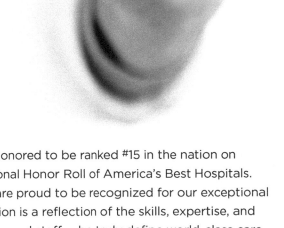

search

far for **nationally** ranked **CARE.**

Out of more than 4,500 hospitals, we're honored to be ranked #15 in the nation on *U.S. News & World Report's* prestigious national Honor Roll of America's Best Hospitals. Ranked #1 in Pennsylvania and Pittsburgh, we are proud to be recognized for our exceptional care and cutting-edge research. This distinction is a reflection of the skills, expertise, and dedication of our extraordinary doctors, nurses, and staff, who truly define world-class care.

To learn more, visit UPMC.com/HonorRoll.

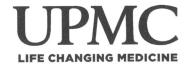

UPMC
LIFE CHANGING MEDICINE

UPMC Presbyterian Shadyside is ranked among America's Best Hospitals by *U.S. News and World Report.*

	COMPLEX SPECIALTY CARE	COMMON PROCEDURES & CONDITIONS
COMPLEX SPECIALTY CARE	● Nationally ranked ● High performing	
COMMON PROCEDURES & CONDITIONS	● High performing ● Average ● Below average	

State Rank Hospital	Cancer	Cardiology & Heart Surgery	Diabetes & Endocrinology	Ear, Nose & Throat	Gastroenterology & GI Surgery	Geriatrics	Gynecology	Nephrology	Neurology & Neurosurgery	Orthopedics	Pulmonology	Urology	Colon Cancer Surgery	Lung Cancer Surgery	Heart Bypass Surgery	Heart Failure	Heart Valve Surgery	Abdominal Aortic Aneurysm	Hip Replacement	Knee Replacement	COPD
PENNSYLVANIA (CONTINUED)																					
21 Excela Health Westmoreland Hospital, Greensburg	–	–	–	–	–	–	–	–	–	–	–	–	●	●	●	●	●	●	●	●	●
21 Geisinger Medical Center, Danville	–	–	–	–	–	–	–	–	–	–	–	–	●	●	●	●	●	●	●	●	●
21 Jeanes Hospital, Philadelphia	–	–	–	–	–	–	–	–	–	–	–	●	●	–	●	●	●	●	●	●	●
21 Jefferson Health-Jefferson Torresdale Hospital, Philadelphia	–	–	–	–	–	–	–	–	–	–	–	●	●	●	●	●	●	●	●	●	●
21 Riddle Hospital, Media	–	–	–	–	–	–	–	–	–	–	–	●	●	●	●	●	–	–	●	●	●
RHODE ISLAND																					
1 Miriam Hospital, Providence	–	–	●	–	●	●	–	●	●	–	●	●	●	●	●	●	–	●	●	●	●
SOUTH CAROLINA																					
1 MUSC Health-University Medical Center, Charleston	●	–	–	●	–	–	●	●	●	●	–	●	●	●	●	●	●	●	●	●	●
2 Bon Secours St. Francis Health System-Greenville	–	–	–	–	–	–	–	–	–	–	–	●	●	●	●	●	●	●	●	●	●
3 Spartanburg Medical Center	–	–	–	–	–	–	–	–	–	–	–	●	●	●	●	●	●	●	●	●	●
4 McLeod Regional Medical Center, Florence	–	–	–	–	–	–	–	–	–	–	–	●	●	●	●	●	●	●	●	●	●
4 Roper St. Francis Hospital, Charleston	–	–	–	–	–	–	–	–	–	–	–	●	●	●	●	●	●	●	●	●	●
6 Prisma Health Greenville Memorial Hospital	–	–	–	–	–	–	●	–	–	–	–	●	●	●	●	●	●	●	–	–	●
6 Providence Hospital, Columbia	–	–	–	–	–	–	–	–	–	–	–	●	●	●	●	●	●	●	●	●	●
8 AnMed Health Medical Center, Anderson	–	–	–	–	–	–	–	–	–	–	–	●	●	●	●	●	●	●	●	●	●
8 Lexington Medical Center, West Columbia	–	–	–	–	–	–	–	–	–	–	–	●	●	●	●	●	●	●	●	●	●
SOUTH DAKOTA																					
1 Avera McKennan Hospital and University Health Center, Sioux Falls	●	–	–	–	–	●	●	●	–	●	–	●	●	–	●	–	–	●	●	●	●
2 Sanford USD Medical Center, Sioux Falls	–	–	–	–	●	–	–	–	–	–	–	●	●	●	●	●	●	●	●	●	●
3 Rapid City Regional Hospital	–	–	–	–	–	–	–	–	–	–	–	●	●	●	●	●	●	●	●	●	●
TENNESSEE																					
1 Vanderbilt University Medical Center, Nashville	●	●	–	●	●	●	–	●	●	●	●	●	●	●	●	●	●	●	●	●	●
2 CHI Memorial Hospital, Chattanooga	–	–	–	–	–	–	–	–	–	–	–	●	●	●	●	●	●	●	●	●	●
2 University of Tennessee Medical Center, Knoxville	–	–	–	–	–	–	–	–	–	–	–	●	●	●	●	●	●	●	●	●	●
4 St. Thomas West Hospital, Nashville	–	–	–	–	–	–	–	–	–	–	–	●	●	●	●	●	●	●	●	●	●
5 Methodist Hospitals of Memphis	–	–	–	–	–	–	–	–	–	–	–	●	●	●	●	●	●	●	●	●	●
5 St. Thomas Midtown Hospital, Nashville	–	–	–	–	–	–	–	–	–	–	–	●	●	●	●	●	●	●	●	●	●
7 Baptist Memorial Hospital-Memphis	–	–	–	–	–	–	–	–	–	–	–	●	●	●	●	●	●	●	●	●	●
7 Bristol Regional Medical Center	–	–	–	–	–	–	–	–	–	–	–	●	●	●	●	●	●	●	●	●	●
7 Holston Valley Medical Center, Kingsport	–	–	–	–	–	–	–	–	–	–	–	●	●	●	●	●	●	●	●	●	●
7 Parkwest Medical Center, Knoxville	–	–	–	–	–	–	–	–	–	–	–	●	●	●	●	●	●	●	●	●	●
7 TriStar Centennial Medical Center, Nashville	–	–	–	–	–	–	–	–	–	–	–	●	●	●	●	●	●	●	●	●	●
12 Maury Regional Hospital, Columbia	–	–	–	–	–	–	–	–	–	–	–	●	–	●	●	–	●	●	●	●	●
12 St. Thomas Rutherford Hospital, Murfreesboro	–	–	–	–	–	–	–	–	–	–	–	●	●	–	●	–	●	●	●	●	●
TEXAS																					
1 Houston Methodist Hospital	●	●	●	–	●	●	–	●	●	●	●	●	●	●	●	●	●	●	●	●	●
2 UT Southwestern Medical Center, Dallas	●	●	●	●	●	●	–	●	●	●	●	●	●	●	●	●	●	●	●	●	●
3 Baylor St. Luke's Medical Center, Houston[24]	●	●	●	–	●	●	–	●	●	●	–	●	●	●	●	●	●	●	●	●	●
4 Baylor University Medical Center, Dallas[25]	–	–	–	–	●	–	●	●	–	●	–	●	●	●	●	●	●	●	●	●	●
5 Memorial Hermann Greater Heights Hospital, Houston	–	–	●	–	●	–	–	–	–	–	–	●	●	●	●	●	●	●	●	●	●
6 Memorial Hermann-Texas Medical Center, Houston	●	–	–	–	●	–	–	–	●	–	–	●	●	●	●	●	●	●	●	●	●
7 Baylor Scott and White Medical Center-Temple	–	–	–	–	–	–	–	–	●	–	●	●	●	●	●	●	●	●	●	●	●
7 St. David's Medical Center, Austin	–	–	–	–	–	–	–	–	–	–	–	●	●	●	●	●	●	●	●	●	●

In complex care specialties, (-) indicates hospital is not nationally ranked or high performing.
In procedures and conditions, (-) indicates care not offered or hospital has too few Medicare patients to be rated.

A footnote indicates that another hospital's results are included, that the hospital has a different name in one or more areas of care, or both.
[24] Dan L Duncan Comprehensive Cancer Center at Baylor St. Luke's Medical Center; Texas Heart Institute at Baylor St. Luke's Medical Center.
[25] Baylor University Medical Center and Baylor Scott and White Heart and Vascular Hospital-Dallas.

▶ **More** @ usnews.com/bestregionalhospitals

State Rank Hospital	CANCER	CARDIOLOGY & HEART SURGERY	DIABETES & ENDOCRINOLOGY	EAR, NOSE & THROAT	GASTROENTEROLOGY & GI SURGERY	GERIATRICS	GYNECOLOGY	NEPHROLOGY	NEUROLOGY & NEUROSURGERY	ORTHOPEDICS	PULMONOLOGY	UROLOGY	COLON CANCER SURGERY	LUNG CANCER SURGERY	HEART BYPASS SURGERY	HEART FAILURE	HEART VALVE SURGERY	ABDOMINAL AORTIC ANEURYSM	HIP REPLACEMENT	KNEE REPLACEMENT	COPD
TEXAS (CONTINUED)																					
9 Houston Methodist Sugar Land Hospital, Sugar Land	–	–	–	–	●	●	–	●	–	●	–	●	●	●	●	●	●	●	●	●	●
9 Memorial Hermann Memorial City Medical Center, Houston	–	–	–	–	–	–	–	–	–	●	–	●	●	●	●	●	●	●	●	●	●
11 Seton Medical Center Austin	–	–	–	–	–	–	–	–	–	●	–	●	●	●	●	●	●	●	●	●	●
11 Texas Health Presbyterian Hospital Dallas	–	–	–	–	–	–	–	●	–	●	–	●	●	●	●	●	●	●	●	●	●
13 Christus Mother Frances Hospital-Tyler	–	–	–	–	–	–	–	–	–	●	–	●	●	●	●	●	●	●	●	●	●
13 Methodist Hospital, San Antonio	–	–	–	–	–	–	–	–	–	●	–	●	●	●	●	●	●	●	●	●	●
15 Doctors Hospital at Renaissance, Edinburg	–	–	–	–	–	–	●	–	–	●	–	●	●	●	●	●	●	●	●	●	●
15 Texas Health Harris Methodist Hospital Fort Worth	–	–	–	–	–	–	–	–	–	●	–	●	●	●	●	●	●	●	●	●	●
17 Baylor Scott and White All Saints Medical Center-Fort Worth	–	–	–	–	–	–	–	–	–	●	–	●	●	–	●	●	●	●	●	●	●
17 BSA Hospital, Amarillo	–	–	–	–	–	–	–	–	–	●	–	●	●	●	●	●	●	●	●	●	●
17 Medical City Dallas	–	–	–	–	–	–	–	–	–	●	–	●	●	●	●	●	●	●	●	●	●
17 Texas Health Harris Methodist Hospital Southwest, Fort Worth	–	–	–	–	–	–	–	–	–	●	–	●	●	–	–	●	–	●	●	●	●
17 UT Health Tyler, Tyler	–	–	–	–	–	–	–	–	–	●	–	●	●	●	●	●	●	●	●	●	●
22 Baptist Medical Center, San Antonio	–	–	–	–	–	–	–	–	–	●	–	●	●	●	●	●	●	●	●	●	●
22 North Cypress Medical Center, Cypress	–	–	–	–	–	–	–	–	–	●	–	●	●	●	●	●	●	●	●	●	●
22 St. David's North Austin Medical Center	–	–	–	–	–	–	–	–	–	●	–	●	●	●	●	●	●	●	●	●	●
22 Valley Baptist Medical Center-Harlingen	–	–	–	–	–	–	–	–	–	●	–	●	●	●	●	●	●	●	–	●	●
UTAH																					
1 University of Utah Hospital, Salt Lake City[26]	●	–	–	–	–	●	–	●	●	–	●	–	●	●	●	●	●	●	●	●	●
2 Utah Valley Hospital, Provo	–	–	–	–	–	–	–	–	●	–	●	–	●	●	●	●	●	●	●	●	●
3 Intermountain Medical Center, Murray	–	–	–	–	–	–	–	–	–	●	●	–	●	●	●	●	●	●	●	●	●
4 Dixie Regional Medical Center, St. George	–	–	–	–	–	–	–	–	–	●	–	●	●	●	●	●	●	●	●	●	●
5 McKay-Dee Hospital, Ogden	–	–	–	–	–	–	–	–	–	●	–	●	●	●	●	●	●	●	●	●	●
VIRGINIA																					
1 University of Virginia Medical Center, Charlottesville	●	–	–	●	●	●	–	●	●	●	●	●	●	●	●	●	●	●	●	●	●
2 Sentara Norfolk General Hospital, Norfolk[27]	●	●	–	●	–	–	–	●	●	●	●	●	●	●	●	●	●	●	–	–	●
3 Carilion Roanoke Memorial Hospital, Roanoke	–	–	●	–	●	–	–	●	●	●	●	●	●	●	●	●	●	●	●	●	●
3 Inova Fairfax Hospital, Falls Church	–	–	–	–	–	–	●	●	●	●	●	●	●	●	●	●	●	●	●	●	●
5 VCU Medical Center, Richmond	–	–	–	–	–	–	–	●	●	●	●	●	●	●	●	●	●	●	●	●	●
6 Bon Secours St. Mary's Hospital, Richmond	–	–	–	–	–	–	–	●	–	●	●	●	●	●	●	●	●	●	●	●	●
6 Virginia Hospital Center, Arlington	–	–	–	–	–	–	–	–	–	●	●	●	●	●	●	●	●	●	●	●	●
8 Centra Lynchburg General Hospital	–	–	–	–	–	–	–	–	–	●	●	–	●	●	●	●	●	●	●	●	●
8 Inova Alexandria Hospital, Alexandria	–	–	–	–	–	–	–	–	–	●	–	–	●	–	●	●	–	●	●	●	●
8 Mary Washington Hospital, Fredericksburg	–	–	–	–	–	–	–	–	–	●	●	–	●	●	●	●	●	●	●	●	●
11 Chippenham Hospital, Richmond	–	–	–	–	–	–	–	–	–	●	●	–	●	●	●	●	●	●	●	●	●
11 Inova Fair Oaks Hospital, Fairfax	–	–	–	–	–	–	–	–	–	●	–	–	●	–	●	●	–	●	●	●	●
11 Winchester Medical Center, Winchester	–	–	–	–	–	–	–	–	–	●	●	–	●	●	●	●	●	●	●	●	●
14 Augusta Health-Fishersville	–	–	–	–	–	–	–	–	–	●	●	–	●	●	●	●	●	●	●	●	●
14 Sentara Leigh Hospital, Norfolk	–	–	–	–	–	–	–	–	–	●	–	–	●	●	●	●	●	●	–	●	●
WASHINGTON																					
1 University of Washington Medical Center, Seattle[28]	●	–	●	●	●	●	●	–	●	●	●	–	●	●	●	●	●	●	●	●	●
2 Virginia Mason Medical Center, Seattle	–	–	–	–	●	●	–	–	–	●	●	●	●	●	●	●	●	●	●	●	●
3 EvergreenHealth Kirkland, Kirkland	–	–	–	–	–	–	●	–	–	●	●	●	●	–	●	●	–	●	●	●	●
3 Providence Sacred Heart Medical Ctr. & Children's Hosp., Spokane	–	–	–	–	–	–	–	–	–	●	●	–	●	●	●	●	●	●	●	●	●

In complex care specialties, (-) indicates hospital is not nationally ranked or high performing.
In procedures and conditions, (-) indicates care not offered or hospital has too few Medicare patients to be rated.

A footnote indicates that another hospital's results are included, that the hospital has a different name in one or more areas of care, or both.
[26]Huntsman Cancer Institute at the University of Utah. [27]Sentara Norfolk General Hospital-Sentara Heart Hospital.
[28]Seattle Cancer Care Alliance/University of Washington Medical Center.

COMPLEX SPECIALTY CARE
- ● Nationally ranked
- ● High performing

COMMON PROCEDURES & CONDITIONS
- ● High performing
- ● Average
- ● Below average

State Rank Hospital	CANCER	CARDIOLOGY & HEART SURGERY	DIABETES & ENDOCRINOLOGY	EAR, NOSE & THROAT	GASTROENTEROLOGY & GI SURGERY	GERIATRICS	GYNECOLOGY	NEPHROLOGY	NEUROLOGY & NEUROSURGERY	ORTHOPEDICS	PULMONOLOGY	UROLOGY	COLON CANCER SURGERY	LUNG CANCER SURGERY	HEART BYPASS SURGERY	HEART FAILURE	HEART VALVE SURGERY	ABDOMINAL AORTIC ANEURYSM	HIP REPLACEMENT	KNEE REPLACEMENT	COPD
WASHINGTON (CONTINUED)																					
5 Providence Regional Medical Center Everett	–	–	–	–	–	–	–	–	–	–	–	–	●	●	●	●	●	●	●	●	●
5 Providence St. Peter Hospital, Olympia	–	–	–	–	–	–	–	–	–	–	–	●	●	●	●	●	●	●	●	●	●
5 Swedish Medical Center-Cherry Hill, Seattle	–	–	–	–	●	–	●	–	–	–	–	●	●	●	●	●	●	–	–	●	●
5 Swedish Medical Center-First Hill, Seattle	–	–	–	–	–	●	–	●	–	–	●	●	●	●	●	–	●	●	●	●	●
9 PeaceHealth Southwest Medical Center, Vancouver	–	–	–	–	–	–	–	–	–	–	–	●	●	●	●	●	●	●	●	●	●
9 PeaceHealth St. Joseph Medical Center, Bellingham	–	–	–	–	–	–	–	–	–	–	–	●	●	●	●	●	●	●	●	●	●
11 Harrison Medical Center, Bremerton	–	–	–	–	–	–	–	–	–	–	–	●	●	●	●	●	●	●	●	●	●
11 Kadlec Regional Medical Center, Richland	–	–	–	–	–	–	–	–	–	–	–	●	●	●	●	●	●	●	●	●	●
11 Legacy Salmon Creek Medical Center, Vancouver	–	–	–	–	–	–	–	–	–	–	–	●	●	●	–	●	–	●	●	●	●
11 Overlake Medical Center, Bellevue	–	–	–	–	–	–	–	–	–	–	–	●	●	●	●	●	●	●	●	●	●
11 St. Joseph Medical Center, Tacoma	–	–	–	–	–	–	–	–	–	–	–	●	●	●	●	●	●	●	●	●	●
16 UW Medicine-Northwest Hospital and Medical Center, Seattle	–	–	–	–	–	–	–	–	–	–	–	●	●	●	●	●	●	●	●	●	●
16 UW Medicine-Valley Medical Center, Renton	–	–	–	–	–	–	–	–	–	–	–	●	●	●	●	●	–	–	–	●	●
18 MultiCare Deaconess Hospital, Spokane	–	–	–	–	–	–	–	–	–	–	–	●	●	●	●	●	●	●	●	●	●
WASHINGTON, D.C.*																					
– MedStar Georgetown University Hospital	●	–	–	–	●	●	–	–	–	–	–	●	●	●	●	●	–	●	●	●	●
– MedStar Washington Hospital Center[29]	–	●	–	–	●	–	–	–	–	–	–	●	●	●	●	●	●	●	●	●	●
– George Washington University Hospital	●	–	–	–	–	–	–	–	–	–	–	●	●	●	●	●	●	●	●	●	●
– Sibley Memorial Hospital	–	–	–	–	–	–	–	●	–	–	–	●	●	●	●	●	●	●	●	●	●
WEST VIRGINIA																					
1 Charleston Area Medical Center, Charleston	–	–	–	–	–	–	–	–	–	–	–	●	●	●	●	●	●	●	●	●	●
2 West Virginia University Hospitals, Morgantown	–	–	–	–	–	–	–	–	–	●	–	●	●	●	●	●	●	●	●	●	●
3 Mon Health Medical Center, Morgantown	–	–	–	–	–	–	–	–	–	–	–	●	●	●	●	●	●	●	●	●	●
3 St. Mary's Medical Center, Huntington	–	–	–	–	–	–	–	–	–	–	–	●	●	●	●	●	●	●	●	●	●
5 Thomas Memorial Hospital, South Charleston	–	–	–	–	–	–	–	–	–	–	–	●	–	–	●	–	–	●	●	●	●
WISCONSIN																					
1 University of Wisconsin Hospitals, Madison	●	●	●	●	●	●	●	●	●	●	●	●	●	●	●	●	●	●	●	●	●
2 Aurora St. Luke's Medical Center, Milwaukee	–	●	–	–	●	●	–	–	–	–	●	●	●	●	●	●	●	●	●	●	●
3 Froedtert Hospital and the Medical College of Wisconsin, Milwaukee	–	–	–	–	●	–	–	–	–	–	●	●	●	●	●	●	●	●	●	●	●
4 Mayo Clinic Eau Claire	–	–	–	–	●	–	–	–	–	–	●	●	●	●	●	●	●	●	●	●	●
5 Aurora Medical Center Grafton	–	–	–	–	–	–	–	–	–	–	–	●	●	●	●	●	●	●	●	●	●
5 Bellin Memorial Hospital, Green Bay	–	–	–	–	–	–	–	–	–	–	–	●	●	●	●	●	●	●	●	●	●
7 Aspirus Wausau Hospital, Wausau	–	–	–	–	–	–	–	–	–	–	–	●	●	●	●	●	●	●	●	●	●
7 Aurora BayCare Medical Center, Green Bay	–	–	–	–	–	–	–	–	–	–	–	●	●	●	●	●	●	●	●	●	●
7 Marshfield Medical Center, Marshfield	–	–	–	–	–	–	–	–	–	–	–	●	●	●	●	●	●	●	●	●	●
7 SSM Health St. Mary's Hospital-Madison	–	–	–	–	–	–	–	–	–	–	–	●	●	●	●	●	●	●	●	●	●
7 UnityPoint Health Meriter, Madison	–	–	–	–	–	●	–	–	●	–	–	●	●	●	●	●	●	●	●	●	●
12 Community Memorial Hospital, Menomonee Falls	–	–	–	–	–	–	–	–	–	●	–	●	●	●	●	●	●	–	●	●	●
13 Aurora Medical Center of Oshkosh	–	–	–	–	–	–	–	–	–	–	–	●	–	–	●	●	–	●	●	●	●
13 Mayo Clinic Health System-Franciscan Healthcare in La Crosse	–	–	–	–	–	–	–	–	–	–	–	●	●	●	●	●	●	●	●	●	●
15 Gundersen Lutheran Medical Center, La Crosse	–	–	–	–	–	–	–	–	–	–	–	●	●	●	●	●	●	●	●	●	●
15 St. Joseph's Hospital, West Bend	–	–	–	–	–	–	–	–	–	●	–	●	●	●	–	●	–	–	●	●	●

In complex care specialties, (-) indicates hospital is not nationally ranked or high performing.
In procedures and conditions, (-) indicates care not offered or hospital has too few Medicare patients to be rated.

A footnote indicates that another hospital's results are included, that the hospital has a different name in one or more areas of care, or both.
[29]MedStar Heart and Vascular Institute.

*These hospitals are displayed without a rank because the D.C. metro area rankings (usnews.com/dchospitals) include hospitals in Virginia and Maryland. These are the four from that list located in the District.

More @ usnews.com/bestregionalhospitals

The #1 hospital in the nation.

Once again, U.S. News & World Report has recognized Mayo Clinic as the #1 hospital in the nation. With the world's top doctors all working together across specialties to give patients the unparalleled care they deserve, Mayo Clinic is a destination for all who may need certainty, options and hope. When you need answers, **You Know Where to Go.**

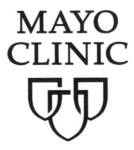

MAYO CLINIC

You Know Where to Go.

CPSIA information can be obtained
at www.ICGtesting.com
Printed in the USA
LVHW071618110919
630734LV00015B/395/P